2005
YEAR BOOK OF
NEONATAL AND
PERINATAL MEDICINE®

The 2005 Year Book Series

Year Book of Allergy, Asthma, and Clinical Immunology™: Drs Rosenwasser, Boguniewicz, Milgrom, Routes, and Weber

Year Book of Anesthesiology and Pain Management™: Drs Chestnut, Abram, Black, Gravlee, Mathru, Lee, and Roizen

Year Book of Cardiology®: Drs Gersh, Cheitlin, Graham, Kaplan, Sundt, and Waldo

Year Book of Critical Care Medicine®: Drs Dellinger, Parrillo, Balk, Bekes, Dorman, and Dries

Year Book of Dentistry®: Drs Zakariasen, Horswell, McIntyre, Scott and Zakariasen Victoroff

Year Book of Dermatology and Dermatologic Surgery™: Drs Thiers and Lang

Year Book of Diagnostic Radiology®: Drs Osborn, Birdwell, Dalinka, Gardiner, Levy, Maynard, Oestreich, and Rosado de Christenson

Year Book of Emergency Medicine®: Drs Burdick, Cydulka, Hamilton, Handly, Quintana, and Werner

Year Book of Endocrinology®: Drs Mazzaferri, Bessesen, Howard, Kannan, Kennedy, Leahy, Meikle, Molitch, Rogol, and Rubin

Year Book of Family Practice®: Drs Bowman, Apgar, Bouchard, Dexter, Miser, Neill, and Scherger

Year Book of Gastroenterology™: Drs Lichtenstein, Burke, Dempsey, Drebin, Ginsberg, Katzka, Kochman, Morris, Nunes, Shah, and Stein

Year Book of Hand Surgery and Upper Limb Surgery®: Drs Berger and Ladd

Year Book of Medicine®: Drs Barkin, Frishman, Klahr, Loehrer, Mazzaferri, Phillips, Pillinger, and Snydman

Year Book of Neonatal and Perinatal Medicine®: Drs Fanaroff, Maisels, and Stevenson

Year Book of Neurology and Neurosurgery®: Drs Gibbs and Verma

Year Book of Nuclear Medicine®: Drs Coleman, Blaufox, Royal, Strauss, and Zubal

Year Book of Obstetrics, Gynecology, and Women's Health®: Dr Shulman

Year Book of Oncology®: Drs Loehrer, Arceci, Glatstein, Gordon, Hanna, Morrow, and Thigpen

Year Book of Ophthalmology®: Drs Rapuano, Cohen, Eagle, Grossman, Hammersmith, Myers, Nelson, Penne, Sergott, Shields, Tipperman, and Vander

Year Book of Orthopedics®: Drs Morrey, Beauchamp, Peterson, Swiontkowski, Trigg, and Yaszemski

Year Book of Otolaryngology-Head and Neck Surgery®: Drs Paparella, Otto, and Keefe

2005

The Year Book of NEONATAL AND PERINATAL MEDICINE®

Editors

Avroy A. Fanaroff, MB BCh (Rand), FRCPE, FRCPCH
Professor & Chair, Department of Pediatrics, Case Western Reserve University School of Medicine; Eliza Henry Barnes Chair of Neonatology, Physician in Chief, Rainbow Babies and Children's Hospital, Cleveland, Ohio

M. Jeffrey Maisels, MB, BCh
Clinical Professor of Pediatrics, Wayne State University School of Medicine, Detroit, Michigan; Clinical Professor of Pediatrics, University of Michigan Medical Center, Ann Arbor, Michigan; Chairman, Department of Pediatrics, William Beaumont Hospital, Royal Oak, Michigan

David K. Stevenson, MD
Harold K. Faber Professor of Pediatrics, Senior Associate Dean for Academic Affairs, Stanford University School of Medicine; Chief, Division of Neonatal and Developmental Medicine, Department of Pediatrics; Director, Charles B. and Ann L. Johnson Center for Pregnancy and Newborn Services, Lucile Salter Packard Children's Hospital at Stanford, Palo Alto, California

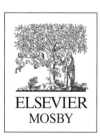

ELSEVIER
MOSBY

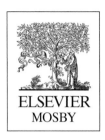

ELSEVIER
MOSBY

Vice President, Continuity Publishing: Timothy M. Griswold
Publishing Director, Continuity: J. Heather Cullen
Associate Developmental Editor: Timothy Maxwell
Senior Manager, Continuity Production: Idelle L. Winer
Senior Issue Manager: Donna M. Skelton
Illustrations and Permissions Coordinator: Dawn Vohsen

Printed in the United States of America
Composition by Thomas Technology Solutions, Inc.
Printing/binding by Sheridan Books, Inc.

Editorial Office:
Elsevier
Suite 1800
1600 John F. Kennedy Blvd.
Philadelphia, PA 19106-3399

International Standard Serial Number: 8756-5005
International Standard Book Number: 0-323-02053-4

Contributing Editors

Ronald L. Ariagno, MD
Professor of Pediatrics, Division of Neonatal and Developmental Medicine, Department of Pediatrics; Director of Pediatric Pulmonary Lab & Pediatric SIDS, Stanford University School of Medicine; Lucile Salter Packard Children's Hospital at Stanford, Palo Alto, California

Daniel Batton, MD
Chief, Division of Newborn Medicine, William Beaumont Hospital, Royal Oak, Michigan

W. E. Benitz, MD
Philip Sunshine Professor; Division of Neonatal and Developmental Medicine, Department of Pediatrics, Stanford University School of Medicine, Director of Nurseries at Lucile Salter Packard Children's Hospital at Stanford, Palo Alto, California

Melvin Berger, MD, PhD
Professor, Pediatrics and Pathology, Case Western Reserve University, Rainbow Babies & Children's Hospital, Division of Pediatric Infectious Diseases, Allergy, Immunology, Rheumatology, Cleveland, Ohio

Richard D. Bland, MD
Professor (Research) of Pediatrics, Division of Neonatal and Developmental Medicine, Department of Pediatrics, Stanford University School of Medicine, Palo Alto, California

R. S. Cohen, MD
Clinical Professor of Pediatrics, Division of Neonatal and Developmental Medicine, Department of Pediatrics, Stanford University School of Medicine, Lucile Salter Packard Children's Hospital at Stanford, Palo Alto, California

Christine Comstock, MD
Director Fetal Imaging, William Beaumont Hospital, Royal Oak, Michigan

David B. DeWitte, MD
Neonatologist, William Beaumont Hospital, Royal Oak, Michigan

Steven M. Donn, MD
Professor of Pediatrics and Director, Neonatal-Perinatal Medicine, University of Michigan Health System, Ann Arbor, Michigan

M. L. Druzin, MD
Charles B. and Ann L. Johnson Professor; Department of Obstetrics and Gynecology; Chief, Division of Maternal Fetal Medicine, Department of Obstetrics and Gynecology, and by courtesy of Pediatrics; Director of Residency, Stanford University School of Medicine, Palo Alto, California

Jonathan M. Fanaroff, MD, JD
Assistant Professor of Pediatrics, Case Western Reserve University, Division of Neonatology, Rainbow Babies & Children's Hospital, Cleveland, Ohio

Lydia Furman, MD
Associate Professor, Pediatrics, Case Western Reserve University School of Medicine, Rainbow Babies & Children's Hospital, Cleveland, Ohio

Bassam Gebara, MD
Clinical Associate Professor of Pediatrics, Wayne State University, Detroit, Michigan; Chief, Division of Pediatric Critical Care Medicine, William Beaumont Hospital, Royal Oak, Michigan

Souheil Gebara, MD
Pediatric Gastroenterology, William Beaumont Hospital, Royal Oak, Michigan

Jeffrey B. Gould, MD, MPH
Robert L. Hess Professor, Division of Neonatal and Developmental Medicine, Department of Pediatrics; Director of Perinatal Epidemiology and Outcomes Research Unit of the Johnson Center, Stanford University School of Medicine, Lucile Salter Packard Children's Hospital at Stanford, Palo Alto, California

Maureen Hack, MD
Professor, Pediatrics, Case Western Reserve University School of Medicine; Director, High Risk Follow-up Program, Rainbow Babies & Children's Hospital, Cleveland, Ohio

Jin S. Hahn, MD
Associate Professor of Neurology and Neurological Sciences and of Pediatrics, and by courtesy, of Neurosurgery, Stanford University School of Medicine, Palo Alto, California

Jonathan Hellmann, MBBCh, FCP(SA), FRCPC
Professor of Paediatrics, University of Toronto; Clinical Director, NICU, The Hospital for Sick Children, Toronto, Ontario, Canada

Susan R. Hintz, MD
Assistant Professor of Pediatrics, Division of Neonatal and Developmental Medicine, Department of Pediatrics, Stanford University School of Medicine, Lucile Salter Packard Children's Hospital at Stanford, Palo Alto, California

Satish C. Kalhan, MD
Professor, Department of Pediatrics; Director, Schwartz Center for Metabolism & Nutrition, Case Western Reserve University School of Medicine at MetroHealth Medical Center, Cleveland, Ohio

Attallah Kappas, MD
Professor Emeritus, The Rockefeller University, New York, New York

Evan J. Kass, MD
Chief, Division of Pediatric Urology, William Beaumont Hospital, Royal Oak, Michigan

Judith M. Klarr, MD
Neonatologist, William Beaumont Hospital, Royal Oak, Michigan

Michaela B. Koontz, MD
Fellow, Pediatric Endocrinology and Metabolism, Rainbow Babies and Children's Hospital, Cleveland, Ohio

Ernest F. Krug III, MDiv, MD
Director, Center for Human Development, William Beaumont Hospital, Royal Oak, Michigan

Ashima Madan, MD
Associate Professor of Pediatrics, Division of Neonatal and Developmental Medicine, Department of Pediatrics, Stanford University School of Medicine, Lucile Salter Packard Children's Hospital at Stanford, Palo Alto, California

Richard J. Martin, MD
Professor, Pediatrics, Reproductive Biology, and Physiology & Biophysics, Case Western Reserve University School of Medicine; Director, Division of Neonatology, Rainbow Babies & Children's Hospital, Cleveland, Ohio

Grace McComsey, MD
Associate Professor, Pediatrics and Medicine, Case Western Reserve University; Chief, Division of Pediatric Infectious Diseases and Rheumatology, Rainbow Babies & Children's Hospital, Cleveland, Ohio

M. Mirmiran, MD, PhD
Senior Research Scientist, Division of Neonatal and Developmental Medicine, Department of Pediatrics, Stanford University School of Medicine, Palo Alto, California

Aideen Moore MB, MD, FRCPC, MHSc
Associate Professor, University of Toronto; Staff Neonatologist, The Hospital for Sick Children, Toronto, Ontario, Canada

Jane Morton, MD
Clinical Professor of Pediatrics, Stanford University School of Medicine, Stanford, California

Mark R. Palmert, MD, PhD
Assistant Professor, Pediatrics and Genetics, Case Western Reserve University School of Medicine; Attending Endocrinologist, Rainbow Babies and Children's Hospital, Cleveland, Ohio

Anna Penn, MD, PhD
Acting Assistant Professor of Pediatrics, Division of Neonatal and Developmental Medicine, Department of Pediatrics Stanford University School of Medicine, Lucile Salter Packard Children's Hospital at Stanford, Palo Alto, California

Cynthia J.E. Pryce, MD
Neonatologist, William Beaumont Hospital, Royal Oak, Michigan

William D. Rhine, MD
Professor of Pediatrics, Division of Neonatal and Developmental Medicine, Department of Pediatrics, Stanford University School of Medicine, Director of Neonatal Intensive Care Unit, Lucile Salter Packard Children's Hospital at Stanford, Palo Alto, California

Ricardo J. Rodriguez, MD
Associate Professor, Pediatrics, Case Western Reserve University School of Medicine, Rainbow Babies & Children's Hospital, Cleveland, Ohio

David N. Rosenthal, MD

Director, Pediatric Heart Failure Program, Lucile Packard Children's Hospital, Palo Alto, California; Associate Professor of Pediatrics, Stanford University School of Medicine, Stanford, California

Barbara J. Stoll, MD

Professor & Chair, Department of Pediatrics, Emory University School of Medicine, Atlanta, Georgia

Philip Sunshine, MD

Professor of Pediatrics Emeritus, Division of Neonatal and Developmental Medicine, Department of Pediatrics, Stanford University School of Medicine, Lucile Salter Packard Children's Hospital at Stanford, Palo Alto, California

Gary Trock, MD

Chief, Division of Pediatric Neurology, William Beaumont Hospital, Royal Oak, Michigan

Krisa Page Van Meurs, MD

Professor of Pediatrics, Division of Neonatal and Developmental Medicine, Department of Pediatrics; Co-Director, Extracorporeal Membrane Oxygenation Program, Stanford University School of Medicine, Lucile Salter Packard Children's Hospital at Stanford, Palo Alto, California

Table of Contents

Journals Represented

Journals represented in this YEAR BOOK are listed below.

Acta Obstetricia et Gynecologica Scandinavica
Acta Paediatrica
American Journal of Clinical Nutrition
American Journal of Epidemiology
American Journal of Human Genetics
American Journal of Neuroradiology
American Journal of Obstetrics and Gynecology
American Journal of Perinatology
American Surgeon
Archives of Disease in Childhood
Archives of Disease in Childhood. Fetal and Neonatal Edition
Archives of Pediatrics and Adolescent Medicine
British Medical Journal
Circulation
Clinical Radiology
European Respiratory Journal
Human Pathology
Intensive Care Medicine
International Journal of Gynaecology and Obstetrics
Journal of Allergy and Clinical Immunology
Journal of Applied Physiology
Journal of Clinical Endocrinology and Metabolism
Journal of Clinical Microbiology
Journal of Infectious Diseases
Journal of Pediatric Gastroenterology and Nutrition
Journal of Pediatric Surgery
Journal of Pediatrics
Journal of Perinatology
Journal of Rheumatology
Journal of the American Medical Association
Lancet
Metabolism: Clinical and Experimental
Neurology
New England Journal of Medicine
Obstetrics and Gynecology
Ophthalmology
Pediatric Infectious Disease Journal
Pediatric Radiology
Pediatric Research
Pediatrics
Proceedings of the National Academy of Sciences
Thoretical Medicine and Bioethics
Transfusion
Ultrasound in Obstetrics and Gynecology

STANDARD ABBREVIATIONS

The following terms are abbreviated in this edition: acquired immunodeficiency syndrome (AIDS), cardiopulmonary resuscitation (CPR), central nervous system (CNS), cerebrospinal fluid (CSF), computed tomography (CT), deoxyribonucleic acid (DNA), electrocardiography (ECG), health maintenance organization (HMO), human immunodeficiency virus (HIV), intensive care unit (ICU), intramuscular (IM), intravenous (IV), magnetic resonance (MR) imaging (MRI), ribonucleic acid (RNA), and ultrasound (US).

NOTE

The YEAR BOOK OF NEONATAL AND PERINATAL MEDICINE® is a literature survey service providing abstracts of articles published in the professional literature. Every effort is made to assure the accuracy of the information presented in these pages. Neither the editors nor the publisher of the YEAR BOOK OF NEONATAL AND PERINATAL MEDICINE® can be responsible for errors in the original materials. The editors' comments are their own opinions. Mention of specific products within this publication does not constitute endorsement.

To facilitate the use of the YEAR BOOK OF NEONATAL AND PERINATAL MEDICINE® as a reference tool, all illustrations and tables included in this publication are now identified as they appear in the original article. This change is meant to help the reader recognize that any illustration or table appearing in the YEAR BOOK OF NEONATAL AND PERINATAL MEDICINE® may be only one of many in the original article. For this reason, figure and table numbers will often appear to be out of sequence within the YEAR BOOK OF NEONATAL AND PERINATAL MEDICINE®.

Introduction

Penning the introduction for the YEAR BOOK OF NEONATAL PERINATAL MEDICINE represents the formal end to the cycle and the culmination of the efforts of a huge team. The cycle starts with the YEAR BOOK staff tearing out the articles from some hundred journals and sending them to the editors for their decision. Articles are selected for inclusion and commentary on the basis of originality, interest, and, of course, addition to the evidence data base. Hence, randomized controlled masked trials always get high priority scores and are almost uniformly selected. The editors then either write the commentaries themselves or assign them to colleagues and friends who continue to willingly give of their time and expertise. Despite the random selection of the articles when it comes time to assemble the book we find that they naturally can be aligned to organ systems, and it has always been gratifying to find the wide varieties of topics that have been covered. The highlights from the literature in the past year are thus gathered together and hopefully serve as a good source of reference as well as new information. The data is provided as a series of appetizers without necessarily including a main course but should satisfy even those with large appetites.

As noted in the feature article in this edition, the passing of Bill Silverman leaves a huge void in the field of medicine in general and neonatal-perinatal medicine in particular. He was not only a pioneer in the field but extremely courageous and unashamedly outspoken. He has inspired and influenced many of the current leaders in the field and through his writing should continue to influence future generations of neonatologists.

This year's selections once again include a number of randomized trials with negative results. Hence, glutamine supplementation, a potent anti-infective agent in adults with burns, was ineffective in reducing hospital-acquired infections in low-birth-weight neonates and morphine administration to ventilated infants was not beneficial but possibly harmful. Trials presented at the annual Pediatric Academic Society meetings suggest that cooling is beneficial for asphyxiated infants, and we look forward to these data being published as well as the true impact of nitric oxide in premature infants. There are a number of selections dealing with the benefits of human breast milk, and the results of some questionnaires have also been included. The new genetics is unraveling a number of new disorders, and we have included, for example, a report on salt wasting and deafness resulting from mutations in two chloride channels, as well as new information on the surfactant genes. There is intriguing information related to differences in the incidence of cryptorchidism in two Scandinavian countries, as well as much information on prematurity and near prematurity.

It is always a pleasurable task to thank our many friends and colleagues who serve as contributors and commentators. They add the spice and flavor to the book, and for that we are grateful. We thank Jonathan Hellman for his continued lead and commentaries on bioethical problems, an ever-important aspect of perinatal-neonatal care. We also acknowledge the excellent support from the Elsevier YEAR BOOK team headed by Nell Wulfart, David Orzechowski, and Tim Maxwell.

Avroy A. Fanaroff, MB, BCh (Rand), FRCPE, FRCPCH

M. Jeffrey Maisels, MB, BCh

David K. Stevenson, MD

Obituary*

WILLIAM SILVERMAN

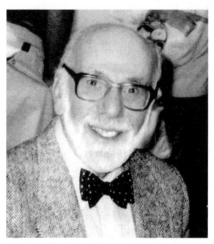

A founding father of neonatology who was a proponent of evidence-based medicine. Born Oct 23, 1917, in Cleveland, OH, USA, he died of renal failure aged 87 on Dec 16, 2004, in Greenbrae, CA, USA.

William Silverman liked to give everyone he knew a badge on which was printed "Semper Plangere"—Latin for "always complain". It was a reflection of how wary he was of medical claims unsupported by strong evidence. As a young faculty member at Columbia University's College of Physicians and Surgeons, in New York, USA, Silverman researched retrolental hyperplasia (retinopathy of prematurity). Although Silverman "proved" in a randomised controlled clinical trial that adrenocorticotropic hormone (ACTH) was an effective treatment for the disease, he was later proven wrong by researchers at Johns Hopkins University. And he found that supplemental oxygen, given to many premature infants at the time, would actually lead to the disease rather than prevent it. This work would make him keenly aware of the importance of evidence in making medical decisions.

His first book, in 1961, was the third edition of *Dunham's Premature Infants*, which had already become a standard text. "He asked the publisher to print it in two print sizes: large for evidence-based material, smaller for that which was his opinion", said John Sinclair, Silverman's protégé and professor emeritus of paediatrics at McMaster University in Hamilton, Canada. The publisher would not comply, and Sinclair had to settle for a warning in the front of the book about the absence of evidence. By 1968, he had become so disillusioned with the way people used data from physiological and laboratory studies to treat premature babies that he resigned from his prestigious chair at Columbia University. He would spend the rest of his career promoting evidence-based medicine, nurturing the careers of countless colleagues worldwide, and championing the cause of children with retinopathy of prematurity through his work with the American Foundation for the Blind.

Dale Phelps, professor of paediatrics and ophthalmology at the University of Rochester, New York, USA, as a young faculty member when she received a letter from Silverman. "I had just submitted my very first presentation on retinopathy of prematurity", she told *The Lancet*. "I got this lovely note—'I wasn't able to attend the presentation, but would love to hear more about your work'." That would begin a correspondence that spanned many years. Silverman had "a huge list of people" to whom he would send notes saying, "think about this, read that, consider doing this", according to Jon E Tyson, director of the Center for Clinical Research and Evidence-Based Medicine at the University of Texas Medical School at Houston, USA. Lawrence M Gartner, professor emeritus of paediatrics and obstetrics/gynaecology at the University of Chicago, USA, met Silverman in the early 1960s when a colleague suggested Gartner visit Silverman at Columbia. That led to Silverman making rounds once a month at the Albert Einstein College of Medicine in New York where Gartner was in charge of the premature unit. "It was absolutely phenomenal, a stirring experience", Gartner told *The Lancet*, because Silverman "always saw the patient as the ultimate person who had to be cared for—his ethical position was beyond that of anyone that I've ever met".

"He was clearly the pioneer" in terms of evidence-based medicine, said David Sackett, founding chair of the Department of Clinical Epidemiology and Biostatistics at McMaster University in Canada and the Founding Director of the Centre for Evidence-Based Medicine at Oxford University, UK. "He played a role in North America that was equal to or even beyond that of Sir Austin Bradford Hill in the UK in terms of introducing randomised trials, because Bill Silverman carried them out in areas where the overwhelming opinion was what was going on was correct. It took an enormous amount of courage to carry out these trials." Silverman was "also very critical of the dominant power within biomedical research—the people who believe that all important answers about human health will come from the laboratory", said Iain Chalmers, editor of the *James Lind Library*. He would often refer to "the divisive effect of reductionist snobbery".

Silverman's last book, *Where's the Evidence?*, arose from his column, "Fumes from the spleen", in *Pediatric and Perinatal Epidemiology* under the pseudonym "Malcontent". He explained in the preface that he used pseudonyms "because I firmly believed W H Auden's remark about writing and writers was doubly relevant in the explication of arguments. An unsigned work, to paraphrase him, forces the reader to respond to the reasoning, not the reasoner."

He is survived by his wife Ruth and his children Daniel, Jennifer, and David.

Ivan Oransky
ivan-oransky@erols.com

William Silverman, MD: Pioneer in Neonatology—Lessons Learned

AVROY A FANAROFF MD AND GILBERT I MARTIN MD

"Sempere Plangere"

This simple Latin term, meaning "Always Complain," was the motto that Bill Silverman used his entire professional career as a reflection of how wary he was of medical claims unsupported by strong evidence.

The passing of Bill Silverman on December 16, 2004, leaves a huge void in the field of medicine in general and in neonatal-perinatal medicine in particular. He was not only a pioneer but extremely courageous and unashamedly outspoken. He exited clinical practice relatively early in his career but remained "our conscience," and was constantly goading us all to look at what we were doing, examine the evidence, and, above all, to keep families involved and informed. Early in his career he was witness to the incredible results with penicillin and other antibiotics. A succession of additional therapeutic miracles and unprecedented medical victories ushered in a new interventionist era. In looking back on that era he noted, "We were so dazzled by the successes, we were blind to an obvious fact. We had woefully little knowledge about the complete biological effects and full social consequences of the uninhibited use of new drugs and innovative technology." These words still ring very true to this day. He was also concerned that in neonatal-perinatal medicine the potentially long delay between the intervention and the detection of harmful effects would result in huge calamities. He equated these deleterious effects to collateral damage in warfare and was deeply disturbed throughout his career by the thousands of children blinded by the small increase in oxygen infused into incubators to eliminate apneic episodes in preterm infants. Another prime example is the infamous DES (diethylstilbestrol) incident wherein millions of pregnant women all over the world were treated with the hormone for more than 30 years, before it was discovered (in 1970) that their offspring were at increased risk for cancer, genitourinary abnormalities, and other adverse outcomes later in their lives.

Bill Silverman was instrumental in performing some of the first randomized trials in neonatal-perinatal medicine. The relative importance of incubator temperature and relative humidity was resolved by Silverman and his colleagues in three sequential analyses. Their study design became a model for further studies in the neonate. In the first study comparing high versus low humidity, they observed a lower mortality and higher temperatures in the high humidity group. In the second study, they controlled humidity and examined the effect of varying only environmental temperature. They noted a striking difference in survival rates. With only a 4°F increase in incubator temperature, they observed a 15% increase in survival .at the higher temperature with the biggest difference affecting the smallest infants. In a further study controlling environmental temperature but varying humidity caused no difference in survival. Applying the appropriate environmental temperature to sick newborns has saved the lives of untold infants and has formed the bedrock of evidence-based medicine for the care of newborn infants. Silverman then turned his attention to the still thorny problem of nosocomial infections. He was devastated when he discovered that in his attempt to prevent these nosocomial infections in preterm infants by a combination of penicillin and sulfonamides more babies died with kernicterus. He thus made us constantly aware, "We cannot always make our patients better, but we can always make them worse!"

Bill Silverman wrote a column titled "Fumes from the Spleen" in the British journal, *Pediatrics and Perinatal Epidemiology*. He signed the column "The Malcontent," believing that an anonymous piece might be reacted to more objectively than a signed one. His e-mail address was fumer@aol.com. The word "fumer" was derived from the title of the column "Fumes From the Spleen". In December 1976 he began submitting quotations, reflections, notes from newspapers and magazines to the journal, *Pediatrics*, under the signature line "Student". He was not the first author to use this pseudonym for William Gossett, a chemist in Ireland who coined the Student's t test, used this signature for the first time in 1908. Dr Tonse Raju (personal communication) in discussing Dr Silverman's "blurbs" summed it up best by saying "an analysis and classification of even a select few of these can provide enough material for a monograph and a source of perspectives on medicine and society in our times, as seen through the eyes of a visionary". His first such contribution as a "Student" read as follows:

> "Two basic inputs are required in making a health decision; one is medical information, and the other is a value system that ranks the desire for health in relation to other wants. Health professionals are trained to supply the individual with medical facts and opinions...... Nevertheless, doctors generally assume that the high priority that they place on health should be shared by others. They find it hard to accept that some people may opt for a brief, intense existence full of unhealthy practices. Such individuals are pejoratively labeled "noncompliant" and pressures are applied on them to recorder their priorities."

Bill Silverman was a prolific contributor to the medical literature as well as the author of several seminal publications. His books, *Retrolental Fibroplasia: A Modern Parable, Human Experimentation: A Guided Step Into The Unkown*, and *Where's the Evidence? Debates in Modern Medicine* are required reading for all health care professionals entering the field of neonatal -perinatal medicine. Bill Silverman was also a sought after lecturer and keynote speaker. My first encounter with him was the enthralling talk that he gave at the neonatal dinner at the Society for Pediatric Research meeting in Atlantic City in 1970. He recounted the tale of the temperature (the importance of thermal regulation in the neonate) and Martin Cooney's exhibits of premature babies in incubators at state fairs. He also gave a remarkable talk on neonatal ethics to a packed auditorium at the Pediatric Academic Society some 30 years later. His choice of language and quotations were remarkable and he was entertaining, stimulating, and always provocative. He forced you to think and reevaluate what you were doing, and you came away from these experiences with a renewed vigor to tackle scientific and ethical problems. In a sense, a prophet, he often quoted the scriptures. A most fitting statement that sums up many of his thoughts and beliefs and is quoted often is: "Teach thy tongue to say I do not know and thou shall progress"

These words are a fitting epitaph to his memory.

1   The Fetus

Transplacental Fetal Treatment Improves the Outcome of Prenatally Diagnosed Complete Atrioventricular Block Without Structural Heart Disease

Jaeggi ET, Fouron J-C, Silverman ED, et al (Univ of Toronto; Univ of Montreal)

Circulation 110:1542-1548, 2004   1–1

Background.—Untreated isolated fetal complete atrioventricular block (CAVB) has a significant mortality rate. A standardized treatment approach, including maternal dexamethasone at CAVB diagnosis and β-stimulation for fetal heart rates <55 bpm, has been used at our institutions since 1997. The study presents the impact of this approach.

Method and Results.—Thirty-seven consecutive cases of fetal CAVB since 1990 were studied. Mean age at diagnosis was 25.6 ± 5.2 gestational weeks. In 33 patients (92%), CAVB was associated with maternal anti-Ro/La autoantibodies. Patients were separated into those diagnosed between 1990 and 1996 (group 1; n=16) and those diagnosed between 1997 and 2003 (group 2; n=21). The 2 study groups were comparable in the clinical presentation at CAVB diagnosis but did differ in prenatal management (treated patients: group 1, 4/16; group 2, 18/21; P<0.0001). Overall, 22 fetuses were treated, 21 with dexamethasone and 9 with β-stimulation for a mean of 7.5±4.5 weeks. Live-birth and 1-year survival rates of group 1 were 80% and 47%, and these improved to 95% for group 2 patients (P<0.01). The 21 patients treated with dexamethasone had a 1-year survival rate of 90%, compared with 46% without glucocorticoid therapy (P<0.02). Immune-mediated conditions (myocarditis, hepatitis, cardiomyopathy) resulting in postnatal death or heart transplantation were significantly more common in untreated anti-Ro/La antibody–associated pregnancies compared with patients treated with steroids (0/18 versus 4/9 live births; P=0.007).

Conclusions.—A standardized treatment approach, including transplacental fetal administration of dexamethasone and beta-stimulation at heart rates <55 bpm, reduced the morbidity and improved the outcome of isolated fetal CAVB.

▶ There is a constant search for noninvasive treatment of the fetus. For the fetus with complete heart block, a disorder with a significant risk of death for the fetus or infant, this study provides at least some encouragement. Now we all know that it is dangerous to read too much into retrospective controls.

Nonetheless, the survival rates rose dramatically for infants with fetal CAVD not associated with other structural heart defects. Also, Doppler echocardiography has emerged as an excellent diagnostic tool in the noninvasive assessment of fetal atrioventricular conduction and its anomalies.

This is an informative series from a single institution where the change to fetal treatment with a combination of dexamethasone and/or β-stimulation predominantly after 1997 was associated with an increase in the number of survivors to 1 year. The beneficiaries of corticosteroids had a 90% 1-year survival compared with only 46% among those not receiving corticosteroids. Those not receiving dexamethasone were also more likely to manifest immune complex disease of the myocardium (myocarditis, cardiomyopathy) and/or liver.

The same team reported for the first time the response of a patient with isolated complete heart block to transplacentally delivered dexamethasone.[1] There was a sustained regression from isolated complete to first-degree heart block. These reports require corroboration but at least provide clinicians with some tools rather than have them stand by helplessly while the fetus becomes hydropic and dies. Corticosteroids remain the old faithful standby when all else fails. In this disorder characterized by immune complexes (see Abstract 12–1) there is a strong rationale for their use. My understanding, too, is that the pacemaker technology has advanced rapidly and that these are becoming feasible for smaller, younger patients.

A. A. Fanaroff, MD

Reference

1. Jaeggi ET, Silverman ED, Yoo SJ, et al: Is immune-mediated complete fetal atrioventricular block reversible by transplacental dexamethasone therapy? *Ultrasound Obstet Gynecol* 23:602-605, 2004.

Screening Performance of First-Trimester Nuchal Translucency for Major Cardiac Defects: A Meta-analysis
Makrydimas G, Sotiriadis A, Ioannidis JPA (Univ of Ioannina, Greece; Tufts–New England Med Ctr, Boston)
Am J Obstet Gynecol 189:1330-1335, 2003   1–2

Objective.—The purpose of this study was to evaluate the screening performance of increased first-trimester nuchal translucency for the detection of major congenital heart defects.

Study Design.—A meta-analysis based on MEDLINE and EMBASE searches (up to June 2002) that assessed the diagnostic performance of increased nuchal translucency for congenital heart defect detection. Weighted sensitivity and specificity estimates (random effects) and summary receiver-operating characteristic curves were obtained.

Results.—Eight independent studies with 58,492 pregnant women were analyzed. There was significant heterogeneity among the studies. Nuchal translucency above the 99th percentile had a sensitivity of 31% and specificity of 98.7% (random effects calculations), with a positive likelihood ratio of 24. Summary receiver-operating characteristic estimates were consistent with these values. The ability of nuchal translucency measurements above this threshold to detect cardiac malformations varied nonsignificantly ($P =$ .64) for different congenital heart defects types (sensitivity range, 25%-55%).

Conclusion.—Nuchal translucency screening is a modestly efficient strategy for congenital heart defect detection; the use of the 99th percentile threshold may capture approximately 30% of congenital heart defects.

▶ This is a meta-analysis of 8 retrospective studies looking at nuchal thickness (NT) of the 10- to 13-week embryo with normal chromosomes as a screening tool for cardiac defects. The sensitivity of increased NT for cardiac defects was 31%. Although some reports have shown a predominance of left-sided heart defects in this positive group, this was not seen in this population. If the ninety-fifth percentile threshold was used, the sensitivity was 37%. The authors then performed a cost analysis in which they assumed that 75% of heart defects will be missed on screening examination but will be detected on a more detailed examination. But this is not usually the case. Screening examinations have a sensitivity of 75% if they include the outflow tracts, and fetal echocardiograms only occasionally reveal more information. This study reminds us that when we are screening for an euploidy and we find a fetus with increased NT, we need to be sure to perform a careful cardiac screen at 18 weeks.

C. Comstock, MD

Pregnancy Outcomes With Increased Nuchal Translucency After Routine Down Syndrome Screening
Cheng C-C, Bahado-Singh RO, Chen S-C, et al (Cathay Gen Hosp, Taipei, Taiwan; Univ of Cincinnati, Ohio)
Int J Gynaecol Obstet 84:5-9, 2004   1–3

Objectives.—The purpose of this study was to evaluate the outcomes of pregnancies with nuchal translucency greater or equal to 3 mm for routine first trimester screening in unselected populations.

Methods.—A total of 2980 pregnant women for first trimester ultrasonography were routinely offered crown-rump length (CRL) and nuchal translucency (NT) for screening for Down syndrome between 11 and 14 weeks' gestation. A complete follow-up was obtained in all cases by a review of medical records.

Results.—Using a cut-off value of 3 mm, the prevalence of increased fetal NT was 0.7% ($n=22$). Among the 22 cases, there were five (227%) chromosomal abnormalities. Of the 17 chromosomally normal pregnancies, four resulted in fetal demise (spontaneous abortion, intrauterine death or termination of pregnancy due to fetal abnormalities). The remaining 13 pregnancies resulted in live births, including one gestational hypertension and one preterm delivery, respectively. The total incidence of an adverse outcome in the group of increased fetal NT was 45.5%.

Conclusions.—In a routine population with first-trimester ultrasonography, fetal NT measuring greater than or equal to 3 mm was associated with a poor pregnancy outcome with not only chromosomal abnormalities and congenital cardiac diseases, but also poor maternal and fetal health or adverse pregnancy outcomes. In addition, this study also demonstrated the necessity for fetal assessment and follow-up in cases where the fetal NT is increased in the first trimester.

▶ This is one of many studies looking at the outcome of fetuses with increased NT in early pregnancy (10-13 weeks). In this paper NT was defined as more than 3 mm, which is the number used in many other publications. Like those, the results here show that the incidence of abnormal chromosomes was high: 22%. The strengths of this report include the unselected population (vs women presenting for genetic testing) and the long-term infant follow-up (to an average age of 21 months). The weakness is the lack of information about the population as a whole and the lack of sensitivity and specificity estimates. How many cases of trisomy 21 occurred in the 2980 patients? How did these results compare with the embryos without NT more than 3 mm?

NT alone has a high false-positive rate. It has recently been combined with a first-trimester serum screening test using pregnancy-associated plasma protein A and β-HCG, which, together with NT, markedly decreases the false-positive rate and increases sensitivity in the detection of aneuploidy. Patients who are positive for this screen then have time to undergo chorionic villus sampling.

C. Comstock, MD

Differential Maturation of the Innate Immune Response in Human Fetuses
Strunk T, Temming P, Gembruch U, et al (Univ of Lübeck, Germany; Univ of Bonn, Germany; Justus Liebig-Univ Giessen, Germany)
Pediatr Res 56:219-226, 2004   1–4

Newborns and especially preterm infants show a unique susceptibility to severe bacterial infections that cause significant morbidity and mortality. As very few data are available on innate immune functions in human fetuses, we conducted a comprehensive study to investigate the expression of several adhesion molecules essentially involved in migration (CD11a, CD11b, CD11c, CD18, and CD62L). Furthermore, phagocytic activity, generation of respiratory burst products, and production of several proinflammatory cytokines were assessed. Various functions of the fetal innate immune system were demonstrated to be essentially different from those observed in term neonates or adults. Expression of several surface markers was significantly diminished on fetal granulocytes. Furthermore, a significantly reduced phagocytic activity of fetal granulocytes and monocytes was found, contrasted by an enhanced generation of reactive oxygen products. In addition, we demonstrate that significant numbers of fetal monocytes are capable of the production of proinflammatory cytokines in response to stimulation. However, the pattern of cytokine production is different from the more mature individuals: the number of IL-6– and tumor necrosis factor-α– positive monocytes were significantly diminished, whereas more IL-8– producing monocytes were found compared with adults. The results of our study add significantly to our understanding of the maturation and impairment of the innate immune response.

▶ Neutrophils play critical roles in the host defense against infection. The increased susceptibility of term as well as preterm babies to bacterial and fungal infection has long suggested that their neutrophils might be a weak link in their innate defense mechanisms. Provision of adequate phagocytic and bactericidal activity at sites of bacterial invasion, as well as at sites of established infection, begins with differentiation and maturation of neutrophil precursors in the bone marrow. Subsequent distinct steps involve activation and attraction of circulating neutrophils, adhesion to and migration out of the circulation, chemotaxis through the tissues, phagocytosis, and ultimately killing of the pathogens. These steps, in turn, depend on cytokines that drive cellular maturation, priming and activation; chemoattractants; adhesion ligands on endothelial cells; and opsonins on the pathogens. Specific receptors on the marrow precursors and circulating cells and appropriate intracellular signaling pathways are necessary for the response to each of these signals.

It has been recognized for some time that even term neonates have limited storage pools of postmitotic neutrophil precursors and that sepsis may rapidly deplete these pools, leading to neutropenia rather than leukocytosis.[1,2] Decreases in complement, the lack of immunoglobulin M antibodies, differences in cytokine production by mononuclear cells, and decreased adhesion molecule expression by endothelial cells all contribute to impaired host defenses in neonates. There also have been several studies demonstrating that neonates' neutrophils are qualitatively different from those in adults, with decreased cellular content of important adhesion molecules and altered responses to stimuli. Interpretation of some of the results has been difficult because it is not clear how to evaluate the extent of activation of the baby's cells during delivery. Strunk et al extend our knowledge of the functional capabilities of neonates' neutrophils by looking earlier in gestation (as early as 21 weeks) than most other studies and by studying intrauterine umbilical vein samples from the fetuses, thus eliminating effects of delivery. Their results are generally consistent with the trends that might have been predicted by previous studies: fetal neutrophils have decreased expression of selectin (CD62L) and integrin (all members of the CD11/CD18 family) adhesion molecules, decreased phagocytic activity, but relatively preserved oxidative burst activity. They also show that lipopolysaccharide stimulation induces less tumor necrosis factor-α and interleukin-6 production by fetal monocytes compared with adults' mononuclear cells. This may also be an extremely important finding, as tumor necrosis factor-α plays a major role in priming circulating neutrophils for increased responses to other stimuli.[3]

We must keep this physiologic immaturity of neutrophil defenses in mind when we consider the risks for, and treatment of, infection in the progressively preterm babies in our neonatal ICUs. The possible relationships among the decrease in the size of the postmitotic neutrophil precursor storage pool, the decrease in content and expression of adhesion molecules, and differences in cytokine production by neonatal mononuclear cells should continue to be actively investigated. Better understanding of what governs the progression of neutrophil precursors through the various stages of maturation and what determines when they are released from the marrow may well improve our ability to strengthen this weak link in the innate host defense mechanisms of preterm babies.

M. Berger, MD, PhD

References

1. Lewis DB, Tu W: The physiologic immunodeficiency of immaturity, in Stiehm ER, Ochs HD, Winkelstein JA (eds): *Immunologic Disorders in Infants and Children*, ed 5. Philadelphia, Elsevier, 2004, pp 687-760.
2. Carr R: Neutrophil production and function in newborn infants. *Br J Haem* 110:18-28, 2000.
3. Berger M, Wetzler E, Wallis RS: Tumor necrosis factor is the major monocyte product that increases complement receptor expression on neutrophils. *Blood* 71:151-158, 1988.

Acute Cardiovascular Effects of Fetal Surgery in the Human
Rychik J, Tian Z, Cohen MS, et al (The Children's Hosp of Philadelphia; Univ of Pennsylvania, Philadelphia)
Circulation 110:1549-1556, 2004   1–5

Background.—Prenatal surgery for congenital anomalies can prevent fetal demise or alter the course of organ development, resulting in a more favorable condition at birth. The indications for fetal surgery continue to expand, yet little is known about the acute sequelae of fetal surgery on the human cardiovascular system.

Method and Results.—Echocardiography was used to evaluate the heart before, during, and early after fetal surgery for congenital anomalies, including repair of myelomeningocele (MMC, n=51), resection of intrathoracic masses (ITM, n=15), tracheal occlusion for congenital diaphragmatic hernia (CDH, n=13), and resection of sacrococcygeal teratoma (SCT, n=4). Fetuses with MMC all had normal cardiovascular systems entering into fetal surgery, whereas those with ITM, CDH, and SCT all exhibited secondary cardiovascular sequelae of the anomaly present. At fetal surgery, heart rate increased acutely, and combined cardiac output diminished at the time of fetal incision for all groups including those with MMC, which suggests diminished stroke volume. Ventricular dysfunction and valvular dysfunction were identified in all groups, as was acute constriction of the ductus arteriosus. Fetuses with ITM and SCT had the most significant changes at surgery.

Conclusions.—Acute cardiovascular changes take place during fetal surgery that are likely a consequence of the physiology of the anomaly and the general effects of surgical stress, tocolytic agents, and anesthesia. Echocardiographic monitoring during fetal surgery is an important adjunct in the management of these patients.

▶ Unique characteristics of the myocardium and specific channels of blood flow differentiate the physiology of the fetus from the newborn. Echocardiography has not only resulted in the early detection of cardiac anomalies, but also added to the understanding of human fetal cardiovascular physiology in the normal and diseased states. Many of the current indications for surgery on the fetus are accompanied by compromised cardiac function with or without the onset of hydrops fetalis. It was, therefore, timely that Rychik et al evaluated the heart before, during and immediately after fetal surgery for a variety of anomalies. This included conditions in which cardiac function would be disturbed as well as repair of myelomeningoceles in which heart function should be normal. It was intriguing to learn that during surgery the heart rate increased, yet cardiac output fell in all the infants, implying that stroke volume has decreased. Ventricular and valvular dysfunction, together with narrowing of the ductus arteriosus, was documented with all the fetal surgical procedures.

As these operative interventions are taking place at critical times for brain development, the consequences of these perturbations in cardiac output may be disastrous. We agree with Rychik et al that "Echocardiographic monitoring during fetal surgery is an important adjunct in the management of these patients."

A. A. Fanaroff, MD

▶ This is an interesting report of the effects of fetal non-cardiac surgery on the fetal cardiovascular system, from a large center with extensive experience in fetal surgery. Cardiovascular derangements are seen in the fetus starting with the uterine incision and continuing throughout the first 24 hours. Most prominently, there is an increase in fetal heart rate during fetal surgery, but a decrease in fetal combined cardiac output (output of left and right ventricles summed). This suggests that despite the obvious fetal stress, the fetus cannot augment or even maintain cardiac output during non-cardiac surgery. Additional abnormalities include the development of fetal ductal constriction, typically lasting 24 hours, and the development of fetal valvular dysfunction (mitral and tricuspid regurgitation), which can be regarded as general markers of fetal myocardial dysfunction in this setting.

The changes described in this report may be manifestations of the fetal stress response to surgery, or may be attributed to the cardiovascular perturbations induced in the mother by the surgical and anesthetic treatment. For example, the development of ductal constriction may be the result of maternal oxygen and indomethacin administration, rather than a generic response. Similarly, the reduced cardiac output may reflect intrinsic limitations of fetal myocardium, or may result from the inhalational anesthetic administered to the mother. Our state of knowledge of this area is quite rudimentary, and this initial report raises as many questions as it answers. Clearly, ongoing cardiovascular evaluation of the fetus is going to be an important component of fetal surgical programs. Currently, this is best achieved with echocardiography.

D. N. Rosenthal, MD

Fetal Middle Cerebral Artery Peak Systolic Velocity in the Investigation of Non-immune Hydrops

Hernandez-Andrade E, Scheier M, Dezerega V, et al (King's College Hosp, London)

Ultrasound Obstet Gynecol 23:442-445, 2004   1–6

Introduction.—Fetal hydrops in red blood cell isoimmunization occurs when the fetal hemoglobin deficit exceeds 6 SD. In this condition, the fetus compensates for anemia by hemodynamic adjustments, which can be evaluated via Doppler US. Measurement of the fetal middle cerebral artery peak systolic velocity (MCA-PSV) provides sensitive prediction concerning the anemic fetus. The potential value of MCA-PSV in the evaluation and management of nonimmune hydrops caused by anemia that demonstrated the same US features as those of immune hydrops was assessed, and the significance of the association between delta MCA-PSV (the difference in SD from the normal mean for gestation) and delta fetal hemoglobin concentration was investigated. The US features and hemoglobin concentration of fetuses with congenital infection were also assessed.

Methods.—Fetal MCA-PSV and fetal hemoglobin concentration in blood obtained by cordocentesis were measured in 16 singleton pregnancies with a diagnosis of nonimmune hydrops fetalis. A detailed US examination revealed moderate or severe ascites, with or without skin edema, and pericardial or pleural effusions in all fetuses. No obvious malformations were observed that could explain the hydrops. In each case, the measured MCA-PSV and hemoglobin concentration were expressed as delta values.

Results.—Of 16 cases of nonimmune hydrops, 7 (43.8%) had parvovirus B19 infection, 1 (14.3%) had α-thalassemia, 1 (14.3%) had primary cardiomyopathy, and 7 (43.8%) had no obvious explanation for hydrops. A significant association was observed between delta MCA-PSV and delta hemoglobin concentration (delta hemoglobin = (delta MCA-PSV + 0.1437)/−0.4154; R^2 = 0.7202; P < .0001) (Fig 3). In 10 cases, the fetal hemoglobin concentration was greater than 4 SD below the normal mean for gestation; in all cases, the MCA-PSV was greater than 2 SD above the normal mean for gestation. A computer search found an additional 9 fetuses with parvovirus B19 infection; in all 9, the predominant US findings were ascites, and the hemoglobin concentration was more than 4 SD below the normal fetus mean. Only 3 of 14 fetuses with cytomegalovirus, toxoplasmosis, coxsackie B, or *Treponema* infection had ascites; 2 of 14 had a hemoglobin deficit of 4 to 6 SD.

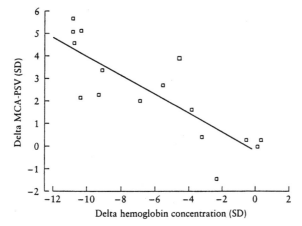

FIGURE 3.—Fetal middle cerebral artery peak systolic velocity (MCA-PSV) plotted against fetal hemoglobin concentration (delta SD). (Courtesy of Hernandez-Andrade E, Scheier M, Dezerega V, et al: Fetal middle cerebral artery peak systolic velocity in the investigation of non-immune hydrops. *Ultrasound Obstet Gynecol* 23:442-445. Copyright 2004 International Society of Ultrasound in Obstetrics & Gynecology. Permission is granted by John Wiley & Sons Ltd on behalf of the ISUOG.)

Conclusion.—In nonimmune hydrops with no obvious structural defects, measurement of MCA-PSV can help detect fetal anemia; this is characterized by tense ascites with dilated heart. Parvovirus B19 infection is the most frequent cause of this disorder. In some cases, intrauterine blood transfusions may reverse the hydrops and result in healthy live births. In hydropic fetuses with no related anemia and normal MCA-PSV, the prognosis is typically poor.

▶ In the past, the management of isoimmunized pregnancies (Rh disease) involved serial amniocenteses to obtain fluid for optical density measurements (Delta OD450) that diagnose fetal anemia by measuring the breakdown products of red blood cells. Recently, MCA-PSV has gradually taken the place of serial amniocenteses in the management of isoimmunized fetuses. In this procedure, the fetal MCA first is identified with color Doppler. The spectral (pulsed) Doppler cursor is then placed near the origin of the MCA and the systolic blood velocity in that artery is measured. Since a high MCA-PSV has reliably distinguished anemic from nonanemic fetuses in immune hydrops, many fewer amniocenteses are now performed.

The question addressed in this article is whether MCA-PSV can aid in the diagnosis and care of fetuses with hydrops from nonimmune causes such as infection. The authors evaluated 16 fetuses with nonimmune hydrops. Since the standard of care in cordocentesis is to determine fetal hematocrit, they obtained MCA-PSVs and then obtained cord blood. They found that only fetuses with abnormally high peak velocities were anemic, and that most of the anemic fetuses were infected with parvovirus. Other infections did not cause anemia, although the fetuses had hydrops.

This article confirms other authors' similar observations that MCA-PSV can detect anemia in nonimmune hydrops. Many fewer cordocenteses, with their attendant problems, will need to be performed in hydropic fetuses since a normal MCA-PSV accurately predicts a normal hematocrit. An abnormally high MCA-PSV will signal a need to confirm anemia by cordocentesis and also will indicate that blood should be ready for fetal transfusion at the time the cordocentesis is performed. MCA-PSV has been a significant diagnostic advance in the treatment of fetal Rh disease and now in nonimmune hydrops.

C. Comstock, MD

Oropharyngeal Fetus in Fetu

Kapoor V, Flom L, Fitz CR (Children's Hosp of Pittsburgh, Pa; Univ of Pittsburgh, Pa)
Pediatr Radiol 34:488-491, 2004   1–7

Background.—Fetus in fetu is a rare entity that usually presents retroperitoneally. A case of an oropharyngeal fetus in fetu was reported.

> *Case Report.*—Premature male fetus, 29.5 weeks' gestation, was delivered because of extreme maternal polyhydramnios. The increased amniotic fluid resulted from the inability of the fetus to swallow, as its oropharynx was obstructed by a large mass, detected by both US and MRI. An urgent ex-utero intrapartum technique (EXIT) was performed, involving a fetal tracheostomy during delivery, while the placenta was in place. The baby weighed 1500 g at birth. An extremely large mass exited the oropharynx through the mouth, with 2 polyps protruding through the nares (Fig 1). The next day, CT scan confirmed a large, heterogeneous mass arising from the hard palate and extending into the oropharyngeal and nasal cavities. Ossified bone resembling vertebrae, ribs, and limbs was detected, consistent with the diagnosis of fetus in fetu. A debulking procedure was performed on day 3 after birth. The resected mass weighed 371 g and was covered by skin. Microscopically, there were neuroepithelial elements, mature brain tissue, hepatoid elements, respiratory- and intestinal-type epithelium, islands of pancreatic tissue, immature and mature cartilage, bony tissue, tooth, salivary gland structures, and squamous epithelium containing hair. The mass also had elements suggestive of yolk sac carcinoma. At 2 weeks of age the residual mass was excised. No immature or yolk sac cells were detected.

Conclusions.—Fetus in fetu usually presents as an abdominal mass; an oropharyngeal presentation is extremely rare. Management is by complete surgical removal, with follow-up monitoring of α-fetoprotein levels to detect malignant degeneration.

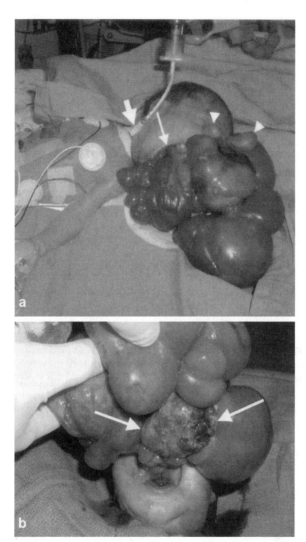

FIGURE 1.—A 29.5-week premature neonate, on day 3 after urgent EXIT delivery due to giant oropharyngeal fetus in fetu. **a,** Large, lobulated mass larger than the neonate's head, protrudes from the oral cavity through a stretched open mouth (*long thin arrow*). Note tracheostomy tube (*short thick arrow*) placed during delivery. *Arrowheads* mark polyploidal components of the mass arising from the nares (hidden by the mass on this image). **b,** View of inferior surface of mass and oral cavity shows mass to be arising from the roof of the oral cavity with an intact tongue and floor of mouth. Large, discolored and ulcerated component of mass (*arrows*) is visible along its inferior surface. (Courtesy of Kapoor V, Flom L, Fitz CR: Oropharyngeal fetus in fetu. *Pediatr Radiol* 34:488-491, 2004. Copyright 2004, Springer-Verlag.)

▶ Every year there is a report of a fetus in fetu, which until I began reviewing articles for this publication, I thought was only a rare occurrence. I guess that it still is a rare occurrence, but it seems like a fetus in one location or another in another fetus is always a part of someone's clinical experience in every year.

Some of these "parasitic" twin circumstances are quite challenging from a practical point of view, and of course, can be lethal depending upon the size and location of the tumor. The fact that the fetus in fetu is uncommonly malignant compared with the teratoma provides little comfort to caretakers and parents depending upon size and location of this unusual retroperitoneal accident of development.

D. K. Stevenson, MD

Antenatal Hydronephrosis: Negative Predictive Value of Normal Postnatal Ultrasound—A 5-year Study
Moorthy I, Joshi N, Cook JV, et al (Guy's and St Thomas' NHS Trust, London; Queen Mary's Hosp for Children, Epsom, England; St Helier NHS Trust, Carshalton, Surrey, England)
Clin Radiol 58:964-970, 2003   1–8

Background.—Fetal hydronephrosis is the most frequently detected abnormality on prenatal US. One institution in London has had a screening program in place since 1991 for the detection of antenatal hydronephrosis. A wealth of literature is available regarding the evaluation of urinary tract abnormalities in infants with antenatal hydronephrosis. However, it would appear that no previous studies have investigated the incidence of abnormality in patients discharged after normal postnatal US. A study was done to determine whether normal postnatal US, when used as part of a rigorous screening protocol for the detection and follow-up of antenatal hydronephrosis, can effectively exclude the majority of infants with congenital urinary tract abnormalities that would otherwise be seen with a urinary tract infection (UTI).

Methods.—A retrospective review was conducted of all babies who had postnatal follow-up of antenatally detected hydronephrosis during a 5-year period at 1 institution (Figs 1 and 2). For the same period, data about all babies seen with a UTI before their first birthday were then analyzed. Cross-referencing of these 2 groups allowed investigators to determine which babies developed a UTI having been previously discharged after normal postnatal US.

Results.—The postnatal follow-up of the antenatal hydronephrosis group included 425 infants. Of these patients, 284 were investigated with US alone. During the same 5-year period, UTI developed in 230 infants before their first birthday. On these babies, only 3 had been previously discharged after normal postnatal US, for a negative predictive value of 98.9% for a normal postnatal US in babies who subsequently had a UTI before their first birthday.

Conclusions.—Careful antenatal and postnatal US was shown to be effective in detecting congenital renal tract abnormalities. It is highly unlikely that infants discharged after a normal postnatal US will still have an undetected urinary tract abnormality. All infants with antenatal hydronephrosis should be started on prophylactic antibiotics at birth, pending further inves-

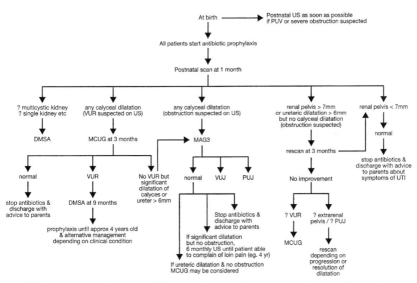

FIGURE 1.—Protocol for postnatal follow-up of antenatal hydronephrosis. (Reprinted by permission of the publisher from Moorthy I, Joshi N, Cook JV, et al: Antenatal hydronephrosis: Negative predictive value of normal postnatal ultrasound—A 5-year study. *Clin Radiol* 58:964-970. Copyright 2003 by Elsevier Science.)

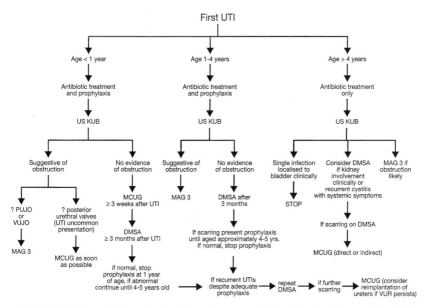

FIGURE 2.—Protocol for investigation of first urinary tract infection. (Reprinted by permission of the publisher from Moorthy I, Joshi N, Cook JV, et al: Antenatal hydronephrosis: Negative predictive value of normal postnatal ultrasound—A 5-year study. *Clin Radiol* 58:964-970. Copyright 2003 by Elsevier Science.)

tigation. A micturating cystourethrogram should be used selectively, and this method should be delayed until the infant is 3 to 4 months old to allow for spontaneous resolution of vesicoureteric reflux.

▶ The authors suggest that by careful US technique, good communication between antenatal and postnatal teams, and meaningful education of parents, we can reduce the number of voiding cystourethrograms (VCUGs) performed for prenatally detected hydronephrosis. The real question to be asked is whether or not this great coordinated effort and the routine use of prophylactic antibiotics for 3 or 4 months is helpful or justified. The authors' own data conclude that vesicoureteral reflux may be discovered in up to 30% of children with prenatally detected hydronephrosis regardless of the degree of hydronephrosis, and a normal US does not exclude its presence.

They go on to state that early detection of vesicoureteral reflux and the prevention of UTI is "crucial in preventing" renal damage. In addition, while it is true that many children with reflux will present in the first year of life with a UTI, it is also true that many will not be detected until they are older. If we are to abandon the routine use of VCUGs in these children, we may lose the best opportunity for early detection and management of vesicoureteral reflux before a UTI occurs.

The VCUG test, when performed in an up-to-date pediatric center, is minimally invasive, requires negligible amounts of ionizing radiation, and carries little risk of inducing UTI. The authors have yet to prove that the routine early detection of vesicoureteral reflux in 30% of these infants is not superior to 3 or 4 months prophylactic antibiotics and waiting for a UTI to occur in children at high risk of vesicoureteral reflux.

E. J. Kass, MD

Intrauterine Repair of Spina Bifida: Preoperative Predictors of Shunt-Dependent Hydrocephalus
Bruner JP, Tulipan N, Reed G, et al (Vanderbilt Univ, Nashville, Tenn; Univ of Massachusetts, Worcester)
Am J Obstet Gynecol 190:1305-1312, 2004   1–9

Objective.—The objective of this study was to determine which factors that are present at the time of intrauterine repair of spina bifida could predict the need for ventriculoperitoneal shunt for hydrocephalus during the first year of life.

Study Design.—One hundred seventy-eight fetuses have undergone intrauterine repair of spina bifida at Vanderbilt University Medical Center since 1997. Among these, 116 fetuses had a postnatal follow-up period of at least 12 months. The primary outcome of the study was the need for a ventriculoperitoneal shunt for hydrocephalus during the first year of life. The following variables were analyzed: maternal demographics (age, race, gravidity, and parity), gestational age at the time of surgery, ventricular size, degree of hindbrain herniation (determined by magnetic resonance imaging in 33 cases), type of defect (myelomeningocele vs myeloschisis), upper level of the lesion, presence of talipes, and intraoperative use of a lumbar drain. Statistical analysis was performed with logistic regression (to test the association of fetal and maternal factors and the need for ventriculoperitoneal shunting), 2-sample t-tests for comparison of means, and receiver operating curves with the use of the probabilities that were generated by the logistic regression for both continuous and categoric versions of the factors.

Results.—Sixty-one of 116 of the fetuses (54%) who underwent operation in utero required the placement of a ventriculoperitoneal shunt before the age of 1 year. The upper level of the lesion (Fig 1) was the strongest predictor of shunt requirement (adjusted odds ratio per 1 level increase with the use of continuous variables [S1 through T10], 1.73 [95% CI, 1.22-2.44]; adjusted odds ratio with the use of upper lesion level ≥L3 vs <L3 as a categorized variable, 5.7 [95% CI, 2.18-14.7]), followed by gestational age at the time of surgery (adjusted odds ratio per 1 week increase with the use of continuous variables, 1.37 [95% CI, 1.06-1.77]; adjusted odds ratio with the use of gestational age ≤25 weeks vs >25 weeks as a categorized variable, 3.3 [95% CI, 1.28-8.24]), and preoperative ventricular size (adjusted odds ratio per 1 unit increase with the use of continuous variables, 1.17 [95% CI, 1.01-1.36]; adjusted odds ratio with the use of ventricular size ≥14 mm vs <14 mm as a categorized variable, 3.5 [95% CI, 1.08-11.16]). Receiver operating curves with the use of the probabilities that were generated by the logistic regression analyses for both the continuous and categoric versions of the factors were compared. The area under the curve was approximately 0.81 for both methods. Thirty-eight of 48 of the fetuses (79%) with an upper level of the lesion ≥L3 required placement of a ventriculoperitoneal shunt, although 25 of 68 of the fetuses (37%) with lesions ≤L4 did not (*P* < .0001). Eighty-four percent of the fetuses with a preoperative ventricular size ≥14 mm (27/

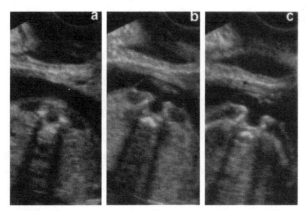

FIGURE 1.—a, The ossification centers are normally arranged in a triangular configuration. b, At 1 level caudad, the lateral ossification centers are widened, and the skin defect becomes visible. This level constitutes the upper level of the lesion. c, One more level down, all ultrasonographic characteristics of the myelomeningocele lesion are fully visible. (Reprinted by permission of the publisher from Bruner JP, Tulipan N, Reed G, et al: Intrauterine repair of spina bifida: Preoperative predictors of shunt-dependent hydrocephalus. *Am J Obstet Gynecol* 190:1305-1312. Copyright 2004 by Elsevier.)

32 fetuses) needed a shunt compared with 41% of the fetuses (34/81 fetuses) with smaller ventricles ($P = .03$). Seventy-one percent of the fetuses who underwent operation at >25 weeks of gestation also required shunt placement (37/52 fetuses); 39% of the fetuses (24/61 fetuses) who were treated ≤25 weeks of gestation did not ($P = .01$). Thirty-five fetuses had a lesion level ≤L4 and a ventricular size <14 mm and underwent operation at ≤25 weeks of gestation. Among these, 8 fetuses (23%) required a ventriculoperitoneal shunt during the first year of life.

Conclusion.—This study suggests that, among fetuses who underwent operation in utero for spina bifida, fetuses with a ventricular size of ≤14 mm at the time of surgery, fetuses who had surgery at ≤25 weeks of gestation, and fetuses with defects that were located at ≤L4 were less likely to require ventriculoperitoneal shunting for hydrocephalus during the first year of life.

▶ The Vanderbilt University Medical Center teams have been the pioneers for the repair of neural tube defects in utero. They have accumulated a considerable experience, enabling them to define the risks and benefits of such a procedure. However, the prospective, randomized, controlled trial, which will finally determine whether the benefits outweigh the potential harm of in utero repair, is still in progress. Bruner et al, in their analysis of 178 patients, indicate that among fetuses who underwent operation in utero for spina bifida, a ventricular size of less than 14 mm at the time of surgery, surgery at 25 weeks or less of gestation, and fetuses with defects that were located at L4 or lower were less likely to require ventriculoperitoneal shunting for hydrocephalus during the first year of life. Notice the positive spin, presenting what was less likely to be associated with an unfavorable outcome rather than the reverse: more likely to need a shunt.

The group had previously reported that intrauterine myelomeningocele repair (IUMR) appears to substantially reduce the incidence of shunt-dependent hydrocephalus when compared with conventional treatment, even when lesion level is taken into account. However, patients with lesions above L3 may not share in this benefit. They also insinuated that IUMR cannot be justified in fetuses older than 25 weeks of gestation.[1] Although the current timing of intrauterine myelomeningocele repair has been found to lessen the degree of herniation of the rhombencephalon and reduce the incidence of shunt-dependent hydrocephalus, it does not statistically improve lower extremity function.[2] Furthermore, fetal repair of neural tube defects inevitably leads to premature delivery. In a case-controlled analysis, Hamdan et al[3] found no difference between short-term complications of prematurity (including respiratory distress and intracranial hemorrhage) after IUMR than those associated with prematurity resulting from other causes.

We can but continue to wait for the completion of the randomized clinical trial to know the next steps.

A. A. Fanaroff, MD

References

1. Tulipan N, Sutton LN, Bruner JP, et al: The effect of intrauterine myelomeningocele repair on the incidence of shunt-dependent hydrocephalus. *Pediatr Neurosurg* 38:27-33, 2003.
2. Tubbs RS, Chambers MR, Smyth MD, et al: Late gestational intrauterine myelomeningocele repair does not improve lower extremity function. *Pediatr Neurosurg* 38:128-132, 2003.
3. Hamdan AH, Walsh W, Bruner JP, et al: Intrauterine myelomeningocele repair: Effect on short-term complications of prematurity. *Fetal Diagn Ther* 19:83-86, 2005.

2 Epidemiology and Pregnancy Complications

Increased Fetal DNA in the Maternal Circulation in Early Pregnancy Is Associated With an Increased Risk of Preeclampsia
Cotter AM, Martin CM, O'Leary JJ, et al (Trinity College Dublin; Coombe Women's Hosp, Dublin)
Am J Obstet Gynecol 191:515-520, 2004   2–1

Background.—Preeclampsia is a leading cause of maternal and perinatal morbidity and mortality. No method exists for reliably determining who will have this polymorphic disease, and treatment is limited to symptomatic management. Preeclampsia can only be resolved by expedited delivery. One central feature of preeclampsia is endothelial cell dysfunction. In addition, defective placentation would appear to be a critical factor. A failure of trophoblastic invasion of the spiral arteries results in placental ischemia, which in turn leads to damage in the maternal vascular endothelium. Trophoblastic invasion is normally completed by 20 weeks' gestation, so it is most likely that the initiating placental pathologic process that leads to preeclampsia occurs long before the development of the clinical syndrome. It would be beneficial, therefore, to develop a test to identify, in early pregnancy, those women at risk of preeclampsia. Whether fetal DNA is present in the maternal circulation in early pregnancy, before preeclampsia is manifest clinically, and whether such a presence could be predictive of the development of preeclampsia were determined.

Methods.—Blood samples were obtained from patients on their first antenatal visit. Study cases included asymptomatic women who subsequently had preeclampsia develop; these patients were matched with control women for parity and gestational age. Fetal DNA in the maternal circulation was quantified with real-time polymerase chain reaction with the use of TaqMan primers and probes directed against SRY gene sequences.

Results.—There were 88 women with preeclampsia matched with 176 control women, all of whom underwent sampling of fetal DNA at a mean gestation (±SD) of 15.7 ± 3.6 weeks. The presence of fetal DNA in the maternal circulation was associated with an 8-fold increase in the risk of having preeclampsia develop.

Conclusions.—An increased amount of fetal DNA was present in the maternal circulation in early pregnancy in women who subsequently had preeclampsia develop. A graded response seemed to exist between the quantity of fetal DNA and the risk of preeclampsia.

▶ The search for the etiology of preeclampsia continues. This is yet another hopeful study that identifies markers easily obtained from pregnant women to determine the level of risk of preeclampsia developing in pregnancy. The authors have shown clearly that fetal DNA is detectable in the maternal circulation and that higher levels of DNA seem to predict the development of preeclampsia in patients in the third trimester. However, there are a number of concerns about these data. The authors themselves point out that the concentration of fetal DNA in maternal whole blood will be greater than in plasma because whole blood will reflect previous pregnancies as well as the ongoing pregnancy and that plasma will be reflective of the current pregnancy. In addition, the predictive reliability is limited to those women carrying male fetuses because it was not possible in this study to distinguish between maternal and fetal karyotypes. Although this is theoretically possible, it was not addressed in this study and remains an issue. The theory that fetal cells and, therefore, DNA in the maternal circulation are involved in some type of inflammatory process that leads to the development of this disease is intriguing, and a number of studies referenced in this article suggest that an inflammatory component is a major contributor in the pathogenesis of this serious illness. We look forward to further studies on this topic, particularly further refinement in the area of whole blood versus plasma and the ability to distinguish between maternal and fetal DNA in the female karyotype.

Unfortunately, this article leaves us with more questions than answers because detection of the group of participants at risk of preeclampsia begs the question about whether there is effective therapy. However, the show must go on, and we should encourage these investigations to continue.

M. L. Druzin, MD

Development of a Large-Scale Obstetric Quality-Improvement Program That Focused on the Nulliparous Patient at Term
Main EK, for the Sutter Health, First Pregnancy and Delivery Clinical Initiative Committee (Sutter Health, Sacramento, Calif; California Pacific Med Ctr, San Francisco; Gould Med Group Modesto, Calif; et al)
Am J Obstet Gynecol 190:1747-1758, 2004   2–2

Background.—In the past several years, the traditional quality indicators in obstetrics have been reappraised. The value of these traditional measures—the total cesarean birth rate and the rate of vaginal birth after cesarean—has been challenged in terms of accurately reflecting a birthing unit's quality of care. An appropriate population and a balanced set of maternal and neonatal measures were identified so that a hospital network obstetric quality improvement program could be established.

Methods.—The site for this study was a large Northern California health care system with more than 40,000 births per year. The investigation was focused on standardized nulliparous patients—those with term, singleton infants in a vertex presentation. Perinatal outcomes and process measures were evaluated and selected by a multidisciplinary task force. Data were collected prospectively and electronically from every hospital and analyzed at a central location. The outcome measures selected for analysis included term, singleton, vertex, and third- or fourth-degree perineal laceration rates, cesarean birth, 5-minute Apgar score of less than 7, and patient satisfaction. The process measures included episiotomy, induction of labor (37-41 weeks), and admittance with cervical dilation of 3 cm or more.

Results.—The completeness of the data collection was improved with each quarter so that, by the end of 2002, the completeness rate for data collection had reached 99.7%. Variation among the system's hospitals was significant for every measure, which is indicative of opportunities for improvement in those areas.

Conclusions.—The use of nulliparity, term gestational age, singleton plurality, and vertex presentation as the major criteria for defining a focus for quality improvement efforts seems to be a balanced and straightforward approach in a large and diverse hospital system. All participants in the system were successfully engaged in the data collection effort.

▶ Quality assessment is the first requisite in any effort to improve quality of care. Operationally, one must decide what to measure and how to account for differences in outcomes that are due to the case mix rather than the quality of care. This case study clearly describes the way in which Northern California's Sutter Health System (more than 40,000 births) approached these issues in developing their systemwide obstetric quality improvement program. The authors present a compelling set of selection criteria for candidate measures, discuss the advantages of using multiple measures of both outcomes and processes, and illustrate their selection process. To minimize differences in the case mix, they used the standardized patient approach, which limited their analysis to nulliparous women with term, singleton infants with vertex presentations. They also present criteria for selecting a standardized population (eg, must be common and raise important management issues in both small and large hospitals). An important consideration when designing a quality improvement program is the size of the dataset required to support an initial assessment and longitudinal follow-up. The Sutter Health System's broad-based program requires the collection of only 20 variables. This article specifically addresses an approach to improving obstetric quality, but it is also an excellent resource for a quality assessment design that can be applied to any medical specialty.

J. B. Gould, MD, MPH

Resistance Exercise Decreases the Need for Insulin in Overweight Women With Gestational Diabetes Mellitus

Brankston GN, Mitchell BF, Ryan EA, et al (Univ of Alberta, Edmonton, Canada)
Am J Obstet Gynecol 190:188-193, 2004   2–3

Objective.—This study examines the effects of circuit-type resistance training on the need for insulin in women with gestational diabetes mellitus.

Study Design.—Thirty-two patients with gestational diabetes mellitus were randomly assigned either to a group that was treated with diet alone or to a group that was treated with diet plus resistance exercise.

Results.—The number of women whose condition required insulin therapy was the same, regardless of treatment. However, a subgroup analysis that examined only overweight women (prepregnant body mass index, >25 kg/m^2) showed a lower incidence of insulin use in the diet-plus-exercise group ($P < .05$). Women in the diet-plus-exercise group were prescribed less insulin ($P < .05$) and showed a longer delay from diagnosis to the initiation of insulin therapy ($P < .05$), compared with the diet-alone group.

Conclusion.—Resistance exercise training may help to avoid insulin therapy for overweight women with gestational diabetes mellitus.

▶ Gestational diabetes mellitus (GDM) is so common (up to 12% of pregnancies) that pregnancy could be regarded as a diabetogenic event. Risk factors for GDM include a strong family history of diabetes mellitus, age, obesity, and physical inactivity. Minority populations are also at higher risk, not only because of family history and genetics, but also because of adaptation to American environmental influences of poor dietary and exercise habits.[1] Women with GDM are at great risk for many pregnancy complications, and their infants are at elevated risk for death and morbidity. Management of GDM has traditionally been through diet and close monitoring of glucose levels, with initiation of insulin therapy when diet alone fails to maintain euglycemia. Because gestational diabetes is characterized by peripheral insulin resistance, exercise becomes a logical intervention and adjunctive therapy. Brankston et al have documented that circuit-type resistance exercise training may help avoid insulin therapy for overweight women with GDM. In fact, they replicate the data of Dye et al,[2] who, on the basis of a population-based registry in New York state, came to a few important conclusions. First, that exercise was associated with reduced rates of GDM only among women with a body mass index greater than 33 (odds ratio, 1.9; 95% confidence interval, 1.2-3.1). Second, surprisingly, because it is usually the noninsured who are at a disadvantage, women of higher socioeconomic status who were obese and did not exercise were at a significantly elevated risk of GDM compared with their counterparts of lower socioeconomic status. We therefore conclude that exercise improves glucose tolerance for overweight women with GDM.

The Sport Medicine Australia statement on the benefits and risks of exercise during pregnancy summarizes the topic extremely well.[3] There are many benefits ranging from weight control, reduced GDM, and improved psychological functioning. Both aerobic exercise and resistant training have been found to be safe; concerns about hyperthermia and neural tube defects in the fetus have been debunked. There is accumulating evidence to suggest that participation in moderate-intensity exercise throughout pregnancy may enhance birth weight. Good diet and exercise are the order of the day from obstetricians to all their pregnant patients.

A. A. Fanaroff, MD

References

1. Fletcher B, Gulanick M, Lamendola C: Risk factors for type 2 diabetes mellitus. *J Cardiovasc Nurs* 16:17-23, 2002.
2. Dye TD, Knox KL, Artal R, et al: Physical activity, obesity, and diabetes in pregnancy. *Am J Epidemiol* 146:961-965, 1997.
3. SMA statement: The benefits and risks of exercise during pregnancy. *Sport Medicine Australia. J Sci Med Sport* 5:11-19, 2002.

Childbearing Beyond Maternal Age 50 and Fetal Outcomes in the United States

Salihu HM, Shumpert MN, Slay M, et al (Univ of Alabama, Birmingham)
Obstet Gynecol 102:1006-1014, 2003   2–4

Objective.—To estimate whether achieving pregnancy beyond maternal age of 50 years compromises fetal well-being and survival.

Methods.—This was a retrospective study on all deliveries in the United States from 1997 to 1999. Four maternal age groups of 20-29 (young), 30-39 (mature), 40-49 (very mature), and 50 or more years (older) were constructed to assess risk gradients for fetal morbidity and mortality.

Results.—A total of 539 deliveries among older mothers (aged 50 and above) were documented (four per 100,000). Among singleton gestations, the risks for low birth weight, preterm, and very preterm were tripled among older mothers, whereas the occurrence of very low birth weight, small size for gestational age, and fetal mortality were approximately doubled compared with those for young mothers. Older mothers also had greater risks for fetal morbidity and mortality than their immediate younger counterparts (40-49 year olds) except for very low birth weight. Among multiple gestations, the differences in risk between older and young mothers were lower than those noted among singletons. Still, compared with young mothers, older mothers had significantly higher risks of low birth weight, very low birth weight, very preterm, and small size for gestational age. Older mothers also had higher risk estimates for multiples than 40–49-year-old gravidas in terms of all fetal morbidity and mortality indices.

Conclusion.—Pregnancy beyond age 50 was associated with increased risks for the fetus. Our findings suggest that this age group is a distinct obstetric high-risk entity that requires special counseling before and after conception.

▶ There are no surprises in looking at the statistics of this report other than the fact there were more than 500 deliveries of women who were aged 50 and older. The fetal morbidity and mortality rates were greater in these older women (the authors' designation). Furthermore, the rates of multiple gestations and prematurity, but not extreme prematurity, were greater than their immediate younger counterparts (aged 40-49 years). The article concludes with the statement that "this age group is a distinct obstetric high-risk entity that requires special counseling before and after conception." My emphasis would be on before conception, but that reflects my bias against pregnancies in women older than 50 years.

Salihu et al[1] also examined the impact of advanced maternal age on survival among quadruplets and quintuplets. I was staggered to learn that between 1995 and 1997 there were 1448 quadruplets and 180 quintuplets delivered in the United States. This is either a tribute to or an indictment of the state of artificial reproductive technology a decade ago. I would anticipate that there are now far fewer megamultiples. In this report older mothers are aged 35 years or older; their mortality rate indexes were compared with those of younger mothers (<35 years old) in terms of early mortality indexes. The neonatal, perinatal, and infant mortality rates were all greater than 2-fold higher in the younger mothers. Stillbirths were also higher in the younger mothers. Hence, advancing maternal age is associated with favorable survival outcomes among quadruplets and quintuplets. The take-home message is that there should be fewer such multiple gestations.

A. A. Fanaroff, MD

Reference

1. Salihu HM, Aliyu MH, Kirby RS, et al: Effect of advanced maternal age on early mortality among quadruplets and quintuplets. *Am J Obstet Gynecol* 190:383-388, 2004.

Clinical Significance of Intra-amniotic Inflammation in Patients With Preterm Premature Rupture of Membranes

Shim S-S, Romero R, Hong J-S, et al (Seoul Natl Univ, Korea)
Am J Obstet Gynecol 191:1339-1345, 2004   2–5

Objective.—This study was conducted to determine the frequency and clinical significance of intra-amniotic inflammation in patients with preterm premature rupture of the membranes.

Study Design.—Amniotic fluid was retrieved from 219 patients with preterm premature rupture of the membranes; the fluid was cultured for aerobic and anaerobic bacteria and mycoplasmas and assayed for neutrophil collagenase, which is also known as matrix metalloproteinase-8. Matrix metalloproteinase-8 was used because previous studies indicated that this was a sensitive and specific index of inflammation and that is correlated with the amniotic fluid white blood cell count. Intra-amniotic inflammation was defined as an elevated amniotic fluid matrix metalloproteinase-8 concentration ($\geq$23 ng/mL). Nonparametric and survival techniques were used for statistical analysis.

Results.—The overall rate of intra-amniotic inflammation was 42% (93/219 samples); proven intra-amniotic infection was detected only in 23% (50/219 samples). Intra-amniotic inflammation with a negative amniotic fluid culture for micro-organisms was found in 23% (51/219 samples) and was as common as proven intra-amniotic infection. Pregnancy outcome was worse in patients with intra-amniotic inflammation and a negative culture than in those patients with a negative culture and without inflammation. There were no differences in the interval-to-delivery or rate of complications between patients with intra-amniotic inflammation and a negative culture and patients with proven amniotic fluid infection.

Conclusion.—We conclude that intra-amniotic inflammation, regardless of culture result, is present in 42% of patients with preterm premature rupture of the membranes and that it is a risk factor for impending preterm delivery and adverse outcome. We propose that intra-amniotic inflammation, rather than infection, be used to classify and treat patients with preterm premature rupture of the membranes.

▶ This report extends previous work from the same investigators and others to yet another group of at-risk patients: those with preterm premature rupture of membranes. Once again inflammation, not infection, correlates with short intervals to delivery, much higher rates of delivery before 34 or 37 weeks' gestation, histologic evidence of chorioamnionitis and funisitis, and increased neonatal morbidity (particularly bronchopulmonary dysplasia). The need for better strategies for recognition and modification of the fetal inflammatory response grows ever more urgent.

W. E. Benitz, MD

The Maternal-Fetal Medicine Units Cesarean Registry: Chorioamnionitis at Term and its Duration—Relationship to Outcomes

Rouse DJ, and National Institute of Child Health and Human Development, Maternal-Fetal Medicine Units Network (Univ of Alabama at Birmingham; et al)
Am J Obstet Gynecol 191:211-216, 2004   2–6

Background.—Chorioamnionitis is a common infection that is associated with risks to both the mother and the neonate. This multicenter, prospective, observational study examined the relationship between chorioamnionitis and its duration to adverse maternal, fetal, and neonatal outcome.

Study Design.—The study group consisted of 21,853 primary cesarean deliveries with a term, singleton neonate. Of these, 1965 were given a diagnosis of chorioamnionitis. Maternal and neonatal adverse outcomes were compared between pregnancies with and without chorioamnionitis. The duration of chorioamnionitis was stratified into 5 intervals and the outcomes compared across these intervals by using the Mantel-Haenszel test for trend.

Findings.—Chorioamnionitis was associated with significantly increased risk of maternal blood transfusion, uterine atony, septic pelvic thrombophlebitis, and pelvic abscess. It was also associated with a 5-minute Apgar score of 3 or less, neonatal sepsis, and seizures. By test of trend, only uterine atony, maternal blood transfusion, maternal admission to intensive care, and 5-minute Apgar score were associated with the duration of chorioamnionitis. By logistic analysis, only uterine atony, 5-minute Apgar score, and neonatal mechanical ventilation within 24 hours of birth were significantly associated with the duration of chorioamnionitis.

Conclusion.—Although chorioamnionitis was associated with increased risk of both maternal and neonatal morbidity, its duration was not related to most adverse outcomes. Therefore, chorioamnionitis is not a reason to terminate labor with cesarean with its added potential for morbidity.

▶ Once again, the importance of chorioamnionitis and its relationship to neonatal outcome is emphasized. The Maternal-Fetal Medicine Units network has the advantages of a multicenter group with common criteria and a good database. The well-recognized maternal and neonatal risks of chorioamnionitis were confirmed by this study. However, the relationship between the duration of clinically diagnosed chorioamnionitis and adverse maternal and fetal neonatal outcomes has not been well studied.

With logistic regression, the only maternal complication of chorioamnionitis was uterine atony, and the only related neonatal complications were Apgar score less than 3 and mechanical ventilation in the first 24 hours after birth. No other maternal and neonatal outcomes were significantly related to duration of chorioamnionitis.

The strength of the study includes the large number of pregnancies and strict criteria for the clinical diagnosis of chorioamnionitis. Weaknesses of these data include the fact that only cesarean deliveries were included and the observational nature of the study. The clinical take-home message for this is that it may be preferable to attempt a vaginal delivery for patients diagnosed with chorioamnionitis. There seems to be no compelling neonatal reason to shorten labor by cesarean section that will lead to greater maternal morbidity.

M. L. Druzin, MD

A Polymorphism in the Promoter Region of TNF and Bacterial Vaginosis: Preliminary Evidence of Gene-Environment Interaction in the Etiology of Spontaneous Preterm Birth

Macones GA, Parry S, Elkousy M, et al (Univ of Pennsylvania, Philadelphia)
Am J Obstet Gynecol 190:1504-1508, 2004   2–7

Introduction.—The rarer of 2 alleles of a polymorphism in the promoter of the tumor necrosis factor (TNF) alpha gene is linked with spontaneous birth after preterm premature rupture of the fetal membranes in some populations. Whether the presence of symptomatic bacterial vaginosis intensifies the risk of spontaneous preterm birth among infants whose mothers have a "susceptible" TNF genotype was determined in a case–control investigation.

Methods.—A total of 125 women who were delivered of their infants before 37 weeks because of ruptured membranes or preterm labor and 250 control subjects who were delivered of their infants after 37 weeks were evaluated. Maternal blood was obtained to determine DNA and the status of the TNF genotype. Antenatal records were reviewed to obtain data regarding symptomatic bacterial vaginosis and other risk factors for preterm birth. Multiple logistic regression analysis was used to assess the interaction between bacterial vaginosis, the TNF genotype, and preterm birth.

Results.—Maternal carriers of the rarer allele (TNF-2) were at significantly higher risk of spontaneous preterm birth (odds ratio, 2.7; 95% CI, 1.7-4.5). The link between TNF-2 and preterm birth was altered by the presence of bacterial vaginosis: women with a susceptible genotype and bacterial vaginosis had higher odds of preterm birth than did control subjects (odds ratio, 6.1; 95% CI, 1.9-21.0).

Conclusion.—Preliminary evidence shows that an interaction between genetic susceptibility (ie, TNF-2 genotype) and environmental factors (ie, bacterial vaginosis) is linked with an increased risk of spontaneous preterm birth.

▶ This article is another one in a plethora of articles looking at gene expression and its relationship to spontaneous preterm birth, preterm premature rupture of the membranes, or both, in some populations. This case-controlled study was performed by identifying DNA from maternal blood analyzed for the TNF genotype. In addition, the presence of symptomatic bacterial vaginosis and its link to those with genetic susceptibilities, the TNF-2 carriers, was investigated. This study clearly showed that the search for a single "silver bullet" for the etiology of preterm labor and premature rupture of the membranes is likely to fail and that multiple interactions between genes, the environment, and many other heretofore unidentified factors will likely be operative in this most vexing of obstetric problems.

Despite limitations, the good news is that our techniques of evaluating genotype and gene expression and the newer science of proteomics will further our knowledge, leading to methods of detection and prevention of this common obstetric problem.

M. L. Druzin, MD

Identification and H₂O₂ Production of Vaginal Lactobacilli From Pregnant Women at High Risk of Preterm Birth and Relation With Outcome

Wilks M, Wiggins R, Whiley A, et al (Barts and the London NHS Trust; Univ of Bristol, England)

J Clin Microbiol 42:713-717, 2004   2–8

Lactobacilli, principally the strains that are hydrogen peroxide (H_2O_2) producing, may have a protective effect against vaginal colonization by pathogenic species such as those that cause bacterial vaginosis. Previous reports have also suggested that H_2O_2-producing lactobacilli in the vagina may protect pregnant women against ascending infection of the chorio-amniotic membranes and uterine cavity. We report the identification and H_2O_2 production of lactobacilli isolated from vaginal swabs collected at 20 weeks' gestation from a population of pregnant women at high risk of preterm birth. We also report the correlation between identification and H_2O_2 production in relation to the outcomes of chorioamnionitis and preterm birth. Lactobacilli were identified by partial 16S rRNA gene sequencing. H_2O_2 production by isolates was determined by a semiquantitative method. The most commonly isolated species were *L. crispatus*, *L. gasseri*, *L. vaginalis* and *L. jensenii*. Amounts of H_2O_2 produced by lactobacilli varied widely. The presence of lactobacilli producing high levels of H_2O_2 in the vagina of this population of pregnant women was associated with a reduced risk of bacterial vaginosis at 20 weeks' gestation and subsequent chorioamnionitis. *L. jensenii* and *L. vaginalis* produced the highest levels of H_2O_2. We postulate that H_2O_2-producing lactobacilli are able to reduce the incidence of ascending infections of the uterus and the subsequent production of proinflammatory molecules which are important in the pathogenesis of chorioamnionitis and preterm birth.

▶ Various forms of lactobacilli and the nutrients (including breast milk) that promote their growth are being intensely studied. Wilks et al introduce us to the H_2O_2-producing vaginal lactobacilli because they may prevent colonization by the pathogens that cause bacterial vaginosis (BV), a major risk factor for prematurity. The authors noted that finding these H_2O_2-producing lactobacilli in the vaginas of this population of pregnant women was associated with a reduced risk of BV at 20 weeks' gestation and subsequent chorioamnionitis.

Letich et al[1] in Vienna performed a meta-analysis to evaluate BV as a risk factor for preterm delivery. Indeed they did. They included women who had been screened for BV, and the outcomes were preterm delivery, spontaneous abortion, maternal or neonatal infection, and perinatal death. Eighteen studies with results for 20,232 patients were included. BV increased the risk of preterm delivery by more than 2-fold. Their neighbors, Hoyme and Saling[2] in Germany, persuaded pregnant women to perform self-measurements of their vaginal pH with test gloves twice a week to screen for any disturbances in the vaginal milieu. If pH was 4.7 or greater or other risk factors were present, they were to see a physician. If these findings were confirmed the women were started on an *L. acidophilus* preparation or, in case of BV, treated with intravaginal clindamycin cream. They have effectively reduced the prematurity rate locally and wish to extend this program to the whole country. My concern is that American women would not readily accept self-evaluation, but I stand to be proven incorrect, especially if the local obstetricians deem this a reasonable and worthwhile approach. It is eminently more logical to attempt to restore the normal vaginal bacteria without resorting to antibiotics therapy. On this topic, Klein and Gibbs[3] summarized recent evidence regarding infection-associated preterm birth with the purpose of making appropriate recommendations. They reported that the routine administration of antibiotics to women with preterm labor and intact membranes is not beneficial; however, antibiotic regimens that include macrolides are recommended for preterm premature rupture of the membranes.

A. A. Fanaroff, MD

References

1. Leitich H, Bodner-Adler B, Brunbauer M, et al: Bacterial vaginosis as a risk factor for preterm delivery: A meta-analysis. *Am J Obstet Gynecol* 89:139-147, 2003.
2. Hoyme UB, Saling E: Efficient prematurity prevention is possible by pH self-measurement and immediate therapy of threatening ascending infection. *Eur J Obstet Gynecol Reprod Biol* 115:148-153, 2004.
3. Klein LL, Gibbs RS: Use of microbial cultures and antibiotics in the prevention of infection-associated preterm birth. *Am J Obstet Gynecol* 190:1493-1502, 2004.

Neonatal Outcome in a Danish National Cohort of 8602 Children Born After *in Vitro* Fertilization or Intracytoplasmic Sperm Injection: The Role of Twin Pregnancy
Pinborg A, Loft A, Andersen AN (Univ of Copenhagen)
Acta Obstet Gynecol Scand 83:1071-1078, 2004   2–9

Background.—In Denmark, 4% of all infants are born after *in vitro* fertilization (IVF) or intracytoplasmic sperm injection (ICSI) and 40% of these children are twins.

Methods.—We investigated neonatal outcome in a complete Danish IVF/ICSI birth cohort including 8602 infants born between 1995 and 2000: 3438 twins (40%) and 5164 singletons (60%). Births conceived after IVF or ICSI were identified by record linkage with the Danish IVF Registry and the National Medical Birth Registry. Data on neonatal outcome were collected from the National Patient Registry.

Results.—IVF/ICSI twins had a 10-fold increased age- and parity-adjusted risk of delivery before 37 completed weeks [odds ratio (OR) 9.9, 95% confidence interval (95% CI) 8.7–11.3] and a 7.4-fold increased risk of delivery before 32 completed weeks (OR 7.4, 95% CI 5.6–9.8) compared with singletons. Correspondingly, ORs of birthweight <2500 g and birthweight <1500 g in twins were 11.8 (95% CI 10.3–13.6) and 5.4 (95% CI 4.1–7.0), respectively. The stillbirth rate was doubled in twins (13.1/1000) compared with singletons (6.6/1000) ($p = 0.002$). The risk of cesarean section and of admittance to a neonatal intensive care unit (NICU) was 4.6- and 1.8-fold higher in IVF/ICSI twins than in singletons. The rate of major malformations was 40.4/1000 in twins and 36.8/1000 in singletons ($p = 0.4$), whereas the total malformation rate (major + minor) was higher in twins (73.7/1000) than in singletons (55.0/1000) ($p = 0.001$). After exclusion of patent ductus arteriosus (PDA), which is strongly associated with preterm birth, no significant differences in any malformation rates were observed between twins and singletons. Apart from the frequency of ICSI children with hypospadias, which reached a significance level of $p = 0.05$, malformation rates in ICSI children were similar to those in IVF children.

Conclusions.—This study indicates that neonatal outcome in IVF/ICSI twins is considerably poorer than in singletons. Thus, the impact is to draw the attention of clinicians to the benefit of elective single embryo transfer (eSET).

Maternal Risks and Perinatal Outcome in a Danish National Cohort of 1005 Twin Pregnancies: The Role of *in Vitro* Fertilization
Pinborg A, Loft A, Schmidt L, et al (Univ of Copenhagen)
Acta Obstet Gynecol Scand 83:75-84, 2004   2–10

Background.—Twin pregnancies constitute 25% of all *in vitro* fertilization (IVF) and intracytoplasmic sperm injection (ICSI) pregnancies There is a lack of knowledge on maternal risks and perinatal outcome of IVF/ICSI twin pregnancies.

Methods.—National survey by questionnaire ($n = 1769$). The study population consisted of all IVF/ICSI twin mothers ($n = 266$) and the two control groups of all IVF/ICSI singleton mothers ($n = 764$) and non-IVF/ICSI twin mothers ($n = 739$) who delivered in Denmark in 1997. The response rate was 89% among IVF twin mothers and overall 81%.

Results.—In terms of maternal risks and perinatal outcome no significant differences were observed between IVF/ICSI twin and non-IVF/ICSI twin pregnancies after stratification for maternal age and parity. Nevertheless, IVF/ICSI twin mothers were more frequently on sick leave (OR 2.5, 95% CI 1.5–4.0) and hospitalized (OR 1.9, 95% CI 1.3–2.8) during pregnancy. Compared with IVF/ICSI singleton pregnancies, IVF/ICSI twin pregnancies were characterized by a higher incidence of preeclampsia (OR 2.4, 95% CI 1.5–4.2) and a higher frequency of sick leave (OR 6.8, 95% CI 4.4–10.5) and hospitalizations during pregnancy (OR 3.5, (95% CI 2.5–4.9); moreover, mean birthweight ($p < 0.001$) and gestational age ($p < 0.001$) were lower. No differences were observed in the incidence of pregnancy-induced hypertension and gestational diabetes between IVF/ICSI twin and singleton pregnancies.

Conclusion.—Although this population study indicates that maternal risks in IVF/ICSI twin pregnancies are comparable with non-IVF/ICSI twin pregnancies, the IVF/ICSI twin mothers were more likely to be on sick leave or hospitalized during pregnancy. Furthermore, maternal risks were higher and obstetric outcome poorer in IVF/ICSI twin vs. IVF/ICSI singleton pregnancies.

▶ In Denmark, 4% of all infants are born after IVF/ICSI, and 40% of these children are twins. Pinborg et al, in this series of reports, provide an excellent perspective on this ever-increasing component of maternal/fetal medicine. National data always trump that from a single center or even a region, and the scope and depth of these reports are very helpful for counseling. The results in of themselves are eminently predictable.

The neonatal outcome in IVF/ICSI twins is considerably poorer than singletons. For starters, the stillbirth rate was doubled in twins (13.1/1000) compared with singletons (6.6/1000) ($P = 0.002$). IVF/ICSI twins had a 10-fold increased chance of delivering prematurely and a 7.4-fold increased risk of delivery before 32 completed weeks compared with singletons. The risks of cesarean section and of admittance to a neonatal ICU were increased substantially. Apart from the frequency of ICSI children with hypospadias, which reached a significance level of $P = 0.05$, malformation rates in ICSI children were similar to those in IVF children. Their primary conclusion is self evident: "draw the attention of clinicians to the benefit of elective single embryo transfer."

In terms of maternal risks and perinatal outcome, no significant differences were observed between IVF/ICSI twin and non-IVF/ICSI twin pregnancies after stratification for maternal age and parity. However, IVF/ICSI twin mothers had a higher incidence of preeclampsia, but not pregnancy-induced hypertension, took more sick leave, and were hospitalized more frequently during pregnancy. Furthermore, their twins were less mature and weighed less. The twins also were more likely to need admission to the neonatal ICU and require a surgical procedure than singletons. You could sum that data to maternal risks were higher and obstetric outcomes poorer in IVF/ICSI twin than IVF/ICSI singleton pregnancies. However, when comparing IVF/ICSI twins to spontaneous dizygotic twins, neonatal outcomes were similar.[1]

At follow-up, no major differences in physical health were observed between IVF/ICSI twins and non-IVF/ICSI twins.[2] But the IVF/ICSI twins had poorer speech development and were more likely to require special needs. Their mothers rated their health poorer. Both IVF/ICSI and non-IVF/ICSI twin parents experienced more marital stress and expressed that twins had more impact on the mother's life compared with singletons. Nevertheless, the only predictor of low divorce/separation risk was IVF/ICSI treatment. My suspicion is that, whereas all these stresses would be the same, in the United States the chances for divorce would be greater. All in all this national dataset is a wonderful resource and reference on the impact of artificial reproduction.

A. A. Fanaroff, MD

References

1. Pinborg A, Loft A, Rasmussen S, et al: Neonatal outcome in a Danish national cohort of 3438 IVF/ICSI and 10,362 non-IVF/ICSI twins born between 1995 and 2000. *Hum Reprod* 19:435-441, 2004.

2. Pinborg A, Loft A, Schmidt L, et al: Morbidity in a Danish national cohort of 472 IVF/ICSI twins, 1132 non-IVF/ICSI twins and 634 IVF/ICSI singletons: Health-related and social implications for the children and their families. *Hum Reprod* 18:1234-1243, 2003.

Accuracy of Sonographically Estimated Fetal Weight in 840 Women With Different Pregnancy Complications Prior to Induction of Labor

Ben-Haroush A, Yogev Y, Bar J, et al (Rabin Medical Center, Petah Tiqva, Israel)
Ultrasound Obstet Gynecol 23:172-176, 2004　　　　　　　　　2–11

Introduction.—No single satisfactory formula has been found for estimating fetal weight, as evidenced by the variety of formulas for this calculation. Even the accuracy of US-based birth weight estimates varies according to the presence of difference complications of pregnancy, including ruptured membranes, fetal growth restriction (FGR), diabetes, suspected fetal macrosomia, and oligohydramnios. The interval between US examination to delivery may also influence accuracy. The single-center experience with sonographically estimated fetal weight (EFW) was assessed shortly before induction of labor in females with pregnancy complications, along with possible variables influencing estimate accuracy.

Methods.—The study included 840 females with singleton pregnancies and cephalic presentation who were admitted for induction of labor between January 1999 and December 2000. All participants underwent detailed US evaluation for EFW, amniotic fluid index, biophysical profile, and placental location. Indications for US evaluation included previous cesarean section, postdate pregnancy, pregnancy-induced hypertension, diabetic pregnancy, suspected large-for-gestational age (LGA) infants, suspected FGR, oligohydramnios, diminished fetal movements, and premature rupture of membranes at or before term. The EFW was calculated after determining fetal abdominal circumference and femur length. After delivery, the birth weight was compared with the EFW.

Results.—The EFW was highly associated with birth weight ($P < .0001$). The mean birth weight was 3207 g; mean absolute weight difference was 227 g (absolute range, 0-1700 g; actual range, -986-$+1700$ g). The mean weight difference was significantly different among patients with LGA infants, FGR infants, and females with preterm premature rupture of membranes (PPROM) (-110 g, $+113$ g, and $+115$ g, respectively; $P < .01$). Stepwise linear regression analysis of the effects of maternal and pregnancy characteristics on the weight difference revealed lower gestational age, higher birth weight, anterior placenta, higher gravidity, and younger maternal age as independent and significant variables linked with greater actual weight difference inaccuracy ($P < .001$), and greater birth weight as the only independent and significant variable associated with greater absolute weight difference ($P = .018$).

Conclusion.—The US EFW is strongly associated with birth weight. Clinicians need to be aware of the risk of overestimation in pregnancies with suspected LGA and underestimation in pregnancies with PPROM and suspected FGR.

▶ This article is an analysis of a hypothetical group of 1,000,000 women. The authors applied known results from recent antenatal testing data to determine which combination of tests for aneuploidy would be most cost effective in the antepartum period.

Interestingly, the design is very similar to that of the FASTER trial (First And Second Trimester Evaluation of Risk), which is a National Institute of Child Health and Human Development-sponsored multisite trial designed to determine the best way to detect trisomy 21 in the antenatal period. That trial concluded in December 2002, and the results will be published soon.

The FASTER trial compares standard of care testing (triple and quad testing) to first trimester testing (nuchal thickness, pregnancy-associated plasma protein A [PAPP-A], and human chorionic gonadotropin [HCG]) and to integrated testing (first trimester testing and quad screen with the results not available until all testing is completed).

The present model, like the FASTER trial, compares the triple, quad, the first trimester, sequential, and integrated screens. Unlike the FASTER trial, it does not consider the serum-only integrated screen but adds a genetic sonogram instead.

The most cost-effective method of prenatal screening in this hypothetical model was the sequential method. In this plan, a first trimester screen is performed (nuchal thickness, PAPP-A, and HCG). The individuals who test positive are offered early testing via chorionic villus sampling. Those who test negative are offered a quad screen in the second trimester. Although this was most cost effective, the loss of normal babies through increased invasive testing was very high, and, therefore, this method of testing is unacceptable.

Integrated screening had the lowest fetal loss rate with little loss in sensitivity. Genetic sonograms, a recent "fashionable" US, do not fare well in this analysis because of their low sensitivity.

One criticism might be that the clinicians are using the wrong numbers in various assumptions, but they wisely ran the numbers using a wide range of possibilities. Another problem in this article is that PAPP-A is very age dependent, and its utility varies greatly, depending on the age at which the first trimester screen was performed. The earlier, the better.

This article goes beyond relating the results of testing by determining what the costs will be in fetal loss, loss of sensitivity, and expenditure of health care dollars. The authors do state that this is not prospective. However, the FASTER trial prospectively examines all but the genetic sonogram and should be published shortly.

C. Comstock, MD

Ultrasound Examination at 37 Weeks' Gestation in the Prediction of Pregnancy Outcome: The Value of Cervical Assessment

Ramanathan G, Yu C, Osei E, et al (King's College Hosp Med School, London)
Ultrasound Obstet Gynecol 22:598-603, 2003   2–12

Objective.—To examine the potential value of routine measurement of cervical length in singleton low-risk pregnancies at 37 weeks of gestation in the prediction of onset and outcome of labor.

Methods.—Cervical length was measured by transvaginal sonography at 37 weeks in 1571 singleton low-risk pregnancies. Outcome measures were gestation at spontaneous onset of labor, post-term delivery, duration of labor and mode of delivery.

Results.—The median cervical length at 37 weeks was 30 mm and there was a significant association between cervical length and gestation at delivery, which increased from a mean of 38 weeks for cervical length of 10 mm to 41 weeks for cervical length of 35 mm. The incidence of delivery after 40 weeks and 10 days was 296 (18.8%) and the incidence increased with cervical length at 37 weeks from 0% to 6%, 35% and 68% for respective cervical lengths of <20, 21-30, 31-40 and 41-50 mm. In the pregnancies with spontaneous onset of labor the incidence of Cesarean section for failure to progress increased from 3.6% to 6.0%, 6.4% and 11.8% for cervical lengths of <20, 21-30, 31-40 and 41-50 mm, respectively. In the pregnancies requiring induction for post-term the incidence of Cesarean section for failed induction or failure to progress increased from 7.5% to 20.1% to 25.0% for cervical lengths of 21-30, 31-40 and 41-50 mm, respectively.

Conclusion.—Measurement of cervical length at 37 weeks can define the likelihood of spontaneous delivery before 40 weeks and 10 days and the risk of Cesarean section in those requiring induction for prolonged pregnancy.

► A prior publication from these investigators had established that the transvaginal sonographic measurement of cervical length was a useful prediction of the likelihood of vaginal delivery within 24 hours of induction. The crucial length was 28 mm with a sensitivity of 0.87 and a specificity of 0.71.[1] The current study was designed to predict how successful the induction of labor would be. Success was defined as a spontaneous vaginal delivery before 40 weeks and 10 days, in contrast to postterm deliveries or those requiring operative intervention. Almost 20% of the infants were delivered beyond 40 weeks and 10 days, and there was an excellent correlation with cervical length. Thus, although a short cervix in the second trimester is predictive of premature onset of labor, an excessively long (41-50 mm) cervix is predictive of delivery beyond term. Cesarean section was also more likely with the very long cervix. Cervical length also predicted whether an operative delivery would be required if and when labor was induced for postterm pregnancies. Predicting outcomes is usually fraught with hazards and uncertainties. Simply measuring cervical length at 37 weeks establishes the likelihood of a prolonged pregnancy and the need for operative intervention. This is useful information for the obstetrician/midwife, and far more information than can be gleaned from the usual manual examination routinely performed at that time. It facilitates planning the best time and mode for delivery.

A. A. Fanaroff, MD

Reference

1. Pandis GK, Papageorghiou AT, Ramanathan VG, et al: Preinduction sonographic measurement of cervical length in the prediction of successful induction of labor. *Ultrasound Obstet Gynecol* 18:623-628, 2001.

Cervical Cerclage for Prevention of Preterm Delivery in Women With Short Cervix: Randomised Controlled Trial

To MS, for the Fetal Medicine Foundation Second Trimester Screening Group (King's College Hosp Med School, London; et al)
Lancet 363:1849-1853, 2004   2–13

Background.—Cervical cerclage has been widely used in the past 50 years to prevent early preterm birth and its associated neonatal mortality and morbidity. Results of randomised trials have not generally lent support to this practice, but this absence of benefit may be due to suboptimum patient selection, which was essentially based on obstetric history. A more effective way of identifying the high-risk group for early preterm delivery might be by transvaginal sonographic measurement of cervical length. We undertook a multicentre randomised controlled trial to investigate whether, in women with a short cervix identified by routine transvaginal scanning at 22-24 weeks' gestation, the insertion of a Shirodkar suture reduces early preterm delivery.

Methods.—Cervical length was measured in 47 123 women. The cervix was 15 mm or less in 470, and 253 (54%) of these women participated in the study and were randomised to cervical cerclage (127) or to expectant management (126). Primary outcome was the frequency of delivery before 33 completed weeks (231 days) of pregnancy.

Findings.—The proportion of preterm delivery before 33 weeks was similar in both groups, 22% (28 of 127) in the cerclage group versus 26% (33 of 126) in the control group (relative risk=0.84, 95% CI 0.54-1.31, p=0.44), with no significant differences in perinatal or maternal morbidity or mortality (Table 2).

Interpretation.—The insertion of a Shirodkar suture in women with a short cervix does not substantially reduce the risk of early preterm delivery. Routine sonographic measurement of cervical length at 22-24 weeks identifies a group at high risk of early preterm birth.

▶ This is an impressive, prospective, randomized trial that proves once again that, although we have the tests and technology to identify women at risk for preterm delivery, we lack the tools to prevent it. Cerclage had no impact on the rate of prematurity in these singleton pregnancies. Newman et al[1] were equally unsuccessful with the use of cerclage at mid-trimester in twin gesta-

TABLE 2.—Primary Analyses of Outcome Measures

	Cerclage (n=127)	Expectant (n=126)	RR (95% CI)	P
Delivery before 33 weeks	28 (22%)	33 (26%)	0·84 (0·54 to 1·31)	0·4411
Gestation at delivery (weeks) (mean [SE])	36·4 (0·42)	35·4 (0·45)	0·95 (−0·26 to 2·15)*	0·1233
GA adjusted BW centile† (median)	41·8 (1·1-99·8)	37·2 (0·7-100)		0·0983
Birthweight‡ (g) (mean [SE])	2769 (85)	2565 (85)	204 (−33 to 441)*	0·0917
Onset of labour				
Spontaneous	92 (72%)	104 (83%)	0·88 (0·77 to 1·00)	0·0692
Iatrogenic	28 (22%)	18 (14%)	1·54 (0·90 to 2·64)	
Indicated after PPROM	7 (6%)	4 (3%)	1·74 (0·52 to 5·78)	
Caesarean section	33 (26%)	23 (18%)	1·42 (0·89 to 2·28)	0·1386
Preterm membrane rupture	23 (18%)	19 (15%)	1·20 (0·69 to 2·09)	0·5171
Maternal pyrexia‡	5 (4%)	1 (1%)	4·92 (0·58 to 41·53)	0·2132
Symptomatic vaginal discharge‡	8 (6%)	1 (1%)	7·87 (1·00 to 62·04)	0·0358
Stillbirth	3 (2%)	5 (4%)	0·60 (0·15 to 2·44)	0·4999
Perinatal deaths§	7 (6%)	10 (8%)	0·69 (0·27 to 1·77)	0·4412
Positive fetal blood culture¶	5/123 (4%)	2/121 (2%)	2·46 (0·49 to 12·43)	0·4464
Bronchopulmonary dysplasia¶	4/123 (3%)	4/121 (3%)	0·98 (0·25 to 3·84)	1·0000
IVH/PVH¶	1/123 (1%)	2/121 (2%)	0·49 (0·05 to 5·35)	0·6204
Retinopathy of prematurity¶	0/123 (0%)	3/121 (2%)	0·14 (0·01 to 2·69)	0·1204

GA=gestational age. BW=birthweight. PPROM=preterm prelabour rupture of membranes. IVH=intraventricular haemorrhage. PVH=periventricular haemorrhage. Data are number (%) unless otherwise indicated.

* Difference in means (95% CI).

†Data missing for one infant in cerclage group and for three infants in expectant group.

‡Outcome data missing for one woman in expectant group.

§Total number of stillbirths and neonatal deaths before hospital discharge.

¶Stillbirths excluded from calculations: missing data for one neonate in cerclage group. Tested where clinically indicated, otherwise assumed to be negative.

(Courtesy of To MS, for the Fetal Medicine Foundation Second Trimester Screening Group: Cervical cerclage for prevention of preterm delivery in women with short cervix: Randomised controlled trial. *Lancet* 363:1849-1853, 2004. Reprinted with permission from Elsevier.)

tions with a shortened cervical length. This failure, together with the failure of antibiotic administration to reduce prematurity in women with bacterial vaginosis, remains a source of great frustration for patients and physicians alike. A 22% prematurity rate indisputably places women with a short cervix in the high-risk category. But all we can do is closely monitor them and ensure that they receive corticosteroids at the first signs of premature labor.

A. A. Fanaroff, MD

Reference

1. Newman RB, Krombach RS, Myers MC, et al: Effect of cerclage on obstetrical outcome in twin gestations with a shortened cervical length. *Am J Obstet Gynecol* 186:634-640, 2002.

Aggressive Tocolysis Does Not Prolong Pregnancy or Reduce Neonatal Morbidity After Preterm Premature Rupture of the Membranes
Combs CA, McCune M, Clark R, et al (Good Samaritan Hosp, San Jose, Calif; Pediatrix Med Group, Fort Lauderdale, Fla)
Am J Obstet Gynecol 190:1723-1731, 2004   2–14

Objective.—This study was undertaken to evaluate whether aggressive tocolysis improves pregnancy outcome after preterm premature rupture of the membranes (PPROM).

Study Design.—Retrospective case-control study of patients with PPROM before 34 weeks of gestation, followed by a prospective cohort study with historical controls. The retrospective phase covered 1995 through 1999 when we used tocolysis aggressively. With the use of survival analysis, we compared latency in our cases with 4 published control series in which tocolysis was never used. On the basis of the results, we adopted a new protocol in mid-2000 limiting tocolysis to 48 hours after betamethasone dosing and we conducted a 2-year prospective evaluation of this new protocol.

Results.—In the retrospective phase, tocolysis was used in 94% of 130 cases and maintained during 84% of 1162 total antenatal patient-days. There was no difference in latency between our cases and the published controls. One or more complications of tocolysis occurred in 18%. In the prospective study, 43% of 63 patients received tocolytics, but these were used at lower doses and were given during only 7% of 770 patient-days. Latency with this very limited tocolytic regimen (median 4.5 days, interquartile range 2.3 to 14.0) was not significantly different than during the last 24 months of aggressive tocolysis (median 3.8 days, 1.8 to 14 days, $P = .16$) and there were no differences in neonatal morbidity.

Conclusion.—Aggressive tocolysis after PPROM causes significant maternal morbidity, but does not increase latency or decrease neonatal morbidity compared with either very limited tocolysis or no tocolysis at all.

▶ It would not be unreasonable to say that, on balance, tocolysis has been one of the most disappointing interventions used in obstetrics. There is no evidence to show that it prolongs gestation to any significant degree. It can be useful in the short term to allow the administration of corticosteroids to the mother (to enhance fetal lung maturation), but, with that exception, its benefits are minimal. In addition, as is shown by these authors, aggressive tocolysis after PPROM can cause significant maternal morbidity with no benefit to the neonate. In a recent review, Mercer[1] notes that although most studies don't demonstrate an increase in maternal or fetal risk when tocolysis is combined with conservative management of PPROM, "neither prophylactic nor therapeutic tocolysis in this setting has been demonstrated to reduce infant morbidity. Hence, tocolytic administration should not be an expected practice." The study of Combs et al supports this conclusion.

M. J. Maisels, MB, BCh

Reference

1. Mercer BM. Preterm premature rupture of the membranes: Diagnosis and management. *Clin Perinatol* 31:765-782, 2004.

Maternal Morbidity and Obstetric Complications in Triplet Pregnancies and Quadruplet and Higher-Order Multiple Pregnancies
Wen SW, Demissie K, Yang Q, et al (Univ of Ottawa, Ontario, Canada; Univ of Medicine and Dentistry of New Jersey, Piscataway)
Am J Obstet Gynecol 191:254-258, 2004   2–15

Background.—The incidence of twinning and higher order multiple pregnancies has markedly increased in industrialized countries over the past 2 decades. Delayed pregnancy and an increased use of assisted reproductive technology are thought to be the greatest contributors to this increase in multiple gestations. Multiple gestation is known to increase the risk of perinatal death and morbidity and, consequently, long-term health sequelae in the offspring. However, less is known about the effect of multiple gestation on the health of the woman. The risk of maternal morbidity and obstetric complications was assessed in women with triplet pregnancies and quadruplet and higher order multiple pregnancies.

Methods.—The 1995 to 1997 Multiple Birth File of the United States was used to compare the outcomes of 152,238 women with twin pregnancies with the outcomes of 5491 women with triplet pregnancies and 423 women with quadruplet or higher order multiple pregnancies.

Results.—After adjustment for confounding factors, the risks of pregnancy-associated hypertension and eclampsia, anemia, diabetes mellitus, abruptio placenta, premature rupture of the membranes, and cesarean delivery were increased in women with triplet pregnancies or quadruplet and higher order multiple gestations compared with women with twin pregnancies (Table 1). A dose–response relationship was observed for pregnancy-associated hypertension, diabetes mellitus, and placental abruption, and women with quadruplet or higher order multiple gestations had higher odds ratios than did women with triplet pregnancies (Table 2).

Conclusions.—The risk of maternal morbidity and obstetric complications is increased in triplet pregnancies and quadruplet or higher order multiple pregnancies compared with that in twin pregnancies. A dose–response relationship was observed for certain outcomes in this study.

TABLE 1.—Comparison of Distribution of Maternal Characteristics Among Women With Twin, Triplet, and Quadruplet and Higher Order Pregnancy

Characteristic	Twin Pregnancy* (%)	Triplet Pregnancy† (%)	Quadruplet or Higher-Order Pregnancy‡ (%)
Mother's race			
White	78.8	89.4	94.8
Black	17.4	8.2	3.3
Other	3.8	2.4	1.9
Mother's age (y)			
<20	7.4	1.7	0.2
20-24	19.1	6.8	5.4
25-29	27.2	23.9	29.8
30-34	28.6	40.2	42.1
≥35	17.7	27.4	22.5
Parity			
1	34.1	51.2	52.7
2	33.3	25.1	27.4
3	18.5	13.5	9.0
≥4	14.1	10.3	10.9
Marital status			
Married	72.0	90.6	97.4
Unmarried	28.0	9.4	2.6
Mother's education (y)			
<12	16.6	5.1	3.1
12	31.8	22.3	24.2
13-15	23.3	25.3	24.9
16	17.5	28.3	29.0
≥17	10.8	19.0	18.8
Prenatal care visit			
First trimester	85.4	93.6	94.6
Second trimester	11.7	5.1	3.7
Third trimester	1.7	0.4	0.5
No visit	1.2	0.9	1.2
Smoking during pregnancy			
Yes	9.7	3.3	1.2
No	70.1	77.5	81.1
Unknown/unavailable§	20.2	19.2	17.7

*N = 152,238 women
†N = 5491 women
‡N = 423 women
§The state of California did not report smoking information.
(Reprinted by permission of the publisher from Wen SW, Demissie K, Yang Q, et al: Maternal morbidity and obstetric complications in triplet pregnancies and quadruplet and higher-order multiple pregnancies. *Am J Obstet Gynecol* 191:254-258. Copyright 2004 by Elsevier.)

TABLE 2.—Comparison of Maternal Health Outcomes Among Women With Twin, Triplet, and Quadruplet and Higher Order Pregnancy

Outcome	Twin (n)	Triplet (n)	Quadruplet or Higher (n)	Triplet vs Twin		Quadruplet vs Twin	
				Crude Odds Ratio (95% CI)	Adjusted Odds Ratio (95% CI)	Crude Odds Ration (95% CI)	Adjusted Odds Ratio (95% CI)
Chronic hypertension	1429 (0.95%)	49 (0.92%)	5 (1.20%)	0.96 (0.71, 1.29)	0.90 (0.68, 1.20)	1.27 (0.46, 3.16)	1.29 (0.53, 3.13)
Gestation hypertension	11692 (7.68%)	567 (10.32%)	48 (11.57%)	1.38 (1.26, 1.52)	1.19 (1.09, 1.31)	1.57 (1.15, 2.15)	1.35 (1.00, 1.83)
Eclampsia	1522 (1.00%)	106 (1.93%)	7 (1.69%)	1.94 (1.58, 2.38)	1.70 (1.38, 2.09)	1.69 (0.24, 3.69)	1.46 (0.69, 3.09)
Anemia	4685 (3.13%)	173 (3.24%)	9 (2.17%)	1.04 (0.88, 1.21)	1.26 (1.08, 1.47)	0.69 (0.33, 1.37)	0.87 (0.45, 1.68)
Diabetes mellitus	5085 (3.34%)	328 (5.97%)	28 (6.75%)	1.84 (1.63, 2.07)	1.56 (1.39, 1.76)	2.10 (1.40, 3.12)	1.81 (1.23, 2.67)
Cardiac disorder	930 (0.62%)	49 (0.92%)	4 (0.96%)	1.48 (1.10, 1.99)	1.14 (0.86, 1.53)	1.56 (0.50, 4.32)	1.21 (0.45, 3.26)
Placental abruption	1842 (1.21%)	86 (1.57%)	8 (1.94%)	1.30 (1.03, 1.63)	1.33 (1.06, 1.66)	1.61 (0.74, 3.34)	1.68 (0.83, 3.38)
Placenta previa	700 (0.46%)	29 (0.53%)	4 (0.99%)	1.16 (0.77, 1.70)	0.97 (0.66, 1.42)	2.15 (0.68, 5.79)	1.90 (0.71, 5.12)
Premature rupture of membrane	9985 (6.66%)	598 (11.17%)	44 (10.65%)	1.76 (1.61, 1.93)	1.68 (1.54, 1.84)	1.67 (1.21, 2.31)	1.63 (1.19, 2.23)
Cord prolapse	856 (0.57%)	31 (0.58%)	3 (0.73%)	1.02 (0.70, 1.48)	1.06 (0.74, 1.53)	1.28 (0.33, 4.09)	1.36 (0.44, 4.25)
Cesarean delivery	77966 (51.21%)	4765 (86.78%)	359 (84.87%)	3.25 (5.77, 6.77)	5.86 (5.42, 6.35)	5.34 (4.06, 7.04)	5.04 (3.86, 6.58)
Labor induction	19176 (12.75%)	157 (2.92%)	13 (3.13%)	0.21 (0.17, 0.24)	0.18 (0.15, 0.21)	0.22 (0.12, 0.39)	0.18 (0.11, 0.32)
Vacuum/forceps	9798 (6.44%)	44 (0.80%)	4 (9.45%)	0.12 (0.08, 0.16)	0.10 (0.07, 0.14)	0.14 (0.04, 0.38)	0.11 (0.05, 0.69)

Note: The risks of maternal morbidity and obstetric complications tend to be higher for women with triplet pregnancies and quadruplet and higher order multiple pregnancies than for women with twin pregnancies.

(Reprinted by permission of the publisher from Wen SW, Demissie K, Yang Q, et al: Maternal morbidity and obstetric complications in triplet pregnancies and quadruplet and higher-order multiple pregnancies. *Am J Obstet Gynecol* 191:254-258. Copyright 2004 by Elsevier.)

▶ The authors report a population-based study that assessed the risk of maternal morbidity and obstetric complications in women with triplet pregnancies and quadruplet or higher order multiple pregnancies. The major strength of the study is its population base. Although troubled in the usual way by being retrospective, the study's size and grouping of twin pregnancies, triplet pregnancies, and quadruplet or higher order multiple pregnancies into cohorts with appropriate matching provide a sobering glimpse of the relationship between multiple gestation pregnancies and the risk of maternal complications. The study even shows a dose–response relationship for the higher multiples. Therefore, a good sense of the escalating morbidity is provided by the article, even though the clarity of the message is tempered by unavoidable selection bias related to the frequent use of assisted reproductive technology for conception of the higher multiples, which further associates with white race, older age, first birth, being married, higher educational level, receiving prenatal care earlier, and being less likely to smoke cigarettes during pregnancy. Some of these latter factors contribute to less risk, but others contribute to higher risk. Thus, the effect of the bias is unclear. The fact that maternal morbidity and obstetric complications such as anemia, diabetes mellitus, gestational hypertension, eclampsia, abruptio placenta, premature rupture of the membranes, and increased cesarean section all occur more frequently in triplet or higher multiple gestation pregnancies after adjustment for various maternal factors is not surprising and tracks well with the morbidity that we observe for the offspring of such pregnancies. The bottom line is that women were not designed to have litters, and risks accrue on both the maternal and the fetal and neonatal sides of the ledger. Because of the impact of assisted reproduction on the risk profile for mothers and babies, the public needs to understand these risks, and parents and society should give some serious consideration to the total costs of assisted reproduction, independent of the ability to pay for the procedure itself. The burden on society in general and on the people who participate in the multiple gestation event is considerable and consequential and not all financial.

D. K. Stevenson, MD

Adverse Outcomes After Preterm Labor Are Associated With Tumor Necrosis Factor-α Polymorphism −863, but Not −308, in Mother-Infant Pairs

Amory JH, Adams KM, Lin M-T, et al (Univ of Washington, Seattle; Fred Hutchinson Cancer Research Ctr, Seattle)
Am J Obstet Gynecol 191:1362-1367, 2004   2–16

Background.—Patients with preterm labor have increased concentrations of proinflammatory cytokines in amniotic fluid and blood. The gene-encoding tumor necrosis factor-α (TNF-α), a pro-inflammatory cytokine, contains several single nucleotide polymorphisms (SNPs) in noncoding regions that are associated with altered TNF-α production. An SNP at −863 is associated with decreased basal synthesis and increased production after stimulation. An SNP at -308 is associated with a higher basal synthesis rate. The association between these 2 SNPs of TNF-α and preterm birth was examined in a prospective study.

Study Design.—The study group consisted of 118 mother-infant pairs with labor prior to 34 weeks' gestation. Primary outcomes consisted of gestational age at birth, chorioamnionitis, TNF-α concentrations in amniotic fluid, and neonatal morbidity. Adverse outcomes were compared to maternal and neonatal SNPs.

Findings.—Mothers who were homozygous for the -863 SNP of TNF-α had significantly earlier delivery, more chorioamnionitis, and greater neonatal morbidity than mothers who were not homozygous for this SNP. The -308 polymorphism was not associated with adverse outcome in this study group.

Conclusion.—An association exists between maternal homozygosity for the -863 SNP of TNF-α and preterm birth, chorioamnionitis, and neonatal complications.

▶ Millions of dollars and hours have been expended in pursuing the Holy Grail of the etiology of preterm labor. The authors of this study are to be congratulated on performing a difficult study on a population of patients with preterm labor prior to 34 weeks' gestation. They have identified a polymorphism that may be associated with preterm delivery and adverse neonatal outcome related to the production of a cytokine, TNF-α. Cytokines have been associated with the onset of preterm labor and adverse outcomes in preterm labor and delivery.

Detection of a polymorphism that detects patients at risk for preterm labor may better identify the group of patients who need intensive surveillance for the onset of preterm labor. The study was not contaminated by the usual selection bias in this type of study, as the patients were prospectively enrolled at between 20 and 34 weeks, with strict definitions of preterm labor and adequate exclusion criteria. Search for a clinically applicable screening test will continue, but this study is an example of how such investigations should be pursued.

M. L. Druzin, MD

3 Genetics and Teratology

Transfer of Fetal Cells With Multilineage Potential to Maternal Tissue
Khosrotehrani K, Johnson KL, Cha DH, et al (Tufts-New England Med Ctr, Boston)
JAMA 292:75-80, 2004   3–1

Background.—Fetal CD34$^+$ cells enter the maternal circulation during pregnancy and persist for decades, resulting in physiologic microchimerism. In the event of maternal injury, fetal cells may develop multilineage capacity in maternal organs. Evidence that fetal microchimeric cells express markers of epithelial, leukocyte, and hepatocyte differentiation within maternal organs was sought.

Methods.—Archived paraffin-embedded tissue section specimens were obtained from 21 women. Ten women had male offspring and were found previously to have high numbers of microchimeric cells. The other 11 women had no previous male pregnancies. Fluorescence in situ hybridization with X and Y chromosome-specific probes was followed by histologic and immunochemical studies with anticytokeratin (AE1/AE3) as a marker of epithelial cells, anti-CD45 as a leukocyte marker, and heppar-1 as a hepatocyte marker.

Findings.—Analysis identified 701 male (XY+) microchimeric cells. Fourteen percent to 60% of the XY+ cells expressed cytokeratin in maternal epithelial tissues, such as thyroid, cervix, intestine, and gallbladder. In hematopoietic tissues, such as lymph nodes and spleen, 90% of XY+ cells were found to express CD45+. Four percent of XY+ cells expressed heppar-1+ in 1 liver sample. Independent observers' analysis of histologic and immunochemical evidence of differentiation was very concordant.

Conclusions.—Microchimeric male cells bearing epithelial, leukocyte, or hepatocyte markers were found in a variety of maternal tissue specimens. These data suggest the presence of fetal cells that may have multilineage ability.

▶ The authors present provocative yet convincing data on the detection of microchimeric male cells, bearing epithelial, leukocyte, and hepatocyte markers, in a variety of maternal tissue specimens. It is not new knowledge that fetal cells can gain access to the maternal circulation—mainly cells of hemato-poietic origin, such as nucleated red blood cells, lymphocytes, and hematopoi-etic stem cells. However, it is new to suggest that fetal cells may have multilineage capacity. The implications for such passage of cells to the mother are unknown, especially with respect to long-term health. Another benefit to pregnancy might be the delivery of a younger population of cells that have dif-ferent capabilities in response to tissue injury. In the case of a male fetus, this is 1 way that a male infant can contribute to his mother's health disposition. It would be nice to think that the contribution is positive, as males are capable of presenting themselves, their mothers, and fathers with so many difficulties beginning in infancy and beyond (the male disadvantage). The fundamental in-timacy of the fetus and mother is further supported by this report of fetal cell microchimerism in the mother. Ultimately, it will be important to understand the progenitor cell population and whether the consequences of such intimacy are positive or negative.

D. K. Stevenson, MD

Meta-analysis of 13 Genome Scans Reveals Multiple Cleft Lip/Palate Genes With Novel Loci on 9q21 and 2q32-35

Marazita ML, Murray JC, Lidral AC, et al (Univ of Pittsburgh, Pa; Univ of Iowa, Iowa City; Univ of Antioquia, Medellin, Colombia; et al)
Am J Hum Genet 75:161-173, 2004   3–2

Background.—Orofacial clefts, particularly cleft lip (CL), cleft palate (CP), and cleft lip with or without cleft palate (CL/P), are common structural birth defects; however the etiology of these defects is complex. The preva-lence at birth is 1/500 to 1/2000, depending on the population. Multidisci-plinary treatment is usually necessary into adulthood in these patients, and both the patients and their families experience health burdens and a variety of psychosocial implications. In recent years, investigators have attempted to locate the genes predisposing to orofacial clefting, using linkage and/or association methods. The purpose of the present study was to identify the genomic regions that contain genes predisposing to CL/P across popula-tions.

Methods.—A total of 13 study populations with genome scans were avail-able for families with isolated, or nonsyndromic (NS), CL/P. Included in these 13 populations were 574 families, with a total of 5990 individual fam-ily members.

Results.—A 10-cM genomic scan of 388 extended multiplex families from 7 diverse populations (a total of 2551 genotyped individuals) demon-strated CL/P genes in 6 chromosomal regions, including a novel region at 9q21. Meta-analyses with the addition of results from an additional 186 families (including 6 populations and 1033 genotyped individuals) showed genomewide significant linkage for 10 more regions, including a novel re-gion at 2q32-35.

Conclusions.—The first genomewide significant linkage results for CL/P are presented, highlighting the power of linkage analysis for the simultaneous detection of multiple genes for a complex disorder.

Interferon Regulatory Factor 6 (*IRF6*) Gene Variants and the Risk of Isolated Cleft Lip or Palate
Zucchero TM, Cooper ME, Maher BS, et al (Univ of Iowa, Iowa City; Univ of Pittsburgh, Pa; HOPE Found, Bacolod City, The Philippines; et al)
N Engl J Med 351:769-780, 2004   3–3

Background.—Cleft lip or palate (or the two in combination) is a common birth defect that results from a mixture of genetic and environmental factors. We searched for a specific genetic factor contributing to this complex trait by examining large numbers of affected patients and families and evaluating a specific candidate gene.

Methods.—We identified the gene that encodes interferon regulatory factor 6 (*IRF6*) as a candidate gene on the basis of its involvement in an autosomal dominant form of cleft lip and palate, Van der Woude's syndrome. A single-nucleotide polymorphism in this gene results in either a valine or an isoleucine at amino acid position 274 (V274I). We carried out transmission-disequilibrium testing for V274I in 8003 individual subjects in 1968 families derived from 10 populations with ancestry in Asia, Europe, and South America, haplotype and linkage analyses, and case-control analyses, and determined the risk of cleft lip or palate that is associated with genetic variation in IRF6.

Results.—Strong evidence of overtransmission of the valine (V) allele was found in the entire population data set ($P<10^{-9}$); moreover, the results for some individual populations from South America and Asia were highly significant. Variation at *IRF6* was responsible for 12 percent of the genetic contribution to cleft lip or palate and tripled the risk of recurrence in families that had already had one affected child.

Conclusions.—DNA-sequence variants associated with *IRF6* are major contributors to cleft lip, with or without cleft palate. The contribution of variants in single genes to cleft lip or palate is an important consideration in genetic counseling.

▶ "Cleft lip with or without cleft palate is one of the most common birth defects and is certainly the most visible. The incidence varies among ethnic groups, ranging from 3.6 per 1000 live births among Native Americans to 2.0 per 1000 among Asians, 1.5 per 1000 among Indians, 1.0 per 1000 among people of European ancestry, and 0.3 per 1000 among Africans. Cleft lip with or without cleft palate is more frequent among boys. In contrast, isolated cleft palate is twice as common among girls and occurs in approximately 0.4 of every 1000 live births in all ethnic groups."[1] For the longest time the etiology of nonsyndromic oral clefts was blandly designated as multifactorial, implying a complex interplay between genetic and environmental factors.

We are indebted to Marazita et al (Abstract 3–2) as well as Zucchero et al (Abstract 3–3) for elucidating the genetic factors that provoke abnormal oral development. Genes or chromosomal rearrangements on many chromosomes can lead to syndromes that include orofacial clefts, with trisomy 13 being the prime example. In these 2 reports the strength and benefits of international collaboration and intense focus on a region of the genome are demonstrated. These are the first genome-wide significant linkage results ever reported for cleft lip and palate, and they represent an unprecedented demonstration of the power of linkage analysis to detect multiple genes simultaneously for a complex disorder. In a review manuscript, Marazita and Mooney[2] summed the situation as follows: "As for nonsyndromic clefting, the large-scale family studies are consistent with one or a few loci exerting major effects on phenotypic expression, although no single gene has been identified as a 'necessary' locus for development of nonsyndromic clefts. Rather, the emerging consensus is that the genetic etiology of nonsyndromic clefting is complex, with several loci showing significant results in at least some studies. Some of these loci may be genes for susceptibility to environmental factors, some may be modifying loci, and some may be 'necessary' loci." Ongoing genetic studies should unravel the complex etiology of cleft palate and other common congenital anomalies.

Parents who have a newborn with a cleft lip, among other things, desperately want to know why it occurred, when will it be repaired, and what the consequences will be. Many parents are now seeking advice on the Internet, where they may also find parental support groups. On the basis of a questionnaire Byrnes et al[3] have determined that parents are dissatisfied with the information that they are receiving concerning clefts. Their questionnaire revealed that "parents wanted informing health professionals to be in greater control of the informing conversation, to show more caring and confidence, to show more of their own feelings, to give parents more of an opportunity to talk and show feelings, to make a greater effort to comfort parents, to provide more information, to initiate more of a discussion about the association between clefts and mental retardation/learning disabilities, and to provide more referrals to other parents during the informing interview." This information should prove helpful when we need to counsel families of a newborn with an oral cleft. Also see Abstracts 8–23 and 10–14.

A. A. Fanaroff, MD

References

1. Mulliken JB: The changing faces of children with cleft lip and palate. *N Engl J Med* 351:745-747, 2004.
2. Marazita ML, Mooney MP: Current concepts in the embryology and genetics of cleft lip and cleft palate. *Clin Plast Surg* 31:125-140, 2004.
3. Byrnes AL, Berk NW, Cooper ME, et al: Parental evaluation of informing interviews for cleft lip and/or palate. *Pediatrics* 112:308-313, 2003.

Long Term Follow Up Study of Survival Associated With Cleft Lip and Palate at Birth

Christensen K, Juel K, Herskind AM, et al (Univ of Southern Denmark, Odense; Natl Inst of Public Health, Copenhagen; Odense Univ, Denmark; et al)
BMJ 328:1405-1406, 2004   3–4

Objective.—To assess the overall and cause specific mortality of people from birth to 55 years with cleft lip and palate.

Design.—Long term follow up study.

Setting.—Danish register of deaths.

Participants.—People born with cleft lip and palate between 1943 and 1987, followed to 1998.

Main Outcome Measures.—Observed and expected numbers of deaths, summarised as overall and cause specific standardised mortality ratios.

Results.—5331 people with cleft lip and palate were followed for 170 421 person years. The expected number of deaths was 259, but 402 occurred, corresponding to a standardised mortality ratio of 1.4 (95% confidence interval 1.3 to 1.6) for males and 1.8 (1.5 to 2.1) for females. The increased risk of mortality was nearly constant for the three intervals at follow up: first year of life, 1-17 years, and 18-55 years. The participants had an increased risk of all major causes of death.

Conclusions.—People with cleft lip and palate have increased mortality up to age 55. Children born with cleft lip and palate and possibly other congenital malformations may benefit from specific preventive health measures into and throughout adulthood.

▶ The fact that there are accurate records available for the population of patients with clefts dating back more than 50 years is both admirable and remarkable. But for the Scandinavian countries it seems to be the standard of care. It is distressing to learn that the mortality rate for patients with cleft lip and palate exceeds the anticipated mortality rate, and that it is constant for the 3 intervals at follow-up: first year of life, 1 to 17 years, and 18 to 55 years. I would have anticipated a higher mortality rate in the first group. Recognizing that there is an increased risk of death mandates closer attention to health maintenance and more rigorous prevention of disease. Clearly, something easier to say than do. To assess whether patients with facial cleft had an increased incidence of psychiatric illness, the Danish Database was once again probed. Patients with facial cleft born between 1936 and 1987 in Denmark were identified, and the admission pattern for these patients with facial cleft was available for the period 1969 through 1993 through the Danish Psychiatric Central registry. Among 6462 patients with facial cleft, 284 (4.4%) were hospitalized for psychiatric illness.

The risk of hospitalized mental disorders in general is increased in patients with cleft palate but not to any substantial degree in patients with cleft lip, with or without cleft palate. Both groups had an increased risk of mental retardation and substance abuse, but the risk for schizophrenia or bipolar illness was not statistically significantly increased compared with the background population. Surprisingly, the authors concluded that there was no evidence that the psychosocial stressors associated with cleft lip with or without cleft palate and its treatment had any substantial impact on the risk for hospitalized mental illness.

So we can add to our data bank the facts that infants born with facial clefts are more likely to require hospitalization for a psychiatric illness and die at a younger age—sobering thoughts and information that I am not sure that I would necessarily share with the parents in the delivery room.

A. A. Fanaroff, MD

Terminal 22q Deletion Syndrome: A Newly Recognized Cause of Speech and Language Disability in the Autism Spectrum
Manning MA, Cassidy SB, Clericuzio C, et al (Stanford Univ, Calif; Univ of California, Irvine; Univ of New Mexico, Albuquerque; et al)
Pediatrics 114:451-457, 2004   3–5

Background.—Cryptic subtelomeric chromosome rearrangements are responsible for 6% to 10% of cases of idiopathic mental retardation. The number of genetic syndromes attributed to these microdeletions has increased as cytogenetic and molecular techniques have become more sophisticated. Eleven new cases of del 22q13.3 were reported to characterize further the clinical phenotype of this recently described syndrome.

Methods.—The study group consisted of 11 patients, aged 5 months to 46 years, who were referred for genetics evaluation because of developmental delay, severe language delay, and dysmorphic features. Of the 11 patients, only 1 was male. There were 5 white patients, 1 Chinese, 1 black, 2 Latina, 1 of mixed race, and 1 of unknown race. Patients received a physical examination, history, and chromosome analysis. Seven patients had a fluorescence in situ hybridization analysis.

Findings.—All 11 patients had delayed motor development, hypotonia, and severe speech and language delay. Dysmorphic facial features included epicanthal folds, large cupped ears, underdeveloped philtrum, lack of cupid's bow, and full supraorbital ridges. Six of the patients had autism-like behaviors. Microscopically visible chromosome deletions were detected in 6 patients, and the remainder were detected by fluorescence in situ hybridization.

Conclusions.—These 11 patients help to characterize the recently reported distal 22q deletion syndrome. This phenotype includes developmental delay, hypotonia, and severely delayed speech. Some patients have behavior in the autism spectrum. Craniofacial features include ear anomalies, short nose, supraorbital fullness, smooth filtrum, and lack of cupid's bow. Referral for genetics evaluation is recommended for patients with these findings.

▶ At first, one might wonder why an article on autism spectrum disorder would be reviewed for this audience? Although chromosome 22 is of great significance for neonatologists (eg, CATCH 22 [Cardiac defects, Abnormal facies, Thymic hypoplasia, Cleft palate, Hypocalcemia, 22nd chromosome deletion], velocardiofacial syndrome), autism is not a common problem in the neonatal ICU. However, prenatal counseling for families with abnormalities involving the 22nd chromosome will come up. In the past, we would focus on looking for cardiac defects. Now, our consult will have to include discussion of this new spectrum of behavioral problems. We may need to start a conversation with our bioethics colleagues, too. What options should be available to a family when chorionic villus sampling identifies this deletion early in gestation? Lastly, those of us who work in developmental follow-up clinics will see children with autism spectrum. High-resolution chromosome analysis may have to be part of that evaluation, too, looking for this and other possibly associated abnormalities (eg, chromosome 15q11-q13 duplication).

R. S. Cohen, MD

Genetic Variation of Infant Reduced Folate Carrier (A80G) and Risk of Orofacial and Conotruncal Heart Defects
Shaw GM, Zhu H, Lammer EJ, et al (March of Dimes Birth Defects Found, Oakland, Calif; Texas A&M Univ, Houston; Children's Hosp, Oakland, Calif)
Am J Epidemiol 158:747-752, 2003   3–6

How folate reduces the risks of congenital anomalies is unknown. The authors focused on a gene involved in folate transport-reduced folate carrier-1 gene (*RFC1*). Using data from a California case-control study (1987-1989 births), the authors investigated whether the risks of orofacial clefts or conotruncal heart defects were influenced by a polymorphism of infant *RFC1* or by an interaction between the *RFC1* gene and maternal periconceptional use of vitamins containing folic acid. A total of 305 liveborn infants with cleft lip with or without cleft palate, 123 with cleft palate, 163 with conotruncal heart defects, and 364 nonmalformed controls were genotyped. Odds ratios of 1.6 (95% confidence interval: 0.9, 2.8) for the *G80/G80* genotype and of 2.3 (95% confidence interval: 1.3, 3.9) for the *G80/A80* genotype were observed relative to the *A80/A80* genotype for conotruncal defects. Among mothers who did not use vitamins, the risk of conotruncal defects was 2.1 (95% confidence interval: 0.7, 5.9) for infants with genotype *G80/G80* compared with those with the *A80/A80* genotype. Among mothers who did use vitamins, the risk was 1.3 (95% confidence interval: 0.7, 2.7). Substantially elevated risks for either cleft group were not observed irrespective of genotype and use/nonuse of vitamins. Thus, this study found modest evidence for a gene-nutrient interaction between infant *RFC1* genotype and periconceptional intake of vitamins on the risk of conotruncal defects.

▶ These authors have extensively studied the problem of neural tube and other defects, such as the role of nutrients and their interactions with genes.[1-3] There is little doubt that folic acid supplementation can effectively reduce the risk of neural tube defects (NTDs); however, the mechanism underlying this beneficial effect remains unclear. Recent evidence suggests that certain folate pathway genes, as well as those related to homocysteine metabolism, might be contributing to this effect. Furthermore, periconceptional dietary intake of choline (choline is involved in 1-carbon metabolism for methylation of homocysteine to methionine), betaine, and methionine also substantially reduces the risk of NTDs.[1]

To elaborate on the mechanism by which folate protects against certain birth defects, Shaw et al focused on a gene involved in folate transport—the reduced folate carrier-1 gene (RFC1). By using the huge California database they constructed a case-control study by which they investigated whether the risks of orofacial clefts or conotruncal heart defects were influenced by a polymorphism of infant RFC1 or by an interaction between the RFC1 gene and maternal periconceptional use of vitamins containing folic acid. They found only a weak correlation for conotruncal abnormalities with the G80/G80 genotype when the mothers did not take additional vitamins.

Numerous studies analyzing 5,10-methylenetetrahydrofolate reductase (MTHFR) variants have resulted in positive associations with increased NTD risk only in certain populations, suggesting that these variants are not large contributors to the etiology of NTDs.[2,3] But with the limited knowledge of the genes involved in regulating NTD susceptibility, at this time it makes little sense for prospective parents to be tested for MTHFR variants or for variants of other known folate pathway genes. This could all change with better understanding of the various gene-nutrient interactions. We have accumulated a lot of data and acquired much knowledge on these devastating defects but still have much to learn.

A. A. Fanaroff, MD

References

1. Shaw GM, Carmichael SL, Yang W, et al: Periconceptional dietary intake of choline and betaine and neural tube defects in offspring. *Am J Epidemiol* 160:102-109, 2004.
2. Finnell RH, Shaw GM, Lammer EJ, et al: Does prenatal screening for 5,10- methylenetetrahydrofolate reductase (MTHFR) mutations in high-risk neural tube defect pregnancies make sense? *Genet Test* 6:47-52, 2002.
3. Zhu H, Wicker NJ, Shaw GM, et al: Homocysteine remethylation enzyme polymorphisms and increased risks for neural tube defects. *Mol Genet Metab* 78:216-221, 2003.

Perinatally Diagnosed Asymptomatic Congenital Cystic Adenomatoid Malformation: To Resect or Not?

Aziz D, Langer JC, Tuuha SE, et al (Hosp for Sick Children, Toronto)
J Pediatr Surg 39:329-334, 2004   3–7

Background.—Management of asymptomatic congenital cystic adenomatoid malformation (CCAM) is controversial. The natural history of untreated asymptomatic CCAM is unknown, although most surgeons recommend resection of these lesions to prevent future infection. The aim of this study was to determine the relative surgical risk of resection compared with the risk of observation for these patients.

Methods.—A retrospective review of hospital records between 1996 and 2002 in a tertiary care pediatric referral center was conducted. All perinatally (prenatal or neonatal) diagnosed CCAMs were included. In addition, patients presenting with late diagnosis of CCAM were also reviewed.

Results.—Forty-eight children had CCAM diagnosed perinatally. Thirteen of these were symptomatic and required surgery within 6 months; these were excluded from the analysis. Of the 35 asymptomatic infants, 6 were operated on electively before 6 months of age (median age, 4.5 months). The other 29 asymptomatic infants were followed up for more than 6 months. Of these, 9 remained asymptomatic and were eventually operated on electively (median age, 13 months). Three (10%) had CCAM infections at 7, 8, and 11 months of age and required resection. The remaining 17 children have not undergone resection and are still asymptomatic (median follow-up, 3 years). An additional 12 patients presented with a late diagnosis of CCAM. All of these presented with complications (infection or pneumothorax) and underwent resection (median age, 6 years). Overall, the complication rate after resection of an asymptomatic CCAM was not significantly different from those of resected CCAM that had already developed infection or pneumothorax ($P = .64$).

Conclusions.—Ten percent of perinatally diagnosed asymptomatic patients had 5 complications requiring surgery during follow-up. The true incidence is probably higher given the relatively short follow-up in our series. Morbidity after resection of a complicated CCAM was not statistically significantly higher than after elective resection for an asymptomatic CCAM. Although conservative management of asymptomatic CCAM may be warranted, a more extended period of follow-up is necessary before this approach can be recommended.

▶ CCAM is by far the most common congenital lung malformation, accounting for approximately 95% of congenital cystic lung diseases, and is usually diagnosed prenatally during routine US evaluation of the fetus. Surgery is required for symptomatic CCAMs, but if the CCAM is asymptomatic, there is a debate about what should be done. The surgeons from the Hospital for Sick Children evaluated their experience with the management of CCAM and they conclude that, in the absence of symptoms, it is reasonable to observe these infants and to intervene surgically if symptoms develop. On the other hand, the length of stay for these infants was significantly longer than those who were operated on before symptoms developed. The other concern is the potential for malignancy, although associations among CCAM, subsequent malignancy, the timing of surgery, and survival are ill defined.

This problem cries out for an appropriately designed, randomized, controlled trial. Discussions of the experience of one or another team of surgeons is all very well but will not get us any closer to understanding the optimal approach to the management of these lesions.

M. J. Maisels, MB, BCh

4 Labor and Delivery

Preterm Meconium Staining of the Amniotic Fluid: Associated Findings and Risk of Adverse Clinical Outcome
Tybulewicz AT, Clegg SK, Fonfé GJ, et al (Royal Hosp for Sick Children, Edinburgh, Scotland; Royal Infirmary, Little France, Edinburgh, Scotland; St James's Univ, Leeds, England)
Arch Dis Child Fetal Neonatal Ed 89:F328-F330, 2004   4–1

Background.—The incidence of preterm meconium staining of the amniotic fluid (MSAF) is uncertain. It may be an indicator of possible listeriosis. It is unclear how great this risk is or whether preterm MSAF is a risk factor for adverse neonatal outcome.

Objective.—To investigate the incidence of preterm MSAF, the incidence of associated maternal and neonatal infection, and the outcomes of the infants at discharge.

Design.—Retrospective case-control study.

Methods.—Infants < 33 weeks gestation with preterm MSAF born in the Simpson Memorial Maternity Pavilion, Edinburgh between 1 January 1994 and 2 January 2001 were matched with the next infant of the same sex and gestation with clear liquor. Maternal and infant characteristics, culture results, placental histology, and clinical outcomes were compared.

Results.—Preterm MSAF was observed in 45/1054 (4.3%) infants below 33 weeks gestation. No maternal or infant listeriosis was identified in cases or controls. There was no significant difference in birth weight, Apgar score, or first pH between cases and controls. Preterm MSAF was associated with prolonged rupture of the membranes (odds ratio (OR) 3.34, 95% confi-

TABLE 4.—Adverse Neonatal Outcomes

	Cases	Controls	Odds Ratio (95% CI)
Number	45	41	
Death	10 (22)	4 (10)	2.64 (0.76 to 9.21)
CLD (36 weeks)	8 (18)	4 (10)	2.0 (0.55 to 7.22)
PVL	1 (2)	1 (2)	0.91 (0.06 to 15.02)
IVH grade 3/4	5 (11)	0 (0)	2.03 (1.62 to 2.53)

Data are number (%).
CLD, Chronic lung disease; PVL, periventricular leucomalacia; IVH, intraventricular haemorrhage.
(Courtesy of Tybulewicz AT, Clegg SK, Fonfé GJ, et al: Preterm meconium staining of the amniotic fluid: Associated findings and risk of adverse clinical outcome. *Arch Dis Child Fetal Neonatal Ed* 89:F328-F330, 2004, with permission from the BMJ Publishing Group.)

dence interval (CI) 1.07 to 10.49), but not maternal hypertension, sepsis, or chorioamnionitis (Table 4). Severe (grade 3/4) intraventricular haemorrhage was significantly more common in infants with preterm MSAF (OR 2.03, 95% CI 1.62 to 2.53). There was no significant difference in mortality. Early onset sepsis was observed in two cases and three controls.

Conclusions.—Preterm meconium staining of the amniotic fluid may be associated with increased risk of intraventricular haemorrhage. It does not appear to be a useful indicator of listeriosis.

▶ Green bile is a healthy sign, but green-tinted amniotic fluid or green gastric aspirates may indicate trouble is brewing. For many years the prevailing teaching was that meconium staining of the amniotic fluid (MSAF) was not seen before 37 weeks' gestation. If the amniotic fluid was meconium stained (green) before that time, clinicians were to consider that the dating of the pregnancy was incorrect, *Listeria* infection was likely, or an upper gastrointestinal obstructive lesion was present. Preterm infants didn't just pass meconium. Tybulewicz et al provide further evidence that meconium staining may be present in up to 5% of preterm infants (<33 weeks' gestation), starting as early as 25 weeks' gestation. Mazor et al[1] reported a similar prevalence in preterm infants. They were unable to make a distinction between thick or thin meconium, but it matters not as NONE of these preterm infants developed meconium aspiration syndrome. Also, none of the infants with MSAF developed *Listeria* sepsis. The 3 cases of *Listeria* sepsis documented over a 7-year period had clear amniotic fluid. Preterm MSAF was associated with prolonged premature rupture of the membranes, but this was not associated with or accompanied by chorioamnionitis. The MSAF infants had a higher prevalence of severe intraventricular hemorrhage but not periventricular leukomalacia. The long-term consequences were unknown in this series, but Spinillo et al[2] observed more cerebral palsy at age 2 among 17 preterm infants with MSAF when compared with 345 preterm infants with clear liquid.

A. A. Fanaroff, MD

References

1. Mazor M, Furman B, Wiznitzer A, et al: Maternal and perinatal outcome of patients with preterm labor and meconium stained amniotic fluid. *Obstet Gynecol* 86:830-833, 1995.
2. Spinillo A, Fazzi E, Capuzzo E, et al: Meconium stained amniotic fluid and risk for cerebral palsy in preterm infants. *Obstet Gynecol* 90:519-523, 1997.

Short-Term Outcome After Active Perinatal Management at 23–25 Weeks of Gestation. A Study From Two Swedish Tertiary Care Centres. Part 1: Maternal and Obstetric Factors

Serenius F, Ewald U, Farooqi A, et al (Umeå Univ, Sweden; Uppsala Univ, Sweden)
Acta Paediatr 93:945-953, 2004   4–2

Aims.—To provide descriptive data on women who delivered at 23–25 wk of gestation, and to relate foetal and neonatal outcomes to maternal factors, obstetric management and the principal reasons for preterm birth.

Methods.—Medical records of all women who had delivered in two tertiary care centres in 1992–1998 were reviewed. At the two centres, policies of active perinatal and neonatal management were universally applied. Logistic regression models were used to identify prenatal factors associated with survival.

Results.—Of 197 women who delivered at 23–25 wk, 65% had experienced a previous miscarriage, 15% a previous stillbirth and 12% a neonatal death. The current pregnancy was the result of artificial reproduction in 13% of the women. In 71%, the pregnancy was complicated either by pre-eclampsia, chorioamnionitis, placental abruption or premature rupture of membranes. Antenatal steroids were given in 63%. Delivery was by caesarean section in 47%. The reasons for preterm birth were idiopathic preterm labour in 36%, premature rupture of membranes in 41% and physician-indicated deliveries in 23% of the mothers. Demographic details, use of antenatal steroids, caesarean section delivery and birthweight differed between mothers depending on the reason for preterm delivery. Of 224 infants, 5% were stillbirths and 63% survived to discharge. On multivariate logistic regression analysis comprising prenatally known variables, reasons for preterm birth were not associated with survival. Advanced gestational duration (OR: 2.43 per wk; 95% CI: 1.59–3.74), administration of any antenatal steroids (OR: 2.21; 95% CI: 1.14–4.28) and intrauterine referral from a peripheral hospital (OR: 2.93; 95% CI: 1.5–5.73) were associated with survival.

Conclusions.—Women who deliver at 23–25 wk comprise a risk group characterized by a high risk of reproductive failure and pregnancy complications. Survival rates were similar regardless of the reason for preterm birth. Policies of active perinatal management virtually eliminated intrapartum stillbirths.

Short-term Outcome After Active Perinatal Management at 23–25 Weeks of Gestation. A Study From Two Swedish Tertiary Care Centres. Part 2: Infant Survival

Serenius F, Ewald U, Farooqi A, et al (Umeå Univ, Sweden; Uppsala Univ, Sweden)

Acta Paediatr 93:1081-1089, 2004   4–3

Aim.—To determine neonatal survival rates based on both foetal (stillborn) and neonatal deaths among infants delivered at 23–25 wk, and to identify maternal and neonatal factors associated with survival.

Methods.—The medical records of 224 infants who were delivered in two tertiary care centres in 1992–1998 were reviewed retrospectively. At these centres, policies of active perinatal and neonatal management were universally applied. Data were analysed by gestational age groups and considered in three time periods. Logistic regression models were used to identify factors associated with survival.

Results.—The rate of foetal death was 5%. Of infants born alive, 63% survived to discharge. Survival rates including foetal deaths in the denominator at 23, 24 and 25 wk were 37%, 61% and 74%, respectively, and survival rates excluding foetal deaths were 43%, 63% and 77%, respectively. Of infants born with 1-min Apgar scores of 0–1, 43% survived. In the total cohort, survival rates including foetal deaths in the denominator increased from 52% in time period 1 to 61% in time period 2 and 74% in time period 3 ($p <$ 0.02). On multivariate logistic regression analysis, higher birthweight (OR: 1.91 per 100 g increment; 95% CI: 1.45–2.52), female gender (OR: 3.33; 95% CI: 1.65–6.75), administration of antenatal steroids (OR: 2.95; 95% CI: 1.46–5.98) and intrauterine referral from a peripheral hospital (OR: 2.35; 95% CI: 1.18–4.68) were associated with survival. Apgar score ≤ 3 at 1 min (OR: 0.46; 95% CI: 0.22–0.95) was associated with decreased survival. The use of antenatal steroids was protective at 23–24 wk (OR: 5.2; 95% CI: 2.0–13.7), but not at 25 wk.

Conclusions.—Active perinatal management that included universal initiation of neonatal intensive care virtually eliminated intrapartum stillbirths and delivery room deaths, and resulted in survival rates that compare favourably with those of recent studies. However, the policies of active care postponed death in non-survivors. Individual variations in outcome in relation to the infant's condition at birth as reflected by the Apgar scores preclude the making of treatment decisions in the delivery room.

Short-term Outcome After Active Perinatal Management at 23–25 Weeks of Gestation. A Study From Two Swedish Perinatal Centres. Part 3: Neonatal Morbidity

Serenius F, Ewald U, Farooqi A, et al (Umeå Univ, Sweden; Uppsala Univ, Sweden)

Acta Paediatr 93:1090-1097, 2004   4–4

Aim.—To determine major neonatal morbidity in surviving infants born at 23–25 weeks, and to identify maternal and infant factors associated with major morbidity.

Methods.—The medical records of 224 infants who were delivered at two tertiary care centres in 1992–1998 were reviewed retrospectively. At these centres, policies of active perinatal and neonatal management were universally applied. Of the 213 liveborn infants, 140 (66%) survived to discharge. Data were analysed by gestational age and considered in three time periods. Logistic regression models were used to identify factors associated with morbidity.

Results.—Of the survivors, 6% had intraventricular haemorrhage grade ≥ 3 (severe IVH) or periventricular leukomalacia (PVL), 15% retinopathy of prematurity $\geq$ stage 3 (severe ROP) and 36% bronchopulmonary dysplasia (BPD). On logistic regression analysis, severe IVH or PVL was associated with duration of mechanical ventilation (odds ratio, OR: 1.53 per 1-wk increment in duration; 95% confidence interval, CI: 1.01–2.33). Severe ROP was associated with the presence of a patent ductus arteriosus (PDA) (OR: 3.31; 95% CI: 1.11–9.90) and birth in time period 3 versus time periods 1 and 2 combined (OR: 6.28; 95% CI: 2.10–18.74). BPD was associated with duration of mechanical ventilation (OR: 2.71 per 1-wk increment in duration; 95% CI: 1.76–4.18) and with the presence of any obstetric complication (OR: 2.67; 95% CI: 1.07–6.65). Gestational age and birthweight were not associated with major morbidity. Of all survivors, 81% were discharged home without severe IVH, PVL or severe ROP.

Conclusions.—Increased survival as a result of active perinatal and neonatal management was associated with favourable morbidity rates compared with those in recent studies. Among survivors born at 23–25 weeks, neither gestational age nor birthweight was a significant determinant of major morbidity.

▶ This is an interesting trio of reports that address the outcome of a regional cohort of infants at 23 to 25 weeks' gestation after the introduction of active perinatal management. The first report chronicles the maternal and obstetric risk factors, which are substantial. These women were characterized by a high risk of reproductive failure (65% miscarriages, 15% stillbirths, and 12% neonatal deaths) and pregnancy complications, including either preeclampsia, chorioamnionitis, placental abruption, or premature rupture of membranes in 71%. The current pregnancy was the result of artificial reproduction in 13% of the women. But the policy of active perinatal management virtually eliminated intrapartum stillbirths and delivery room deaths and resulted in a 63% overall survival rate to discharge; 43% of infants born with an Apgar score of 0 to 1 survived. (Remember postdischarge deaths during the first year of life are not uncommon in a cohort such as this.) On multivariate logistic regression analysis higher birth weight, female gender, administration of antenatal corticosteroids, and birth at the tertiary center all increased the chances for survival. Survival rates, including fetal deaths in the denominator at 23, 24, and 25 weeks, were 37%, 61%, and 74%, respectively. This compares favorably with U.S. data of 30% (23 weeks), 59% (24 weeks), and 72% (25 weeks) for a similar period. Furthermore, the Swedish cohort was not characterized by an increase in the major neonatal morbidities. Håkansson (Abstract 14–6) by using the Swedish National Data Base, compared the outcomes from the North of Sweden (the proactive group) to the less active South over a prolonged period of time (1984-1999). In infants with a gestational age of 22 to 25 weeks, the proactive policy was significantly associated with more live births, fewer infant deaths on the first day of life, more operative deliveries, fewer infants with extremely low Apgar scores, a higher degree of centralized management, and increased number of infants alive at 1 year with no evidence of increased morbidity.

Although the data tend to speak for themselves, the time period under consideration is 7 years ago; since then we have seen little improvement in the survival rates even with proactive (aggressive) management. Many questions remain unanswered, and resuscitating infants at 22 to 23 weeks' gestation will remain in that category.

A. A. Fanaroff, MD

Perinatal Intervention and Neonatal Outcomes Near the Limit of Viability
Louis JM, Ehrenberg HM, Collin MF, et al (Case Western Reserve Univ, Cleveland, Ohio)
Am J Obstet Gynecol 191:1398-1402, 2004   4–5

Background.—Infants born extremely premature pose particular challenges to the obstetrician and neonatologist. The survival and morbidity rates of preterm infants are known to worsen with earlier gestational age at delivery, but the outcomes of fetuses who are delivered near the limit of viability continue to evolve. Survival after delivery near the limit of potential viability is associated with significant short- and long-term morbidity. Morbidity is known to increase with declining gestational age across the spectrum of preterm birth, but concerns have been expressed that increasing resuscitative efforts for the periviable fetus might increase the survival rate at the expense of increased morbidity in survivors. Trends in the level of obstetric and neonatal intervention near the limit of viability were evaluated, and perinatal morbidity and mortality rates were assessed over time.

Methods.—A retrospective chart review was conducted of live-born infants who were delivered at 23 to 26 weeks of gestation and who weighed between 500 and 1500 g between 1990 and 2001 at an urban tertiary care center. The maternal charts were reviewed for clinical characteristics and the antenatal and intrapartum course. The neonatal charts were reviewed for short-term morbidities that included respiratory distress syndrome, intraventricular hemorrhages, necrotizing enterocolitis, and retinopathy of prematurity, as well as survival. The study group was further divided into 2 cohorts: group 1 (1990 to 1995) and group 2 (1996 to 2001); these groups were compared for the obstetricians' willingness to intervene, neonatal resuscitation efforts, infant mortality rates (in gestational age subgroups), and short-term morbidity. Multivariate analyses, with control for obstetricians' willingness to intervene, neonatal resuscitation, cohort, and gestational age, were performed to evaluate infant survival in the entire cohort and morbidity in the survivors.

Results.—Records were evaluated for a total of 260 mothers and 293 newborn infants. Comparison of the 2 cohorts (group 1 vs group 2) found increases over time in the following: intent to intervene for a fetal indication (70% vs 89%), cesarean delivery for malpresentation (20% vs 42%), and survival (54% vs 70%). The pregnancies in group 1 were less likely to have received antenatal steroids (7.7% vs 60%) or surfactant (39% vs 73%). The survival rate increased with advancing gestational age at delivery (24%, 51%, 68%, and 85% at 23, 24, 25, and 26 weeks of gestation, respectively). However, the incidences of necrotizing enterocolitis, retinopathy of prematurity, intraventricular hemorrhages, respiratory distress syndrome, sepsis, and bronchopulmonary dysplasia did not decline significantly with increasing gestational age after an adjustment was made for other factors.

Conclusions.—Obstetric intervention and aggressive neonatal resuscitation has increased for fetuses delivered between 23 and 26 weeks of gestation. However, although survival in these infants has increased over time and with advancing age at delivery, the short-term morbidity in survivors is similar, regardless of their gestational age.

▶ The authors suggest, from an obstetric perspective, what some of us have suggested for awhile—that obstetric intervention and aggressive neonatal resuscitation resulting in a brief delay in delivery of infants between 23 and 26 weeks' gestational age may improve the chance of survival but may not necessarily affect short-term morbidity in survivors. This observation is discouraging and should make us pause to consider the consequences of our decision making for the babies and their families around this time in gestation. Nonetheless, our dilemma remains: we are not usually able to tell whether a particular individual will be the one who develops the likely complications. Some may escape unscathed and may develop normally. Moreover, an absolute correlation does not exist between short-term complications observed within the first month of life and long-term neurodevelopmental outcomes. Short-term surrogates, such as the presence of intraventricular hemorrhaging, are poor harbingers of long-term injuries and disabilities. Much of the practice of neonatology in this realm of prematurity should be considered investigational and should be subjected to rigorous study.

D. K. Stevenson, MD

Fetal Infants: The Fate of 4172 Infants With Birth Weights of 401 to 500 Grams—The Vermont Oxford Network Experience (1996-2000)

Lucey JF, Rowan CA, Shiono P, et al (Univ of Vermont, Burlington; Vermont Oxford Network, Burlington; Univ of Oxford, England; et al)
Pediatrics 113:1559-1566, 2004   4–6

Introduction.—Significant improvements in the survival of extremely low birth weight infants have been observed during the past decade. The limits of care and the impact of treatment in extremely low birth weight infants were assessed in a population of infants who previously rarely survived.

Methods.—Demographic and clinical data for infants with birth weights of 401 to 500 g who were entered into the Vermont Oxford Network Database between 1996 and 2000 were reviewed.

Results.—A total of 4172 extremely low birth weight infants with a mean gestational age of 23.3 weeks who were born at 346 participating centers were evaluated. Overall, 17% of infants survived until discharge. A total of 2186 infants (52%) died in the delivery room (DR), and 1986 (48%) were admitted to a neonatal ICU (NICU) (Fig 1). Compared with those who died in the DR, infants who survived the DR and who were admitted to the NICU were more likely to be female (58% vs 48%), to be small for gestational age (56% vs 11%), to have received prenatal steroids (61% vs 12%), and to have been delivered by cesarean section (55% vs 5%). Thirty-six percent of infants admitted to the NICU survived to discharge. The mean age of the 690 survivors of the NICU was 25.3 weeks. Significant morbidity was observed among survivors in the NICU (Table 5).

Conclusion.—A substantial proportion of marginally viable infants survive. They have a high incidence of serious morbidities while in the NICU. There is very little data concerning the long-term outcome in these infants since the medical and developmental status of few of these infants has been carefully documented. Parents need to be informed concerning the high incidence of serious problems in extremely low birth weight infants.

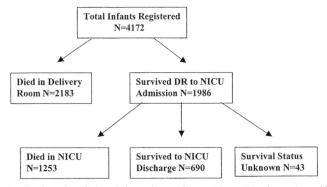

FIGURE 1.—Total number of inborn infants who were born at 401 to 500 g: disposition. *Abbreviations: DR,* Delivery room; *NICU,* neonatal ICU. (Reproduced with permission of *Pediatrics,* courtesy of Lucey JF, Rowan CA, Shiono P, et al: Fetal infants: The fate of 4172 infants with birth weights of 401 to 500 grams— The Vermont Oxford Network Experience (1996-2000). *Pediatrics* 113:1559-1566, 2004.)

TABLE 5.—Outcomes of NICU Survivors

Outcome	NICU Survivors
RDS	651/690 (94%)
Pneumothorax	77/690 (11%)
PDA	358/690 (52%)
Indomethacin	447/690 (65%)
Surgical PDA ligation	96/690 (14%)
Coagulase-negative staph sepsis	255/687 (37%)
Late bacterial sepsis	184/687 (27%)
Nosocomial infection	366/687 (53%)
Fungal infection	76/687 (11%)
Necrotizing enterocolitis	60/690 (9%)
Cranial ultrasound obtained	677/690 (98%)
IVH (grades 1-4)	179/677 (26%)
Severe IVH (grades 3-4)	55/677 (8%)
ROP examination performed	670/690 (97%)
ROP	598/670 (89%)
Severe ROP	268/670 (40%)
Chronic lung disease at 36 wk	498/673 (74%)

Abbreviations: NICU, Neonatal ICU; *RDS,* respiratory distress syndrome; *PDA,* patent ductus arteriosus; *IVH,* intraventricular hemorrhage; *ROP,* retinopathy of prematurity.

(Reproduced with permission of *Pediatrics,* courtesy of Lucey JF, Rowan CA, Shiono P, et al: Fetal infants: The fate of 4172 infants with birth weights of 401 to 500 grams—The Vermont Oxford Network Experience (1996-2000). *Pediatrics* 113:1559-1566, 2004.)

▶ The authors describe, on behalf of their colleagues and members of the Vermont Oxford Network, the enrollment in their Network of the smallest, most immature infants, observing that these marginally viable babies are surviving in surprisingly large absolute numbers (17% of many thousands). This article of a non–population-based cohort only tees up the most important issue for all of us in the field of neonatology, which is related to knowing and assuming responsibility for the long-term neurodevelopmental follow-up of these vulnerable people. Even without apparent injuries, these infants may have compromised neurodevelopmental outcomes, and severe disabilities may occur in 40% to 50% of these fetuses displaced from the womb. Certainly, many deaths occur in the DR and in the first day of life. However, some infants do continue to receive intensive care through the first month of life, ultimately dying later. Proportionally, this is not a large number, but it does reflect prolonged suffering for some—death is the final outcome and a dreadful "return on investment." In many respects, such care of the "fetal" newborn could be considered investigative, and a legitimate question might be whether these individuals should all be considered participants in a research endeavor, designed to determine the safety and efficacy of intensive care applied to this part of the population. Such a suggestion is a challenging one, at the very least bringing into sharp relief the tension between the inalienable rights of very small, immature citizens and fetuses whose biology is most conducive to intrauterine life, not extrauterine existence; these fetuses have become newborns with no clear avenue toward long-term intact survival without the actions of physicians (sustained iatrogenesis), who do not know what is best to ensure not only survival but also survival of people, who ultimately will need all their faculties to succeed in a very challenging world.

D. K. Stevenson, MD

The Risks of Underwater Birth
Pinette MG, Wax J, Wilson E (Maine Med Ctr, Portland)
Am J Obstet Gynecol 190:1211-1215, 2004   4–7

Background.—Estimates show that more than 150,000 water births occurred worldwide between 1985 and 1999. The literature was reviewed to identify possible complications of water birth.

Methods and Findings.—An extensive literature search using PubMed identified 74 articles on water births. No benefits for the neonate were reported. Several studies suggested some benefit in maternal pain management, but there was no clear evidence that immersion in water decreases the risk of perineal tears, duration of labor, or analgesia use. Sixteen articles reported complications associated with underwater birth. The complications reported were fresh water drowning, neonatal hyponatremia, neonatal waterborne infectious disease, cord rupture with neonatal hemorrhage, hypoxic ischemic encephalopathy, and death. There were no adequately controlled trials of delivery underwater compared with delivery in air.

Conclusion.—Water birth may be associated with potential complications that do not occur with birth in air. The rates of these complications are probably low but have yet to be defined.

▶ The authors summarize their review of the risks of underwater birth by concluding that there is a lack of evidence to suggest the benefit of underwater birth and increasing evidence to suggest poor outcomes that might be attributable to the procedure. Birth is risky enough. If a clear benefit cannot be shown for the newborn, then why add any risk for a parental preference?

That true underwater birth can be technically performed safely is not disputed, but nature seems ultimately geared toward the establishment of an air-liquid interface in the lungs of a spontaneously breathing newborn infant. The likelihood of transitional attempts at breathing fresh water should be diminished, not enhanced. If underwater birth is encouraged, alveolar collapse and the engagement of a neonatologist would be an unintended consequence.

The fact that most underwater births occur in fresh water, in fact, can complicate things further. If large amounts of such fluid are absorbed quickly, it could result in electrolyte abnormalities that might contribute to hemolysis or exacerbate third-space problems in the context of associated hypoxic-ischemic events. At any rate, an old adage might be appropriate to consider in this context: "Just when you thought it was safe to get back in the water. . ."

D. K. Stevenson, MD

Duration of Intubation Attempts During Neonatal Resuscitation

Lane B, Finer N, Rich W (Univ of California, San Diego)

J Pediatr 145:67-70, 2004   4–8

Objective.—Since the American Academy of Pediatrics Neonatal Resuscitation Program recommends that intubation should be completed in approximately 20 seconds, we measured the duration of neonatal intubation attempts by different operators, using video recordings of neonatal resuscitations.

Study Design.—We used an ongoing quality improvement program to measure the duration of intubation attempts.

Results.—The mean duration for the 50 successful intubations, including 6 for meconium, was 27.3 seconds compared with 29.8 seconds for unsuccessful attempts (not significant) (Figure). Fifteen infants were successfully intubated on each of the first and second attempts, 10 on the third attempt, and 10 required more than 3 attempts. The mean duration of successful intubation was 31.9 seconds for PL-1's, 27.5 seconds for PL-2/3's, and 23.6 seconds for fellows. Overall intubations were more successful for a duration of 30 seconds or less compared with 20 seconds or less (72% vs 38%; $\chi^2 =$ 10.3, *P*= 001). No infant decompensated between 20 and 30 seconds. Ten successful and 12 failed attempts took longer than 40 seconds.

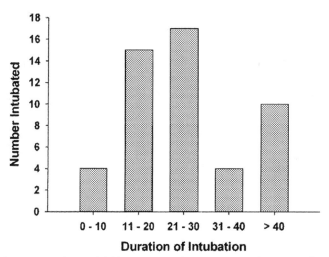

FIGURE.—Duration of successful delivery room intubations, represented in 10-second intervals. (Reproduced by permission of the publisher from Lane B, Finer N, Rich W: Duration of intubation attempts during neonatal resuscitation. *J Pediatr* 145:67-70. Copyright 2004 by Elsevier.)

Conclusions.—We recommend that a duration of 30 seconds is a reasonable guideline for neonatal intubation during resuscitation.

▶ Dr Finer and his group have conducted a unique quality improvement process at the University of California San Diego Medical Center to monitor delivery room resuscitation. Analysis of the video recordings permits evaluation of all aspects of resuscitation. In this case they wanted to know how long it took to intubate a depressed neonate. It is not surprising that the fellows were more efficient than the PL2s, who were, in turn, more efficient than the PL1s. The neonatal resuscitation program textbook recommends a limit of 20 seconds for the process of intubation, but in this study the authors show that in the ongoing process of intubation, no infant developed bradycardia between 20 and 30 seconds, indicating that if the heart rate is continuously assessed (as it must always be) and if no bradycardia occurs, then the intubation attempt can continue up to at least 30 seconds. This is important because a success rate at 30 seconds of 72% versus 38% at 20 seconds suggests that it is worth waiting an additional 10 seconds to complete a successful intubation.

M. J. Maisels, MB, BCh

Delivery Room Continuous Positive Airway Pressure/Positive End-Expiratory Pressure in Extremely Low Birth Weight Infants: A Feasibility Trial
Finer NN, for the National Institute of Child Health and Human Development Neonatal Research Network (Univ of California, San Diego; et al)
Pediatrics 114:651-657, 2004   4–9

Objective.—Although earlier studies have suggested that early continuous airway positive pressure (CPAP) may be beneficial in reducing ventilator dependence and subsequent chronic lung disease in the extremely low birth weight (ELBW) infant, the time of initiation of CPAP has varied, and there are no prospective studies of infants who have received CPAP or positive end-expiratory pressure (PEEP) from initial resuscitation in the delivery room (DR). Current practice for the ELBW infant includes early intubation and the administration of prophylactic surfactant, often in the DR. The feasibility of initiating CPAP in the DR and continuing this therapy without intubation for surfactant has never been determined prospectively in a population of ELBW infants. This study was designed to determine the feasibility of randomizing ELBW infants of <28 weeks' gestation to CPAP/PEEP or no CPAP/PEEP during resuscitation immediately after delivery, avoiding routine DR intubation for surfactant administration, initiating CPAP on neonatal intensive care unit (NICU) admission, and assessing compliance with subsequent intubation criteria.

Methods.—Infants who were of <28 weeks' gestation, who were born in 5 National Institute of Child Health and Human Development Neonatal Research Network NICUs from July 2002 to January 2003, and for whom a decision had been made to provide full treatment after birth were randomized to receive either CPAP/PEEP or not using a neonatal T-piece resuscitator (NeoPuff). Infants would not be intubated for the sole purpose of surfactant administration in the DR. After admission to the NICU, all nonintubated infants were placed on CPAP and were to be intubated for surfactant administration only after meeting specific criteria: a fraction of inspired oxygen of >0.3 with an oxygen saturation by pulse oximeter of <90% and/or an arterial oxygen pressure of <45 mm Hg, an arterial partial pressure of carbon dioxide of >55 mm Hg, or apnea requiring bag and mask ventilation.

Results.—A total of 104 infants were enrolled over a 6-month period: 55 CPAP and 49 control infants. No infant was intubated in the DR for the exclusive purpose of surfactant administration. Forty-seven infants were intubated for resuscitation in the DR: 27 of 55 CPAP infants and 20 of 49 control infants. Only 4 of the 43 infants who had a birth weight of <700 g and 3 of the 37 infants of <25 weeks' gestation were resuscitated successfully without positive pressure ventilation, and no difference was observed between the treatment groups. All infants of 23 weeks' gestation required intubation in the DR, irrespective of treatment group, whereas only 3 (14%) of 21 infants of 27 weeks' required such intubation. For infants who were not intubated in the DR, 36 infants (16 CPAP infants and 20 control infants) were subsequently intubated in the NICU by day 7, in accordance with the protocol. Overall, 80% of studied infants required intubation within the first 7 days of life. The care provided for 52 (95%) of 55 CPAP infants and 43 (88%) of the 49 control infants was in compliance with the study protocol, with an overall compliance of 91%.

Conclusions.—This study demonstrated that infants could be randomized successfully to a DR intervention of CPAP/PEEP compared with no CPAP/PEEP, with intubation provided only for resuscitation indications, and subsequent intubation for prespecified criteria. Forty-five percent (47 of 104) of infants <28 weeks' gestation required intubation for resuscitation in the DR. CPAP/PEEP in the DR did not affect the need for intubation at birth or during the subsequent week. Overall, 20% of infants did not need intubation by 7 days of life. This experience should be helpful in facilitating the design of subsequent prospective studies of ventilatory support in ELBW infants.

▶ This feasibility pilot conducted in 5 NICHD Neonatal Research Network centers provides new information regarding the need for intubation for resuscitation in the DR. Infants aged 23 to 27 weeks were randomly assigned to either CPAP in the DR or no CPAP. Infants were intubated in the DR only for resuscitation, and both groups were placed on CPAP in the neonatal ICU. In the neonatal ICU, specific criteria for intubation and surfactant administration were followed. The overall rate of intubation in the DR was 45% and appeared to be directly related to gestational age and birth weight; all infants born at 23 weeks required intubation in the DR, while intubation was required in 14% of infants born at 27 weeks. The use of CPAP did not appear to influence the percentage of infants requiring intubation (49% vs 41%), but the composition of the CPAP and control groups was not equivalent, with a lower mean birth weight and lower rate of antenatal steroid use in the infants in the CPAP arm.

In the neonatal ICU, the CPAP infants surprisingly had a lower pH and higher $PaCO_2$ on admission. By 7 days of age, 80% of all infants were intubated. Most were apparently intubated for reaching an FiO_2 greater than 0.3 and not for elevated $PaCO_2$ or apnea. A higher threshold for intubation may be necessary to test whether CPAP benefits the very low birth weight infant given this experience. The rates of adverse outcomes of death, CLD, pneumothorax, and intubation were all higher in the CPAP group, but these differences may be caused by the lower birth weight and use of antenatal steroids.

This pilot feasibility study achieved excellent protocol compliance (91%). The small number of infants still extubated at 7 days will be a barrier to testing the hypothesis of whether CPAP in the DR without prophylactic surfactant benefits the very low weight infant.

K. P. Van Meurs, MD

5 Infectious Disease and Immunology

Trends in Sepsis-Related Neonatal Mortality in the United States, 1985-1998
Lukacs SL, Schoendorf KC, Schuchat A (Ctrs for Disease Control and Prevention, Hyattsville, Md; Ctrs for Disease Control and Prevention, Atlanta, Ga)
Pediatr Infect Dis J 23:599-603, 2004   5–1

Background.—In the United States, bacterial sepsis affects up to 32,000 live births annually. In the 1990s, intrapartum antibiotic prophylaxis (IAP) was recommended to prevent maternal-infant transmission of group B *Streptococcus* (GBS), a leading cause of sepsis occurring in the first week of life (early onset sepsis). Since IAP has been used, early onset GBS disease declined 70%; however, increased antibiotic use associated with IAP might lead to more severe or antimicrobial resistant etiologies of sepsis. To understand the influence of IAP on neonatal sepsis, in general, we evaluated neonatal mortality from sepsis before and after IAP recommendations were issued.

Methods.—Using the National Center for Health Statistics Linked Birth/ Infant Death Datasets, we compared trends in sepsis-related early neonatal mortality (<7 days) and late neonatal mortality (7-27 days) among singleton United States births from 1985 through 1991 to 1995 through 1998 [data beyond 1998 not included because of International Classification of Diseases (ICD)-10/ICD-9 coding differences]. We compared trends in mortality between the 2 time periods by estimating the average annual percent change in mortality using log linear regression and stratified by gestational age.

Results.—Combined early and late neonatal mortality from sepsis averaged 39.6/100,000 live births from 1985 through 1991 and 31.8/100,000 live births from 1995 through 1998. Early neonatal mortality from sepsis averaged 24.9/100,000 live births from 1985 through 1991 and 15.6 from 1995 through 1998; late neonatal mortality averaged 14.8/100,000 live births from 1985 through 1991 and 16.2 from 1995 through 1998. Early neonatal mortality declined more steeply after IAP recommendations were issued, 5.0% annually from 1995 through 1998 versus 3.0% annually from 1985 through 1991. Late neonatal mortality increased more from 1995 through 1998, 5.0% annually compared with 0.5% from 1985 through 1991.

Conclusions.—Lower mortality rates and greater declines in early neonatal mortality from sepsis during 1995-1998 indicate greater survival of infants beyond 7 days of life and suggest an association with GBS disease prevention efforts. Thus these findings provide some evidence for continuing IAP for GBS-colonized women. Our findings of apparent increasing trends in late neonatal mortality from sepsis necessitate follow-up with clinical studies.

▶ The National Center for Health Statistics Linked Birth/Infant Death Dataset are useful for monitoring changes in infant mortality rate. Furthermore, it is comforting to find that the widespread use of intrapartum antibiotic prophylaxis for GBS-colonized women has been accompanied by a measurable decline in mortality rates from sepsis. On the other hand, this dataset only covers the time period through 1998, and it will be interesting to see if the newer guidelines have an even greater impact.[1] There is still considerable anxiety as to whether the widespread use of IAP will be accompanied by a change in the causes of neonatal sepsis with antibiotic-resistant organisms predominating. The data of Rentz et al[2] are encouraging in this regard.

A. A. Fanaroff, MD

References

1. Schrag S, Gorwitz R, Fultz-Butts K, et al: Prevention of perinatal group B streptococcal disease. Revised guidelines from CDC. *MMWR Recomm Rep* 16:51:1-22, 2002.
2. Rentz AC, Samore MH, Stoddard GJ, et al: Risk factors associated with ampicillin-resistant infection in newborns in the era of group B streptococcal prophylaxis. *Arch Pediatr Adolesc Med* 158:556-560, 2004.

Factors Associated With Hand Hygiene Practices in Two Neonatal Intensive Care Units
Cohen B, Saiman L, Cimiotti J, et al (Oceanside High School, NY; Columbia Univ, New York)
Pediatr Infect Dis J 22:494-498, 2003   5–2

Objective.—To determine whether hand hygiene practices differ between levels of contact with neonates; to characterize the hand hygiene practices of different types of personnel; and to compare hand hygiene practices in neonatal intensive care units (NICUs) using different products.

Methods.—Research assistants observed staff hand hygiene practices during 38 sessions in two NICUs. Patient touches were categorized as touching within the neonates' environment but only outside the Isolette (Level 1), touching within the Isolette but not the neonate directly (Level 2) or directly touching the neonate (Level 3). Hand hygiene practices for each touch were categorized into five groups: cleaned hands and new gloves; uncleaned hands and new gloves; used gloves; clean hands and no gloves; uncleaned hands and no gloves.

Results.—Research assistants observed 1472 touches. On average each neonate or his or her immediate environment was touched 78 times per shift. Nurses ($P = 0.001$), attending physicians ($P = 0.02$) and physicians-in-training ($P = 0.03$) were more likely to use appropriate practices during Level 3 touches, but only 22.8% of all touches were with cleaned and/or newly gloved hands. The mean number of direct touches by staff members with cleaned hands was greater in the NICU using an alcohol-based hand rub than in the NICU using antimicrobial soap ($P < 0.01$).

Conclusions.—Hand hygiene was suboptimal in this high risk setting; administrative action and improved products may be needed to assure acceptable practice. In this study use of an alcohol-based product was associated with significantly improved hand hygiene and should be encouraged, as recommended in the new CDC hand hygiene guideline.

Combined Use of Alcohol Hand Rub and Gloves Reduces the Incidence of Late Onset Infection in Very Low Birthweight Infants

Ng PC, Wong HL, Lyon J, et al (Chinese Univ of Hong Kong; Prince of Wales Hosp, Hong Kong)
Arch Dis Child Fetal Neonatal Ed 89:F336-F340, 2004   5–3

Objective.—To assess the incidence of late onset (> 72 hours) infection and necrotising enterocolitis (NEC) in very low birthweight (VLBW) infants in two 36 month periods using two hand hygiene protocols: conventional handwashing (HW; first 36 month period); an alcohol hand rub and gloves technique (HR; second 36 month period).

Method.—VLBW infants admitted to the neonatal intensive care unit during the period December 1993-November 1999 were eligible. A new hand hygiene protocol using alcohol handrub and gloves was introduced in December 1996. Each patient's case record was reviewed retrospectively by two independent investigators using a standard data collection form. The incidence of NEC and systemic infections, including bacterial or fungal septicaemia, meningitis, and peritonitis, in the two periods were compared.

Results.—The HW and HR groups contained 161 and 176 VLBW infants respectively. The incidence of late onset systemic infection decreased from 13.5 to 4.8 episodes (including NEC)/1000 patient days after introduction of the HR regimen, representing a 2.8-fold reduction. Similarly, the incidence of Gram positive, Gram negative, and fungal infections decreased 25-fold, 2.6-fold, and 7-fold respectively. There was also a significant reduction in the incidence of NEC in the HR group (p < 0.0001). Subgroup analysis revealed that the incidence of methicillin resistant *Staphylococcus aureus* (MRSA) septicaemia was significantly decreased in the second 36 month period (p = 0.048). The clinical data suggest that infants in the HW group had significantly earlier onset of sepsis (p < 0.05) and required oxygen supplementation for longer (p < 0.05) than those in the HR group. Significantly more VLBW infants were discharged from the neonatal intensive care unit without ever being infected (p < 0.0001), and also significantly fewer infants had more than one episode of infection in the HR group (p < 0.0001).

Conclusion.—The introduction of the HR protocol was associated with a 2.8-fold reduction in the incidence of late onset systemic infection, and also a significant decrease in the incidence of MRSA septicaemia and NEC in VLBW infants. This decrease in infection rate was maintained throughout the second 36 month period.

▶ The article by Cohen et al (Abstract 5–2), like many before it, documents beyond any level of doubt that hand hygiene is suboptimal in this high-risk setting. The fact that infants are touched more than 70 times per shift and appropriate hand hygiene is carried out less than 25% of the time should come as a loud wake-up call for all nursery personnel. Hand hygiene is not rocket science or even advanced technology. The authors suggest "administrative action and improved products may be needed to assure acceptable practice." Wrong! They are needed. In Cohen et al's study the use of an alcohol-based product was associated with significantly improved hand hygiene and should not only be encouraged but has been recommended in the new Centers for Disease Control and Prevention hand hygiene guideline.

Nosocomial sepsis has always been considered an inevitable consequence of prematurity. Infection not only increases the rates of morbidity and mortality, but also substantially increases the costs. It is necessary to change the culture in the nursery from a focus on early detection of infection to prevention. Care providers must accept the premise that medical care is a complex system and infection represents a system breakdown. The prevailing consensus that most acquired sepsis is preventable, and the implementation of policies based on available evidence will reduce the rate of infection has been substantiated by the results. Hand hygiene policies including education, monitoring (policing), elimination of false nails and hand jewelry in the nursery, and liberal use of waterless hand disinfectants are critical to the success of the endeavor. Other key elements include the early introduction and increased use of human milk for enteral nutrition and aggressive removal of central venous catheters. Use of maximum sterile barrier precautions by personnel trained and skilled in central catheter insertion, followed by meticulous care in preventing catheter hub contamination, will reduce the incidence of catheter-related sepsis. Applying these few, simple changes has helped many nurseries significantly lower their rates of hospital-acquired infections.

Kennedy et al[1] surveyed the nursery health care workers (HCW) in St Louis regarding catheter insertion and care as well as hand hygiene. They found a disconnect existed between central venous catheter knowledge and beliefs and practice. HCW did not know the relationship between bacterial hand counts and rings and fingernails and did not believe rings or long or artificial fingernails increased the risk of nosocomial infections. Sixty-one percent of HCWs regularly wore at least 1 ring to work; 56% wore their fingernails shorter than the fingertip, and 8% wore artificial fingernails. Furthermore, there was a lackadaisical approach to maximal sterile barrier precautions when inserting central lines. These data emphasize the need for continuing education for all HCW.

Ng et al (Abstract 5–3) introduced a policy of an alcohol hand rub and the use of gloves to their nursery in Hong Kong in 1996. This was associated with a 2.8-fold reduction in the incidence of late-onset systemic infection and a significant decrease in the incidence of MRSA septicemia and NEC in VLBW infants. Won et al[2] in Taiwan reported that improved compliance with hand-washing was associated with a significant decrease in overall rates of nosocomial infection and respiratory infections in particular. Their conclusion was "Washing hands is a simple, economical, and effective method for preventing nosocomial infections in the NICU." So, to follow the Nike slogan, "Let's just DO IT."

A. A. Fanaroff, MD

References

1. Kennedy AM, Elward AM, Fraser VJ: Survey of knowledge, beliefs, and practices of neonatal intensive care unit healthcare workers regarding nosocomial infections, central venous catheter care, and hand hygiene. *Infect Control Hosp Epidemiol* 25:747-752, 2004.
2. Won SP, Chou HC, Hsieh WS, et al: Handwashing program for the prevention of nosocomial infections in a neonatal intensive care unit. *Infect Control Hosp Epidemiol* 25:742-746, 2004.

Labor Promotes Neonatal Neutrophil Survival and Lipopolysaccharide Responsiveness

Molloy EJ, O'Neill AJ, Grantham JJ, et al (Mater Misericordiae Univ, Dublin; Coombe Women's Hosp, Dublin; Univ College, Dublin)
Pediatr Res 56:99-103, 2004   5–4

Labor is a mild proinflammatory state that is associated with fetal leukocytosis. Elective cesarean section has been linked with increased neonatal morbidity, which may be partially immune mediated. We hypothesized that labor may alter neutrophil phenotype and thereby decrease neonatal complications. We characterized neutrophil function and survival in normal neonates after either uncomplicated vaginal delivery (VD) or elective cesarean section (CS) without labor. Spontaneous neutrophil apoptosis is delayed in cord blood neutrophils of neonates after normal labor (VD) compared with CS, as assessed by propidium iodide DNA incorporation using flow cytometry. This demonstrates their ability to maintain an inflammatory response. CD11b expression on neonatal neutrophils after CS is decreased, providing further evidence of altered activation or priming. Lipopolysaccharide responsiveness, characterized by CD11b and apoptosis, is similar in VD and adults, but CS-derived neutrophils are unresponsive. Baseline TLR-4 levels are elevated in CS in contrast to the other groups, although expression is not up-regulated by lipopolysaccharide co-incubation. Neonatal neutrophil survival and function are altered by labor and may increase antibacterial function and neutrophilia. This suggests that labor of any duration may be immunologically beneficial to the normal term neonate.

▶ It is well known that labor primes (increases the responsiveness to subsequent stimuli without actually activating) or activates the neonate's neutrophils. Priming or activation of neutrophils is generally associated with resistance to apoptosis. This is thought to result in increased survival of neutrophils at sites of infection compared with cells removed from blood without stimulation in the laboratory. Molloy et al extend to apoptosis previous observations on the effects of labor on neonatal neutrophil priming and survival. As expected, neutrophils from babies delivered vaginally after labor are more resistant to apoptosis than those from babies delivered by cesarean section without labor. The differences are not great, however, and might well be overshadowed by effects of cytokines and chemoattractants in vivo if the baby becomes infected. Whether the differences demonstrated by Molloy et al are clinically significant remains to be seen. Furthermore, as pointed out by the authors, it cannot be predicted whether these differences are beneficial, by increasing the host defense capabilities of the neutrophils, or detrimental, by increasing their ability to cause tissue damage in inflammatory conditions. The extent to which these differences in neutrophil function may contribute to or actually account for differences in the prognosis or outcomes of cesarean section versus vaginal delivery thus remain unclear.

M. Berger, MD, PhD

Is Interleukin-6 −174 Genotype Associated With the Development of Septicemia in Preterm Infants?

Harding D, Dhamrait S, Millar A, et al (Univ of Bristol, England; Royal Free and Univ College London Med School; Univ of Nottingham, England)
Pediatrics 112:800-803, 2003   5–5

Objective.—Systemic infection affects one quarter of preterm infants. Defense from infection is in part mediated by the cytokine interleukin-6 (IL-6). We tested the hypothesis that the IL-6 −174 GG genotype, associated with lower IL-6 response to inflammation, is also associated with the development of septicemia in preterm infants.

Methods.—The study group comprised 157 infants who were born at ≤32 weeks. Genotype distribution (34% [54] GG, 46% [72] GC, 20% [31] CC) and C allele frequency (0.43; 95% confidence interval [CI]: 0.37-0.48) were similar to the UK adult population. Among the patients who developed bacterially confirmed septicemia (n = 51 [33%]), there was a significantly higher prevalence of the IL-6 −174 GG genotype than that observed in those who did not develop infection (47% vs 28% for GG: odds ratio [OR]: 2.3; 95% CI: 1.1-4.5). This association remained statistically significant (OR: 2.7; 95% CI: 1.2-6.3) after multiple binary logistic regression adjustment for other significant predictors of the development of septicemia. Late infection alone was similarly associated with GG genotype (septicemia 47% vs no septicemia 29% for GG: OR: 2.2; 95% CI: 1.1-4.3).

Conclusions.—Variation in the IL-6 gene seems to influence the defense against bacterial pathogens in the very preterm infant.

▶ Systemic illness and infection in preterm infants is the end result of a battle won by sheer weight of numbers and virulence of the invading organisms over the limited host defense. Thus, during their initial hospitalization, almost 50% of infants with birth weights below 750 g and 25% between 751 and 1000 g will have a documented infection.[1] An integral part of the host defense is IL-6. Harding et al therefore tested, and through the available data, substantiated the hypothesis that the IL-6 −174 GG genotype, associated with lower IL-6 response to inflammation, is associated with the development of septicemia in preterm infants.

Through quality improvement programs stressing hand hygiene, rapid removal of central venous lines, and rapid transition to enteral nutrition, considerable strides can be made in the prevention of infection.[2,3]

Identification of neonates at risk for sepsis has traditionally been based on history together with measurement of the white blood count and cytokines, including lipoprotein binding protein; IL-1, IL-6, IL-8, and IL-10; tumor necrosis factor-α; procalcitonin; and C-reactive protein, either single or in varying combinations. In the not too distant future we should be in a position to determine a number of genetic markers that render preterm infants more susceptible to infection. We will then have to develop selected strategies to prevent infection in these vulnerable infants.

A. A. Fanaroff, MD

References

1. Stoll BJ, Hansen N, Fanaroff AA: Late-onset sepsis in very low birth weight neonates: The experience of the NICHD Neonatal Research Network. *Pediatrics* 110:285-291, 2002.
2. Cohen B, Saiman L, Cimiotti J, et al: Factors associated with hand hygiene practices in two neonatal intensive care units. *Pediatr Infect Dis J* 22:494-499, 2003.
3. Ng PC, Wong HL, Lyon DJ, et al: Combined use of alcohol hand rub and gloves reduces the incidence of late onset infection in very low birthweight infants. *Arch Dis Child Fetal Neonatal Ed* 89:F336-F340, 2004.

Tumor Necrosis Factor α −308 Polymorphism Associated With Increased Sepsis Mortality in Ventilated Very Low Birth Weight Infants
Hedberg CL, Adcock K, Martin J, et al (Louisiana State Univ, Shreveport; Univ of Mississippi, Jackson)
Pediatr Infect Dis J 23:424-428, 2004   5–6

Background.—Sepsis commonly complicates the clinical course of critically ill very low birth weight infants, with as many as 30% developing hospital-acquired bacteremia. The tumor necrosis factor α (TNF-α) −308

G/A single nucleotide polymorphism (SNP) is associated with adverse outcome in septic adult patients.

Methods.—One hundred seventy-three mechanically ventilated very low birth weight infants were genotyped for the TNF-α –308 G/A SNP.

Results.—One hundred twenty (69%) infants were homozygous GG, 45 (26%) were heterozygous AG and 8 (5%) were homozygous AA; 2 of 120 (2%) infants developed early bacteremia in the GG group, and 1 of 53 (2%) developed early bacteremia in the AA/AG group ($P = 0.919$). One or more episodes of late bacteremia/fungemia developed in 59 of 120 (49%) infants with the GG genotype and 23 of 53 (43%) infants with the AG/AA genotype ($P = 0.484$). Endotracheal tube colonization rates were 65 of 120 (54%) for infants with the GG genotypes and 28 of 53 (53%) for infants with the AG/AA genotypes ($P = 0.871$). Nosocomial pneumonia developed in a similar number of infants in both genotype groups (9 of 120 infants vs. 3 of 53 infants; $P = 0.461$). Mortality from sepsis was 3 times greater in infants with the AA/AG genotypes than in those with the GG genotype (10% *vs.* 3%; $P = 0.038$). This difference in sepsis mortality was even greater when only bacteremic/fungemic infants are considered (4 of 59 infants *vs.* 6 of 23 infants; $P = 0.026$).

Conclusions.—These data suggest that the TNF-α –308 A allele does not affect the development of sepsis in ventilated premature infants but may increase mortality once sepsis develops.

▶ As noted in the commentary accompanying Abstract 2–13, bloodstream infections are extremely common in low birth weight infants. Also, there was a correlation between the IL-6-174 GG genotype, associated with lower interleukin-6 response to inflammation and the development of septicemia in preterm infants. There was a significantly higher prevalence of the IL-6-174 GG genotype (47%) than that observed in those who did not develop infection (28%; odds ratio, 2.3; 95% confidence interval, 1.1-4.5). Furthermore, sepsis has adverse long-term developmental sequelae, including both neurodevelopmental and growth impairment.[1] Working along the same theme, Hedberg et al have studied the TNF-α –308 G/A single nucleotide polymorphism in ventilated newborns at risk for sepsis. Although they did not find a correlation between polymorphisms of this gene, they did not come up entirely empty handed as the mortality rate from sepsis was 3-fold higher in infants with the AA/AG genotypes than those with the GG genotype. This is a very small series and should only be considered in this context. But it is intriguing and adds support and interest (if not a great deal of data) to the concept of genetic susceptibility to sepsis and the outcome from sepsis.

A. A. Fanaroff, MD

Reference

1. Stoll BJ, Hansen NI, Adams-Chapman I, et al: National Institute of Child Health and Human Development Neonatal Research Network: Neurodevelopmental and growth impairment among extremely low-birth-weight infants with neonatal infection. *JAMA* 292:2357-2365, 2004.

Measurement of Interleukin 8 in Combination With C-Reactive Protein Reduced Unnecessary Antibiotic Therapy in Newborn Infants: A Multicenter, Randomized, Controlled Trial

Franz AR, for the International IL-8 Study Group (Univ of Ulm, Germany; et al)
Pediatrics 114:1-8, 2004   5–7

Objective.—Neonatal bacterial infections carry a high mortality when diagnosed late. Early diagnosis is difficult because initial clinical signs are nonspecific. Consequently, physicians frequently prescribe antibiotic treatment to newborn infants for fear of missing a life-threatening infection. This study was designed to test the hypotheses that a diagnostic algorithm that includes measurements of interleukin 8 (IL-8) and C-reactive protein (CRP) 1) reduces antibiotic therapy and 2) does not result in more initially missed infections compared with standard management that does not include an IL-8 measurement.

Methods.—Term and preterm infants who were <72 hours of age and had clinical signs or obstetric risk factors suggesting neonatal bacterial infection but stable enough to wait for results of diagnostic tests were enrolled into the study. A total of 1291 infants were randomly assigned to receive antibiotic therapy according to the guidelines of each center (standard group) or to receive antibiotic therapy when IL-8 was >70 pg/mL and/or CRP was >10 mg/L (IL-8 group). The primary outcome variables were 1) the number of infants treated with antibiotics and 2) the number of infants with infections missed at the initial evaluation.

Results.—In the IL-8 group, fewer infants received antibiotic therapy than in the standard group (36.1% [237 of 656] vs 49.6% [315 of 635]). In the IL-8 group, 24 (14.5%) of 165 infants with infection were not detected at the initial evaluation, compared with 28 (17.3%) of 162 in the standard group.

Conclusions.—The number of newborn infants who received postnatal antibiotic therapy can be reduced with a diagnostic algorithm that includes measurements of IL-8 and CRP. This diagnostic strategy seemed to be safe.

▶ The ability to identify the presence of a bacterial infection in a neonate (and therefore, the need for antibiotic therapy) would certainly help us reduce the use of antibiotics in this population. Because IL-8 arises early in the course of neonatal bacterial infections, the authors hypothesized that measurements of IL-8 and CRP will reduce the need for antibiotic therapy but will not result in more missed infections when compared with standard management that does not include IL-8 measurement. Their randomized, controlled trial shows that by applying their diagnostic strategy and algorithm they were able to reduce the number of infants receiving antibiotics without increasing the number of infants whose infection remained undiagnosed. This is a practical and useful approach provided it is restricted to stable infants and excludes those who are sick or at very high risk. An absolute reduction of antibiotic usage of 13.5% (relative reduction of 27%) is both statistically and clinically significant.

M. J. Maisels, MB, BCh

Does Human Milk Reduce Infection Rates in Preterm Infants? A Systematic Review

de Silva A, Jones PW, Spencer SA (Univ Hosp of North Staffordshire, Stoke on Trent, England; Keele Univ, Staffordshire, England)
Arch Dis Child Fetal Neonatal Ed 89:F509-F513, 2004   5–8

One of the reasons for advocating human milk (HM) feeding for preterm infants is the belief that this provides the infant with a degree of protection from infection. Providing fresh HM for such infants is challenging for mothers and staff, and consequently it is important that its benefits are rigorously evaluated. Therefore a systematic review was undertaken to assess all publications concerned with human milk feeding and infection in very low birth weight (VLBW) preterm infants. Nine studies—six cohort and three randomised controlled trials (RCT)—were assessed using predefined criteria. Methodological problems included poor study design, inadequate sample size, failure to adjust for confounding variables, and inadequate definitions of HM feeding and outcome measures. In conclusion, the advantage of HM in preventing infection in preterm, (VLBW) infants is not proven by the existing studies. Recommendations are made regarding the methodology required for further study of this important topic.

▶ There is no doubt about the multitude of benefits conveyed by HM both in the term and preterm infant, but our enthusiasm must be tempered by the cold light of data when analyzed by a disinterested observer. These authors conclude that we have yet to demonstrate that HM is effective in preventing infection in VLBW infants. They draw attention to the significant methodological flaws in all the published cohort studies, including the failure to account for important confounders. Inadequate sample sizes are also listed as an important problem. In addition, 4 of the 9 studies reviewed were performed in countries where the risk of infection is substantially higher than it is in the United States or Western Europe.

Nevertheless, even with a small sample size, if a significant difference is found, the difference is still significant. A small sample size might exaggerate (by chance) the magnitude of the differences found, but a small sample size can only be blamed for failing to find a significant difference. Thus, the finding of a significantly lower incidence of sepsis in 4 U.S. studies in which the odds ratios ranged from 0.24 to 0.38 is difficult to ignore. An odds ratio of 0.24 implies that the infants who received HM were 76% less likely to develop sepsis than those who did not.

I agree with the authors that the time is ripe for a large cohort study that will provide a more conclusive answer to this question. Such a study is well within the capability of the current National Institute of Child Health and Human Development neonatal network group of neonatal ICUs. Until this study is done, however, I will retain my bias in favor of HM for VLBW infants.

M. J. Maisels, MB, BCh

Are Complete Blood Cell Counts Useful in the Evaluation of Asymptomatic Neonates Exposed to Suspected Chorioamnionitis?
Jackson GL, Engle WD, Sendelbach DM, et al (Univ of Texas, Dallas; Parkland Health and Hosp System, Dallas)
Pediatrics 113:1173-1180, 2004   5–9

Objective.—Chorioamnionitis complicates 1% to 10% of pregnancies and increases the risk of neonatal infection. Women with chorioamnionitis receive intrapartum antibiotics, often resulting in inconclusive neonatal blood cultures. Peripheral neutrophil values are used frequently to assist in the diagnosis of neonatal infection and to determine duration of antibiotics; we sought to determine the utility of this approach.

Methods.—A prospective observational study was performed in 856 near-term/term neonates who were exposed to suspected chorioamnionitis. Each received antibiotics for 48 hours unless clinical infection or positive blood cultures occurred. Peripheral neutrophils were measured serially and analyzed using the reference ranges of Manroe et al; an additional analysis of only the initial neutrophil values used the normal ranges of Schelonka et al. Results of neutrophil analyses were not used to determine duration of therapy. Fifty percent of asymptomatic neonates were seen postdischarge to ascertain recurrent infection. Local patient charges were examined.

Results.—Ninety-six percent of neonates were asymptomatic and had negative cultures, and antibiotics were discontinued at 48 hours. A total of 2427 neutrophil counts were analyzed. Although abnormal neutrophil values were more frequent in infected or symptomatic neonates, 99% of asymptomatic neonates had ≥ 1 abnormal value. The specificity and negative predictive values for abnormal neutrophil values ranged between 0.12 and 0.95 and 0.91 and 0.97, respectively; sensitivity was 0.27 to 0.76. Significant differences in interpretation of the initial neutrophil values were noted, depending on the normal values used. Follow-up was performed for 373 asymptomatic neonates until 3 weeks' postnatal age. Eight required rehospitalization; none had evidence of bacterial infection. If neutrophil values had been used to determine duration of antibiotics, then local costs would have increased by 76,000 dollars to 425,000 dollars per year.

Conclusions.—Single or serial neutrophil values do not assist in the diagnosis of early-onset infection or determination of duration of antibiotic therapy in asymptomatic, culture-negative neonates who are ≥ 35 weeks' gestation and are delivered of women with suspected chorioamnionitis.

▶ The Centers for Disease Control and Prevention, American Academy of Pediatrics, and other responsible organizations issue guidelines based on the best available evidence or, when evidence is not available, on a consensus of the members of the expert committee generating the guidelines. Ongoing and critical evaluation of these recommendations is therefore a necessary and often enlightening undertaking. These authors show that when a woman has received antibiotics for suspected chorioamnionitis before delivery, obtaining a complete blood cell count on the infant is not helpful. It could even be harmful (if the count is considered abnormal) by unnecessarily prolonging the use of antibiotics. This will increase the risk of subsequent resistance and the cost of care. They recommend extending antibiotic therapy for 4 to 7 days in neonates who have clinical evidence of infection or a positive blood culture. This makes good sense. It also makes sense to abandon knee-jerk lab tests. I cannot remember the last time I made an important change in my therapy based on the complete blood cell count in a well-looking infant whose mother had received antibiotics.

M. J. Maisels, MB, BCh

Features of Invasive Staphylococcal Disease in Neonates
Healy CM, Palazzi DL, Edwards MS, et al (Baylor College of Medicine, Houston; The Woman's Hosp of Texas, Houston)
Pediatrics 114:953-961, 2004   5–10

Introduction.—Most clinical descriptions of invasive staphylococcal disease (ISD) in neonates date from before the mid-1980s, when neonatal viability and intensive care differed markedly from current standards. The contemporary incidence, clinical characteristics, and outcome of infants with ISD were evaluated in a retrospective cohort investigation of a neonatal ICU (NICU).

Methods.—All infants in the NICU with ISD between January 2000 and June 2002 were evaluated. Confirmed ISD was considered to be clinical sepsis and *Staphylococcus aureus* (SA) isolated from 1 or more blood cultures (BCs) or a sterile body site excluding urine or coagulase-negative staphylococci (CoNS) isolated from 2 or more BC or for 1 BC and a sterile body site. Probable ISD was considered to be CoNS isolated from 1 BC or a sterile body site for which clinical and laboratory data reviewed by 3 infectious disease specialists demonstrated that antimicrobial treatment was appropriate. Confirmed and combined confirmed plus probable cases were evaluated.

Results.—A total of 149 episodes were found (139 confirmed [39 SA, 44 CoNS], 66 probable) in 137 infants (mean gestational age [GA], 27.6 weeks [22.4-36.4 weeks]; mean birth weight, 981 g [350-2995 g]). Four infants (3%) had early-onset infection (2 SA, 2 CoNS). The median age at start of infection was similar (17 days for SA, 18 days for CoNS). Intravascular catheters were in situ in 38% of infants in the SA group and 43% in the CoNS group. The CoNS infections were more likely than SA infections to be linked with very low birth weight (<1500 g), lower GA, and history of more intravascular catheters and concurrent total parenteral nutrition (catheter and parenteral nutrition days were similar). Multivariate analysis (after correcting for birth weight, complications of prematurity, and hypoxia at the time of sepsis evaluation) was significantly linked with CoNS and hypotension with SA infections; other clinical characteristics were similar. Methicillin-resistant SA was responsible for 8% of SA infections. Among infants with ISD, SA was more commonly involved at 2 or more sites than CoNS. More focal complications (primarily bone and joint) were observed with SA than

TABLE 4.—Clinical Manifestations of ISD Episodes

	Confirmed (*n* [%])			Confirmed and Probable (*n* [%])		
	SA (*n* = 39)	CoNS (*n* = 44)	*P* Value	SA (*n* = 41)	CoNS (*n* = 108)	*P* Value
Bacteremia	25 (64)	44 (100)	<.001	26 (62)	101 (94)	<.001
Skin and soft tissue	29 (74)	19 (43)	.007	31 (76)	36 (33)	<.001
Bone and joint*	5 (13)	2 (5)	.25	6 (14)	2 (2)	.006
Endocarditis/endocarditis equivalent†	1 (3)	3 (7)	.62	1 (2)	3 (3)	.99
Pneumonia	3 (8)	2 (5)	.66	3 (7)	14 (13)	.4
Peritonitis	1 (3)	1 (2)	.99	1 (2)	6 (6)	.67
Meningitis	1 (3)	0	.47	1 (2)	7 (7)	.46

*Confirmed by radiology and culture.
†Endocarditis equivalent; portal vein thrombosis.
(Courtesy of Healy CM, Palazzi DL, Edwards MS, et al: Features of invasive staphylococcal disease in neonates. *Pediatrics* 114:953-961, 2004. Reproduced by permission of *Pediatrics*.)

with CoNS; this resulted in a 2- to 3-fold higher SA-associated morbidity rate (Table 4). Death directly attributable to either organism was similar between groups (5% for SA, 5% confirmed, 3% for confirmed/probable CoNS).

Conclusion.—It appears that CoNS occurred in smaller, more premature infants than SA and was associated with intravascular catheters in a minority of cases. Hypoxia and hypotension were the only presenting characteristics that differentiated CoNS and SA. The SA-associated morbidity was marked, yet did not have a higher risk of death (5%) than CoNS.

▶ This contemporary retrospective study in a single NICU does debunk some well-entrenched historic misconceptions. It describes the 2 most common modern-era causes of late-onset sepsis in their NICU: CoNS and SA. While the incidence remains low, the mortality rate in very low birth weight infants is still cause for concern.

Attempts to clinically differentiate CoNS from SA were unsuccessful and probably unnecessary, as initial therapy is identical (vancomycin and an aminoglycoside). But it is certainly necessary to switch to the appropriate antibiotic once sensitivities are known.

Morbidity and mortality rates were very similar and belie the common practice of mandatory intravascular catheter removal as standard practice.

This particular unit may not be representative, as it had high rates of NICU admissions and use of prenatal antibiotics and postnatal steroids. Perhaps early enteral feedings, early continuous positive airway pressure, IV immunoglobulin, and so forth may decrease the risk of developing late-onset infection.

J. M. Klarr, MD

Defective Neutrophil Oxidative Burst in Preterm Newborns on Exposure to Coagulase-Negative Staphylococci

Björkqvist M, Jurstrand M, Bodin L, et al (Örebro Univ, Sweden)
Pediatr Res 55:966-971, 2004   5–11

The neutrophil oxidative burst is a product of the regulated assembly of the multicomponent oxidase enzyme. Our aim was to compare the oxidative burst in term ($n = 10$) and preterm newborns <31 wk gestational age ($n = 10$) after stimulation with coagulase-negative staphylococci *in vitro*. Strains of *Streptococcus epidermidis* with different invasive and slime-producing properties, one strain of *S. haemolyticus*, and one strain of group B-streptococcus were investigated. A whole-blood flow cytometric assay using the oxidation of hydroethidine to ethidium bromide was used. The oxidative activity in unstimulated neutrophil granulocytes [polymorphonuclear leukocytes (PMNLs)] was similar in term and preterm newborns, but the preterm newborns showed a significantly lower capacity to upregulate the oxidative burst intensity after bacterial stimulation ($p = 0.004$). In the term but not in the preterm group, the oxidative burst intensity after bacterial stimulation correlated with the baseline oxidative burst intensity. After bacterial stimulation, there was a trend toward a greater percentage of activated neutrophils in the term group than in the preterm group, but the difference was less pronounced than that in oxidative burst intensity. Significant differences in oxidative burst response to different bacterial strains were observed ($p < 0.001$), but the differences could not be correlated exclusively to invasive capacity or slime-producing properties. It is concluded that the baseline oxidative activity is similar in term and preterm PMNLs but that preterm PMNLs have a decreased capacity to increase the oxidative burst in response to bacterial stimulation.

▶ PMNLs are qualitatively and quantitatively the most effective killing phagocytes of the host defense. PMNLs use both oxygen-independent and oxygen-dependent mechanisms of microbial killing. The oxygen-dependent killing begins with membrane penetration, receptor binding, and phagocytosis of the invading organism. A respiratory burst ensues and reactive oxygen intermediates are synthesized. Defects in chemotaxis, adhesion, phagocytosis, and microbicidal activity have been reported in preterm infants. Björkqvist et al have looked for and found significant differences in oxidative burst response to different bacterial strains between term and preterm infants. They noted that the baseline oxidative activity is similar in term and preterm PMNLs, but that preterm PMNLs have a decreased capacity to increase the oxidative burst in response to bacterial stimulation. Furthermore, the differences could not be correlated exclusively to invasive capacity or slime-producing properties. Add this to the already impressive list of reasons why preterm infants are more susceptible to bloodstream infections.

Further evidence of vulnerability includes abnormalities of human leukocyte antigen (HLA) and impaired responses to toll-like receptor (TLR)-4 and TLR-3 ligands in human cord blood.[1,2] Presentation of HLA molecules is an important part of an efficient immune response, and the TLR-4 signaling pathway plays an essential role in host defense against gram-negative bacteria while TLR-3–mediated signaling is critically involved in antiviral immunity. Birle et al[1] documented that HLA-DR expression on monocytes as determined by flow cytometry was lower during the first week of life of term and preterm neonates with and without signs of infection than those of adults. Newborns with respiratory distress syndrome, but without signs of infection, also showed reduced HLA-DR expression. On the other hand maternal conditions such as preeclampsia, prenatal treatment with steroids, and mode of delivery had no influence on the expression of HLA-DR. They concluded that low HLA-DR expression on monocytes contributes to impaired neonatal host defense, especially in preterm neonates.

A. A. Fanaroff, MD

References

1. Birle A, Nebe CT, Gessler P: Age-related low expression of HLA-DR molecules on monocytes of term and preterm newborns with and without signs of infection. *J Perinatol* 23:294-299, 2003.
2. De Wit D, Tonon S, Olislagers V, et al: Impaired responses to toll-like receptor 4 and toll-like receptor 3 ligands in human cord blood. *J Autoimmun* 21:277-281, 2003.

Level of Maternal IgG Anti–Group B Streptococcus Type III Antibody Correlated With Protection of Neonates Against Early-Onset Disease Caused by This Pathogen

Lin F-YC, Weisman LE, Azimi PH, et al (Natl Insts of Health, Bethesda, Md; Dept of Health and Human Services, Bethesda, Md; Baylor College of Medicine, Houston; et al)
J Infect Dis 190:928-934, 2004   5–12

The present study estimates the level of maternal immunoglobulin (Ig) G anti–group B streptococcus (GBS) type III required to protect neonates against early-onset disease (EOD) caused by this pathogen. Levels of maternal serum IgG anti–GBS type III, measured by enzyme-linked immunosorbent assay, in 26 case patients (neonates with EOD caused by GBS type III) and 143 matched control subjects (neonates colonized by GBS type III who did not develop EOD) of ≥34 weeks gestation were compared. The probability of EOD decreased with increasing levels of maternal IgG anti–GBS type III ($P = .01$). Neonates whose mothers had ≥10 µg/mL IgG anti–GBS type III had a 91% lower risk for EOD, compared with those whose mothers had levels of <2 µg/mL. A vaccine that induces IgG anti–GBS type III levels of ≥10 µg/mL in mothers can be predicted to offer a significant degree of protection against EOD caused by this pathogen.

▶ This multicenter study brings quantitative precision to a qualitative relationship that was recognized 3 decades ago: babies born to women with low levels of type-specific protective antibodies are more likely to develop invasive disease caused by GBS. The primary conclusion of this article, which focuses on EOD caused by type III GBS, is that vaccines that induce production of type-specific antibodies with maternal serum levels of 10 µg/mL or greater are predicted to confer substantial type-specific protection against early-onset GBS disease in their infants. A key caveat is identified in the discussion, however. The type-specific antibody level was less than 2 µg/mL in 42% of the mothers of babies with early-onset GBS disease. It is very unlikely that these low antibody levels are a consequence of a lack of antigen exposure, suggesting that these women, like other adults with low preimmunization antibody levels, may respond poorly to GBS vaccines. If so, population-based immunization strategies may fail in precisely those individuals who are at greatest risk. A great deal of difficult work remains to be done before immunization can replace intrapartum antibiotic prophylaxis as the mainstay of early-onset GBS prevention.

W. E. Benitz, MD

Risk Factors Associated With Ampicillin-Resistant Infection in Newborns in the Era of Group B Streptococcal Prophylaxis

Rentz AC, Samore MH, Stoddard GJ, et al (Univ of Utah, Salt Lake City)
Arch Pediatr Adolesc Med 158:556-560, 2004   5–13

Objectives.—To document the trend of ampicillin-resistant infections in newborns weighing at least 1500 g and to determine factors associated with ampicillin-resistant neonatal early-onset infection in the era of routine group B streptococcal prophylaxis.

Design.—Case-control study.

Setting.—Referral hospital with level I through level III nurseries.

Patients.—Newborns aged 0 to 7 days with cultures positive for bacterial infection, born from January 1994 to August 2002 (n = 53). Random controls were matched to admission year and nursery level (n = 159).

Main Outcome Measures.—Trends of and factors associated with ampicillin-resistant infections.

Results.—Trends in our institution were the same as those found in some recent reports, a decrease in group B streptococcal early-onset infections without a concomitant increase in gram-negative early-onset infections. Specifically, when stratified by birth weight, newborns weighing at least 1500 g had no increase in gram-negative pathogens in the eras both before and after group B streptococcal prophylaxis (0.8 per 1000 live births to 0.3 per 1000 live births; incidence ratio, 2.3 [95% confidence interval, 0.5-10.9]). No increase in ampicillin resistance was seen during the same 3 periods (50%, 60%, and 50%, respectively; $P = .97$). Independent risk factors associated with ampicillin-resistant early-onset infection were intrapartum antibiotics for a 24-hour duration or longer (odds ratio, 4.8 [95% confidence interval, 1.0-23.3]) and clinical chorioamnionitis (odds ratio, 9.2 [95% confidence interval, 2.6-32.9]).

Conclusions.—No increase in early-onset infections with gram-negative or ampicillin-resistant pathogens was detected. Ampicillin-resistant early-onset infection was associated with intrapartum antibiotics given for 24 hours or longer prior to delivery and with clinical chorioamnionitis. Ampicillin sodium and gentamicin sulfate remain appropriate initial antibiotic therapies for early-onset infection in newborns weighing at least 1500 g and without these risk factors.

▶ Intrapartum antibiotic use has increased in recent years for both prophylaxis of neonatal disease and therapy of maternal disease. National programs to reduce vertical transmission of group B streptococcal disease, by using intrapartum penicillin, have been successful. Although it is generally believed that short-term intrapartum exposure to antibiotics in labor is safe, concerns have been raised about a possible change in the types of pathogens associated with early-onset sepsis (switch to a predominance of gram-negative organisms) and the emergence of antibiotic-resistant organisms. In studies from the NICHD Neonatal Research Network, gram-negative organisms were responsible for the majority of early-onset infections among very low birth weight infants (401-1500 g), and ampicillin resistance in *Escherichia coli* isolates was common (85%).[1]

Rentz et al studied infants weighing at least 1500 g at birth and found a reduction in early-onset group B streptococcal disease, with no increase in gram-negative infections over time (1994-2002). Although there was no overall increase in ampicillin-resistant pathogens, these investigators found that prolonged maternal intrapartum antibiotics before delivery (at least 24 hours) and clinical chorioamnionitis were risk factors for resistance. The verdict is out on the microbiologic safety of prolonged maternal antibiotics. Although it is known that antibiotics reduce maternal and neonatal sequelae from maternal chorioamnionitis, the clinical diagnosis of chorioamnionitis is far from clear cut. Further studies are needed to address the appropriateness of prolonged antibiotic use in labor and potentially preventable causes of antibiotic resistance.

B. J. Stoll, MD

Reference

1. Stoll BJ, Hansen N, Fanaroff AA, et al: Changes in pathogens causing early-onset sepsis in very-low-birth-weight infants. *N Engl J Med* 347:240-247, 2002.

The Effect of Prophylactic Ointment Therapy on Nosocomial Sepsis Rates and Skin Integrity in Infants With Birth Weights of 501 to 1000 g
Edwards WH, for the Vermont Oxford Network Neonatal Skin Care Study Group (Children's Hosp of Dartmouth, Lebanon, NH: et al)
Pediatrics 113:1195-1203, 2004   5–14

Objective.—Extremely low birth weight infants have a high risk of developing nosocomial bacterial sepsis (NBS). Immature fragile skin may represent an inadequate protective barrier to bacteria colonizing the skin. We conducted a randomized, multicenter trial to determine whether prophylactic application of an emollient ointment would result in a lower incidence of death and/or NBS in the first 28 days of life, compared with routine skin care.

Methods.—Infants of birth weight 501 to 1000 g and gestational age ≤30 weeks were assigned randomly to receive generalized application of ointment twice a day through day 14 (prophylactic group [P]) or local application of ointment to the site of injury (routine skin care [R]). The study was conducted at 53 neonatal intensive care units that were members of the Vermont Oxford Network.

Results.—Included in the analysis were 1191 infants (P: 602; R: 589). No difference was found in the combined primary outcome of NBS or death (33.6% P vs 30.3% R; relative risk [RR]: 1.10; 95% confidence interval [CI]: 0.89, 1.27). The incidence of death was no different between the groups (10.8% P vs 12.1% R; RR: 0.87; 95% CI: 0.59, 1.25). More infants in the prophylactic group had NBS (25.8% P vs 20.4% R; RR: 1.26; 95% CI: 1.02, 1.54), predominantly in the lower birth weight infants (501-750 g) and for infections caused by coagulase-negative staphylococci. Infants in the prophylactic group had better skin condition on days 1 to 14 of life and less skin injury on days 15 to 28 of life. There was no difference between groups in other complications of prematurity.

Conclusions.—Prophylactic application of ointment did not lead to a difference in death and/or NBS in the first 28 days of life. There may be an increase in the risk of NBS associated with this practice.

▶ The idea that a simple and inexpensive intervention might improve outcomes for ELBW infants is always very attractive. The fragility of the skin of extremely premature newborns makes it both a target for nosocomial bacterial infection as well as a less than effective barrier to the external environment. In addition, skin breakdown occurs when adhesive tape is removed. Thus, the idea that the protective function of the skin might be preserved or improved by applying an ointment is very appealing. Unfortunately, in this large, well-designed, randomized, controlled trial, the prophylactic application of an emollient ointment not only had no effect on mortality rate, but it actually increased the risk of NBS. As the authors note, we will need to develop some "other strategies for supporting epidermal barrier function during maturation in ELBW infants."

M. J. Maisels, MB, BCh

Single-Dose Perinatal Nevirapine Plus Standard Zidovudine to Prevent Mother-to-Child Transmission of HIV-1 in Thailand

Lallemant M, for the Perinatal HIV Prevention Trial (Thailand) Investigators (Institut de Recherche Pour le Développement, Paris; et al)

N Engl J Med 351:217-228, 2004   5–15

Background.—Although zidovudine prophylaxis decreases the rate of transmission of the human immunodeficiency virus (HIV) type 1 substantially, a large number of infants still become infected. We hypothesized that the administration, in addition to zidovudine, of a single dose of oral nevirapine to mothers during labor and to neonates would further reduce transmission of HIV.

Methods.—We conducted a randomized, double-blind trial of three treatment regimens in Thai women who were receiving zidovudine therapy during the third trimester of pregnancy. In one group, mothers and infants received a single dose of nevirapine (nevirapine-nevirapine regimen); in another, mothers and infants received nevirapine and placebo, respectively (nevirapine-placebo regimen); and in the last, mothers and infants received placebo (placebo-placebo regimen). The infants also received one week of zidovudine therapy and were formula-fed. The end point of the study was infection with HIV in the infants, established by virologic testing.

Results.—Between January 15, 2001, and February 28, 2003, a total of 1844 Thai women were enrolled. At the first interim analysis, the independent data monitoring committee stopped enrollment in the placebo-placebo group. Among women who delivered before the interim analysis, the as-randomized Kaplan-Meier estimates of the transmission rates were 1.1 percent (95 percent confidence interval, 0.3 to 2.2) in the nevirapine-nevirapine group and 6.3 percent (95 percent confidence interval, 3.8 to 8.9) in the placebo-placebo group (P<0.001). The final per-protocol transmission rate in the nevirapine-nevirapine group, 1.9 percent (95 percent confidence interval, 0.9 to 3.0), was not significantly inferior to the rate in the nevirapine-placebo group (2.8 percent; 95 percent confidence interval, 1.5 to 4.1). Nevirapine had an effect within subgroups defined by known risk factors such as viral load and CD4 count. No serious adverse effects were associated with nevirapine therapy.

Conclusions.—A single dose of nevirapine to the mother, with or without a dose of nevirapine to the infant, added to oral zidovudine prophylaxis starting at 28 weeks' gestation, is highly effective in reducing mother-to-child transmission of HIV.

► It has been a decade since the landmark ACTG 076 study was reported, showing a significant decrease in vertical HIV transmission with the use of zidovudine monotherapy. Since then, several studies have demonstrated that more intensive treatments of mothers further reduced transmission rates to less than 2%. Unfortunately, the cost of these regimens is prohibitive in developing countries, leading to the current unacceptable rates of HIV transmission to newborns Lallemant et al enrolled 1844 HIV-infected pregnant women in

Thailand in this randomized, double-blind, placebo-controlled study. All women were receiving zidovudine therapy, starting in the third trimester. The authors investigated whether single doses of nevirapine, given to the mother at the onset of labor with or without a single dose given to the newborn infant, would further delay vertical transmission. All infants received a 1-week course of zidovudine. Breastfeeding was not allowed. After an early analysis showing a significantly higher rate of transmission for the group in which neither mother nor infant received nevirapine compared with the group in which both mother and baby received nevirapine (6.3% vs 1.1%, respectively; $P < .001$), the former arm was discontinued. In the final analysis, the transmission rate was 1.9% in the nevirapine-nevirapine group and 2.8% in the nevirapine-placebo group ($P > .05$). This fact that a single dose of nevirapine added to a short course of zidovudine in pregnant women can further reduce the rate of HIV transmission is great news for developing countries. Unfortunately, the downside of this successful addition of nevirapine includes issues of toxicity and resistance. Nevirapine has been associated with significant hepatotoxicity—at times fatal—when given to HIV-infected pregnant women, specifically those with CD4 cell count greater than 250 cells/mm^3 at the initiation of therapy. Although hepatotoxicity has not yet been described with single doses of nevirapine, it remains a reason for caution. An even more concerning issue is the emergence of resistance after single doses of nevirapine—as high as 15% to 40% in some studies. This may jeopardize the efficacy of nevirapine-based regimens in decreasing vertical transmission in future pregnancies. Similarly, recent data showed that resistance to single-dose nevirapine may jeopardize the mother's virologic response to future antiretroviral therapy. In this regard, Jourdain et al[1] showed that virologic response of women with nevirapine-containing regimens was independently associated with prior receipt of nevirapine during labor. Since the use of nonnucleoside reverse transcriptase inhibitors such as nevirapine is very common and, at times, the only option in developing countries, the resistance issue is of concern and should be balanced against minimizing the risk of mother-to-infant transmission of this deadly virus.

G. McComsey, MD

Reference

1. Jourdain G, Ngo-Giang-Huong N, Le Coeur S, et al: Intrapartum exposure to nevirapine and subsequent maternal responses to nevirapine-based antiretroviral therapy. *N Engl J Med* 351:229-340, 2004.

Marginal Increase in Cost and Excess Length of Stay Associated With Nosocomial Bloodstream Infections in Surviving Very Low Birth Weight Infants

Payne NR, Carpenter JH, Badger GJ, et al (Children's Hosps and Clinics, Minneapolis; Vermont Oxford Network, Burlington; Univ of Vermont, Burlington; et al)
Pediatrics 114:348-355, 2004   5–16

Objective.—Nosocomial bloodstream infections (NBIs) are associated with serious morbidity and prolonged length of stay (LOS) in very low birth weight (VLBW) infants. However, the marginal costs and excess LOS associated with these infections have never been measured in different birth weight (BW) categories after adjustment for many of the potentially confounding demographic variables, comorbidities, and treatments. The objective of this study was to measure the marginal cost and excess LOS caused by NBIs in surviving VLBW infants in different BW categories.

Methods.—This retrospective study examined data previously collected as part of the Neonatal Intensive Care Quality Improvement Collaborative

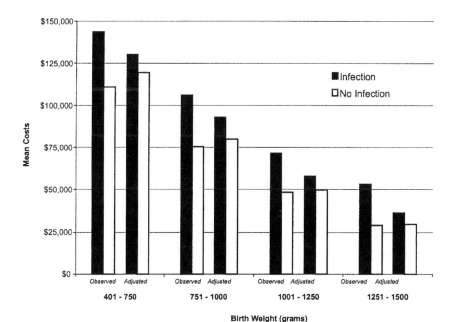

FIGURE 2.—Mean costs for infants with and without NBI. Observed values are those obtained before adjustment for potentially confounding demographic factors, interventions, and comorbidities. Adjusted values represent the results after adjusting for potentially confounding factors. Infected infants in the 3 higher BW categories incurred significantly higher treatment costs before and after adjustment (*P* < .05). Differences in mean costs in the 401 to 750 BW category were significant before adjustment but not after adjusting for covariates (*P* = .01). All means presented correspond to the geometric mean. (Courtesy of Payne NR, Carpenter JH, Badger GJ, et al: Marginal increase in cost and excess length of stay associated with nosocomial bloodstream infections in surviving very low birth weight infants. *Pediatrics* 114:348-355, 2004. Reprinted by permission of *Pediatrics*.)

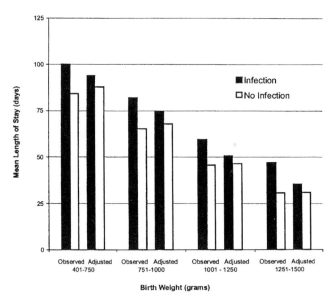

FIGURE 3.—Mean LOS for infants with and without NBI. Observed values are those obtained before adjustment for potentially confounding demographic factors, interventions, and comorbidities. Adjusted values represent the results after adjusting for potentially confounding factors. Infected infants in all 4 BW categories incurred significantly higher LOS before and after adjustment ($P < .05$). All means presented correspond to the geometric mean. (Courtesy of Payne NR, Carpenter JH, Badger GJ, et al: Marginal increase in cost and excess length of stay associated with nosocomial bloodstream infections in surviving very low birth weight infants. *Pediatrics* 114:348-355, 2004. Reprinted by permission of *Pediatrics*.)

2000 and the Vermont Oxford Network clinical outcomes database. Univariate analyses and multiple regression were used to examine the effect of NBIs on hospital costs and LOS. Seventeen neonatal intensive care units that participated in the Neonatal Intensive Care Quality Improvement Collaborative 2000 submitted both clinical and financial data on their VLBW infants who were born from January 1, 1998, to December 31, 1999. This study included data from both university and community hospitals.

Results.—NBIs occurred in 19.7% of 2809 patients included in this study. NBI was associated with significantly increased treatment costs for infants with BW 751 to 1500 g (Fig 2). The marginal costs of NBIs, as estimated by multiple regression, varied from 5875 dollars for VLBW infants with a BW of 401 to 750 g to 12 480 dollars for those with BW of 751 to 1000 g. LOS was significantly increased in all BW categories. The excess LOS estimated by multiple regression varied from 4 days in VLBW infants with a BW of 1001 to 1251 g to 7 days in those with a BW of 751 to 1000 g (Fig 3).

Conclusions.—NBIs are associated with increased hospital treatment costs and LOS but by varying amounts depending on the BW (Table 4). Preventing a single NBI could reduce the treatment costs of a VLBW infant by at least several thousand dollars. These savings are a greater percentage of the total treatment costs in VLBW infants with BW 1001 to 1500 g than in smaller infants.

TABLE 4.—Estimated Mean Costs and LOS for Infants With and Without
NBI After Adjusting for Potential Confounding Variables
Using Multiple Regression

BW, g	Mean Costs, $				Mean LOS, Days			
	No NBI	NBI	Difference	*P* Value	No NBI	NBI	Difference	*P* Value
401-750	123 012	128 887	5875	.141	88	94	6	.029
751-1000	81 580	94 060	12 480	.009	68	75	7	.006
1001-1250	50 784	60 367	9583	.002	47	51	4	.010
1251-1500	30 411	36 687	6276	.001	31	36	5	.006

*Values for mean cost and mean LOS correspond to geometric means.
(Courtesy of Payne NR, Carpenter JH, Badger GJ, et al: Marginal increase in cost and excess length of stay associated with nosocomial bloodstream infections in surviving very low birth weight infants. *Pediatrics* 114:348-355, 2004. Reprinted by permission of *Pediatrics*.)

▶ It would be surprising if NBIs in our VLBW population did not increase the cost and LOS. It is surprising, however, that NBIs are more costly in those infants with BWs between 751 and 1000 g versus those with BWs of 401 to 750 g, although LOS increased more in the lower than in the higher BW group. These investigators used data from 17 hospitals and, based on their results, they estimate that NBIs added almost $1 million to the cost of treating surviving VLBW infants in the United States in 1999 dollars. A relatively modest reduction in these infections would result in an enormous saving in health care expenditure in the United States alone. Reducing nosocomial infections is a fundamental goal of any form of hospitalized care, and nowhere is this more important than in our neonatal ICUs. We know how to do it, but we need to mobilize our resources and refocus our attention on the basic approaches to preventing NBIs in this vulnerable population. One can only echo the author's conclusion that reducing NBIs is "clinically important, financially prudent, and medically possible" and should be a "national priority."

M. J. Maisels, MB, BCh

6 Cardiovascular System

Autoimmune Response in Mothers of Children With Congenital and Post-natally Diagnosed Isolated Heart Block: A Population Based Study
Julkunen H, Miettinen A, Walle TK, et al (Helsinki Univ Hosp, Finland; Scripps Research Inst, La Jolla, Calif)
J Rheumatol 31:183-189, 2004   6-1

Objective.—To study the autoimmune response in mothers of children with isolated congenital heart block (CHB) and heart block (HB) diagnosed postnatally.

Methods.—We reviewed the Finnish hospital registries for patients born between 1950 and 2000 and diagnosed with isolated HB before the age of 16 years. Clinical data and sera for the determination of autoantibodies were available from 67 mothers of children with CHB and from 37 mothers of children with postnatally diagnosed HB 9.9 years and 22.6 years (mean) after the index delivery, respectively. Maternal antibodies to 52 kDa and 60 kDa SSA and 48 kDa SSB were determined by time-resolved fluoroimmunoassay (TR-FIA) and by immunoblotting. Other marker antibodies for connective tissue diseases (CTD) were determined by immunoblot and/or by immunofluorescence. The control group comprised 136 mothers with primary Sjögren's syndrome (SS), systemic lupus erythematosus (SLE), or other CTD with healthy children.

Results.—Sixty of our 67 mothers (90%) of children with CHB had antibodies to SSA or SSB by the methods initially used in this study. When retests and tests performed previously were taken into account, only 3 (4%) of the 67 mothers did not have any autoantibodies. Two (3%) of the 67 mothers had antibodies to dsDNA and one (1%) each to Jo-1/HRS, RNP-70 kDa, and histone proteins. Of 37 mothers of children with postnatally diagnosed HB, only 3 (8%) had any autoantibodies. Increased risk of having a child with CHB was indicated by maternal primary SS and high levels of anti-SSA and anti-SSB by all assays, whereas low risk was indicated by maternal SLE or other CTD and undetectable or low levels of the antibodies. No single anti-SSA or anti-SSB test was clearly superior to others, but in general, immunoblots were more specific than TR-FIA.

Conclusion.—Maternal autoimmune disorder is almost always associated with CHB but only rarely with postnatally diagnosed HB. Anti-SSA and anti-SSB are marker antibodies for mothers of children with CHB, and an increased risk of having an affected child is indicated by maternal primary SS and high titer antibodies to SSA and SSB.

▶ Rheumatic autoimmune diseases affect women, particularly during their childbearing age. If the maternal disease is characterized by the presence of IgG isotype autoantibodies, these can cross the placenta and affect the fetus. This is typically the case of the so-called neonatal lupus erythematosus (NLE). A similar mechanism has been shown in infants of patients with immune thrombocytopenic purpura (ITP) and, less frequently, in those from mothers with antiphospholipid syndrome (APS) where the placenta bears the brunt of the pathology, resulting in a growth-restricted infant. Although the precise pathogenic mechanism of antibody-mediated injury remains unknown, antibodies alone appear to be insufficient to cause disease, and fetal factors are likely contributory. In vivo and in vitro evidence support a pathologic cascade involving apoptosis of cardiocytes, surface translocation of Ro and La antigens, binding of maternal autoantibodies, secretion of profibrosing factors (eg, TGF beta) from the scavenging macrophages and modulation of cardiac fibroblasts to a myofibroflast scarring phenotype.[1] The neonatal lupus syndromes (NLS), although quite rare, carry significant mortality and morbidity if there are cardiac manifestations. These include varying degrees of block identified in utero and even late onset cardiomyopathy. Unfortunately, there is documentation that incomplete blocks (including those improving in utero with dexamethasone) can progress postnatally, despite the clearance of the maternal antibodies from the neonatal circulation.[2] The incidence of CHB is 1 per 20,000 live births, and neonatal lupus accounts for approximately 80% of the cases.

The report from Julkunen et al is truly a remarkable testimony to the health care system in Finland. The investigators were able to review records for over 50 years, identify more than 100 patients with HB, including 67 with CHB and 37 diagnosed postnatally, and established a control group with connective tissue disorders, but no heart disease. Not only that, but there were samples available for antibody analysis. They found a strong correlation between maternal autoimmune disorder and CHB, but only rarely was a maternal rheumatic disorder associated with postnatally diagnosed HB. They concluded that anti-SSA and anti-SSB are marker antibodies for mothers of children with CHB and the higher the antibody titer the greater chance of an affected fetus. Buyon et al[1] commented that although anti-SSA/Ro-SSB/La antibodies are detected in more than 85% of mothers whose fetuses are identified with CHB in a structurally normal heart, when clinicians applied this testing to their pregnant patients, the risk for a woman with the candidate antibodies to have a child with CHB was at or below 1 in 50. We need to explore further what protects the fetus, despite antibody passage in mothers with lupus erythematosus, hyperthyroidism, immune thrombocytopenia, and even myasthenia gravis. In all these disorders, roughly 10% to 15% of the fetuses will be affected, despite abundant antibody transfer during gestation. We also need to find more effective therapies and establish the role of corticosteroids and IV immunoglobulin for CHB.

A. A. Fanaroff, MD

References

1. Buyon JP, Rupel A, Clancy RM: Neonatal lupus syndromes. *Lupus* 13:705-712, 2004.
2. Eronen M, Miettinen A, Walle TK, et al: Relationship of maternal autoimmune response to clinical manifestations in children with congenital complete heart block. *Acta Paediatr* 93:803-809, 2004.

Abnormal Heart Rate Characteristics Are Associated With Neonatal Mortality

Griffin MP, O'Shea TM, Bissonette EA, et al (Univ of Virginia Health System, Charlottesville; Wake Forest School of Medicine, Winston-Salem, NC)
Pediatr Res 55:782-788, 2004   6–2

Introduction.—Estimating the risk of in-hospital mortality in the newborn intensive care unit can provide important information for health-care providers, and illness severity scores have been devised to provide mortality risk estimates. Calculation of illness severity scores is time-consuming, and the information used to predict mortality is collected only for the first 12 to 24 h of life. A noninvasive continuous measure that uses information collected throughout the hospitalization and that requires no data entry could be less costly and more informative. We have previously shown that the abnormal heart rate characteristics (HRC) of reduced variability and transient decelerations accompany neonatal illness such as late-onset sepsis. We hypothesized that more frequent and severe abnormal HRC are associated with an increased risk of death. We tested this hypothesis in two ways. Using data on infants older than 7 d of age, we first determined the association of the HRC index with death in the next week Second, we devised a cumulative HRC score and determined its association with in-hospital death. There were 37 deaths in the 685 patients. The major findings were 1) the HRC index showed highly significant association with death in the succeeding 7 d (receiver-operating characteristic area > 0.7, $p < 0.001$), and 2) the cumulative HRC was highly significantly associated with neonatal in-hospital mortality (receiver-operating characteristic area > 0.80, $p < 0.001$). In both analyses, HRC added information to birth weight, gestational age, and postnatal age ($p < 0.01$). The HRC index provides independent information about the risk of neonatal death in the upcoming 7 d, and the cumulative HRC is an estimate of the risk of in-hospital neonatal mortality.

▶ These investigators used single-processing methods to collect continuous ECG and HRC data. By using sophisticated statistical analysis, the authors calculated an HRC index and a cumulative HRC score and showed that these indexes are significantly associated with the risk of death in the succeeding 7 days and with neonatal in-hospital death. At a very basic level, we have long been aware that reduced heart rate variability is a bad sign suggesting that there is a problem with the autonomic nervous system. The assessment of this type of risk is not only useful from a clinical perspective, but also in designing clinical trials where balanced assignment of risk in the study and control groups is important. These investigators have extended their observations to include the use of the HRC index in predicting the likelihood of sepsis in the neonate,[1] an observation that could significantly change the way that we practice.

M. J. Maisels, MB, BCh

Reference

1. Griffin PM, Lake D, Moorman JR: Heart rate characteristics and laboratory tests in neonatal sepsis. *Pediatrics* 115:937-941, 2005.

Bradycardia and Desaturation During Skin-to-Skin Care: No Relationship to Hyperthermia
Bohnhorst B, Gill D, Dördelmann M, et al (Hannover Med School, Germany; Univ of Tuebingen, Germany)
J Pediatr 145:499-502, 2004   6–3

Objective.—We recently found increased temperature and increased bradycardia and desaturation during skin-to-skin care (SSC). We wanted to determine if these effects were related.

Study Design.—Twenty-two infants (median gestational age at birth 28.5 weeks [range 24-31], median age at study 25.5 days [range 10-60 days], median birth weight 1025 g [range 550-1525 g], median weight at study 1320 g [range 900-2460 g]) underwent three 2-hour recordings of breathing movements, nasal airflow, heart rate, and pulse oximeter saturation (SpO_2): at thermoneutrality (TN) during incubator care, at TN during SSC, and at elevated temperature (ET) during incubator care. Core temperature was measured via a rectal probe. Recordings were analyzed for the summed rate of bradycardia and desaturation (heart rate <2/3 of baseline; $SpO_2 \leq 80\%$).

Results.—Rectal temperature remained unchanged during SSC and increased by 0.6 degrees C during ET ($P < .001$). The summed rate of bradycardia and desaturation was increased during SSC but not during ET (TN: median 2.2/hour (range, 0-19), ET: median 1.7/hour (range, 0-13), SSC: 3.0/hour (0-25), $P < .02$ SSC vs ET).

Conclusion.—Bradycardia and desaturation were increased during SSC, even at constant rectal temperature, whereas ET had no effect on these events. Moderate hyperthermia did not increase respiratory instability in preterm infants.

▶ From relatively humble beginnings 20 years ago, and with the encouragement of a small band of devotees, skin-to-skin (kangaroo) care of preterm infants is gaining widespread international acceptance. Apart from providing a gentler, kinder environment for neonatal intensive care, it offers the promise of greater parental involvement, promotes breastfeeding, and provides a unique source of warmth for the infant. Of course, these benefits cannot come at the expense of cardiorespiratory stability, and most available data are somewhat anecdotal. Bohnhorst et al sought to determine whether episodic apnea, bradycardia, and desaturation are influenced by skin-to-skin care, and whether any increase in such episodes might be attributed to hyperthermia. Increase in environmental temperature has, for many years, been considered a cause for neonatal apnea, although this study did not support that observation. There was also no increase in the incidence of apnea or bradycardia episodes during skin-to-skin care, and this is encouraging for the advocates of this technique. However, over short periods of monitoring, as in this study, there is a great variability in the incidence of short apneas and accompanying bradycardia, and many infants will have no apnea at all. Therefore, it is not surprising that the incidence of these episodes was not significantly affected by kangaroo care. The investigators did notice an increase in the number of desaturation episodes, although the mean nadir in oxygen saturation was not greater. Those findings suggest that respiratory stability has the potential for being compromised during skin-to-skin care, although the long-term significance of episodic desaturation in preterm infants is unknown. All of which demonstrate that this nursing technique requires vigilance on the part of caregivers, may not be appropriate for all infants, and deserves systematic study as reported here.

R. J. Martin, MD

Cerebrovascular Effects of Rapid Volume Expansion in Preterm Fetal Sheep

Mayock DE, Gleason CA (Univ of Washington, Seattle)
Pediatr Res 55:395-399, 2004   6–4

Preterm human infants are often treated with volume expansion during their initial stabilization. There are limited data regarding the cerebral vascular effects of this therapeutic approach. The effects of blood volume expansion on cerebral vascular reactivity and oxygen metabolism in very immature animals have not been determined. We examined the effects of volume expansion, with and without hypoxia, on cerebral blood flow and metabolism in unanesthetized, chronically catheterized, preterm fetal sheep. Rapid volume expansion with i.v. dextran increased circulating blood volume. Arterial blood pressure did not increase, nor did cerebral blood flow. However, volume expansion resulted in lower arterial Hb concentration and, consequently, oxygen content without a compensatory increase in cerebral blood flow. Cerebral oxygen delivery fell significantly. Induction of severe hypoxia after volume expansion resulted in an increase in cerebral blood flow, as expected, but the increase in flow was not enough to maintain cerebral oxygen delivery. Rapid volume expansion in normovolemic preterm fetal sheep is associated with decreased cerebral oxygen delivery, and this is further compromised when oxygen content is decreased.

▶ There is a general agreement that systemic hypotension is a common condition in extremely low birth weight, early-gestation infants. How common (approximately 33%) cannot be answered precisely because there is no consensus on the definition or the threshold for therapeutic intervention. Furthermore, the optimal means of restoring normal circulating blood volume, blood pressure, and cardiac output have yet to be determined. Whether crystalloids or colloids are preferable is also unclear in newborns. In their Cochrane review, Osborn and Evan[1] commented "There is no evidence from randomized trials to support the routine use of early volume expansion in very preterm infants without cardiovascular compromise. There is insufficient evidence to determine whether infants with cardiovascular compromise benefit from volume expansion. There is insufficient evidence to determine what type of volume expansion should be used in preterm infants (if at all), or for the use of early red cell transfusions." Although many hypotensive babies are hypovolemic, there are many other causes for hypotension and they should all be considered, including defining the hemodynamics echocardiographically, before pushing volume. Because systemic hypotension is associated with increased mortality rate as well as both short- and long-term morbidity, volume expansion, dopamine, and dobutamine have been the agents most commonly used to treat hypotension. Although volume expansion is liberally used in newborn intensive care, little is known about its effects on hemodynamics or outcomes. Ewer et al,[2] using data that were obtained from anonymous regional case notes of Project 27/28, a British National case-controlled study run by the Confidential Enquiry into Stillbirths and Deaths in Infancy, reported that newborns who received 30 mL/kg volume expansion in the first 48 hours of life were more likely to die than those who received fewer than 30 mL/kg (odds ratio, 4.5; 95% confidence interval, 1.2-17.2). More is not necessarily better!

Mayock and Gleason, by studying the effects of volume expansion with and without hypoxia in immature lambs, provide some insight into this problem. They note that rapid volume expansion in normovolemic preterm fetal sheep did not affect blood pressure or cerebral blood flow but was associated with decreased cerebral oxygen delivery. This was further compromised when oxygen content was decreased. We can but speculate on the long-term consequences of these findings in human beings but should be cautious about overaggressive volume correction with crystalloids or colloids, which might cause hemodilution and reduce oxygen delivery to the brain.

Corticosteroids have added a new wrinkle to the management of hypotension. Many hypotensive preterm infants have low cortisol levels, and corticosteroids are being increasingly used to prevent or treat hypotension in these babies. Corticosteroid therapy has resulted in improved blood pressure and circulation but with many complications, including the unanticipated spontaneous gut perforation and the long-term problem of the increased incidence of cerebral palsy and intellectual impairment.[3,4]

In view of these significant problems with therapy, there is an imperative to better study this problem, define hypotension (based on hemodynamic measurements which are feasible and reproducible), and determine the optimal therapy.

A. A. Fanaroff, MD

References

1. Osborn DA, Evans N: Early volume expansion for prevention of morbidity and mortality in very preterm infants. *Cochrane Database Syst Rev* 2:CD002055, 2004.
2. Ewer AK, Tyler W, Francis A, et al: Excessive volume expansion and neonatal death in preterm infants born at 27-28 weeks gestation. *Paediatr Perinat Epidemiol* 17:180-186, 2003.
3. Watterberg KL, Gerdes JS, Cook KL: Impaired glucocorticoid synthesis in premature infants developing chronic lung disease. *Pediatr Res* 50:190-195, 2001.
4. Watterberg KL, Gerdes JS, Cole C, et al: Prophylaxis of early adrenal insufficiency to prevent bronchopulmonary dysplasia: A multicenter trial. *Pediatrics* 114:1649-1657, 2004.

Maternal Age and Other Predictors of Newborn Blood Pressure
Gillman MW, Rich-Edwards JW, Rifas-Shiman SL, et al (Harvard Med School, Boston; Univ of Rochester, NY)
J Pediatr 144:240-245, 2004   6–5

Objective.—To investigate perinatal predictors of newborn blood pressure.

Study Design.—Among 1059 mothers and their newborn infants participating in Project Viva, a US cohort study of pregnant women and their offspring, we obtained five systolic blood pressure readings on a single occasion in the first few days of life. Using multivariate linear regression models, we examined the extent to which maternal age and other pre- and perinatal factors predicted newborn blood pressure level.

Results.—Mean (SD) maternal age was 32.0 (5.2) years, and mean (SD) newborn systolic blood pressure was 72.6 (9.0) mm Hg. A multivariate

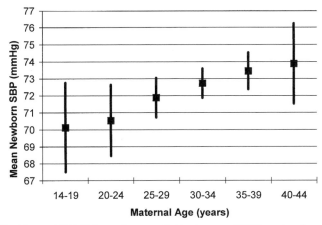

FIGURE.—Mean and 95% CI for newborn systolic blood pressure (SBP) by maternal age group. Data from 1059 mothers and newborns participating in Project Viva. (Reprinted by permission of the publisher from Gillman MA, Rich-Edwards JW, Rifas-Shiman SL, et al: Maternal age and other predictors of newborn blood pressure. *J Pediatr* 144:240-245. Copyright 2004 by Elsevier.)

TABLE 5.—Increment in Newborn Systolic Blood Pressure (mm Hg)
for Each Increase of 5 Years of Maternal Age,
From Mixed Linear Models

Model Covariates	Change in SBP (mm Hg)	95% CI
Maternal age (5 y)	0.8	0.2, 1.4
Birth weight (kg)	2.9	1.6, 4.2
Primigravida vs not	0.2	−1.0, 1.4
Prepregnancy BMI (kg/m²)	0.01	−0.1, 0.1
3rd trimester SBP (10 mmHg)	0.9	0.2, 1.6
Infant age when BP measured (24 h)	2.4	1.7, 3.0
Heart rate (10 bpm)	0.3	−0.04, 0.7

BMI, Body mass index; *SBP*, systolic blood pressure; *CI*, confidence interval.
Data from 1059 mothers and newborns participating in Project Viva.
(Reprinted by permission of the publisher from Gillman MA, Rich-Edwards JW, Rifas-Shiman SL, et al: Maternal age and other predictors of newborn blood pressure. *J Pediatr* 144:240-245. Copyright 2004 by Elsevier.)

model showed that for each 5-year increase in maternal age, newborn systolic blood pressure was 0.8 mm Hg higher (95% CI, 0.2, 1.4) (Figure). In addition to maternal age, independent predictors of newborn blood pressure included maternal third trimester blood pressure (09 mm Hg [95% CI, 0.2, 1.6] for each increment in maternal blood pressure); infant age at which we measured blood pressure (2.4 mm Hg [95% CI 1.7, 3.0] for each additional day of life); and birth weight (2.9 mm Hg [95% CI, 1.6, 4.2] per kg) (Table 5).

Conclusions.—Higher maternal age, maternal blood pressure, and birth weight were associated with higher newborn systolic blood pressure. Whereas blood pressure later in childhood predicts adult hypertension and its consequences, newborn blood pressure may represent different phenomena, such as pre- and perinatal influences on cardiac structure and function.

▶ There is evidence of an association between prenatal events such as advanced maternal age and diabetes and hypertension during pregnancy and blood pressure levels in childhood and adolescence. Thus, an evaluation of prenatal events on newborn blood pressure is certainly warranted. The relationship between maternal age and systolic blood pressure is quite striking, although there is no ready explanation for this observation. While it is true that changes in newborn blood pressure may well reflect the development of cardiac structure and function during fetal life, we don't know if neonatal blood pressures are associated with subsequent blood pressures.

The key to the observations of these investigators might lie in the placenta. We need additional data to define the relationship between neonatal blood pressure and the subsequent development of hypertension or other cardiovascular disease.

M. J. Maisels, MB, BCh

Independent Factors Associated With Outcomes of Parachute Mitral Valve in 84 Patients

Schaverien MV, Freedom RM, McCrindle BW (Univ of Toronto)
Circulation 109:2309-2313, 2004   6–6

Background.—Parachute mitral valve (PMV) is defined as a unifocal attachment of the mitral valve chordae to a single or dominant papillary muscle and may cause subvalvar obstruction. We sought to determine factors associated with outcomes.

Method and Results.—Patients (n=84; 64% male) who presented between 1977 and 2001 at a median age of 3 days (range, birth to 5.4 years) were assessed with PMV (without atrioventricular septal defect). Associated cardiac anomalies in 99% included aortic coarctation in 68%, atrial septal defect in 54%, ventricular septal defect in 46%, aortic valve stenosis in 32%, subaortic stenosis in 20%, and left ventricular hypoplasia in 19%, with complex anomalies in 14%. Noncardiac anomalies were noted in 32%. Survival (n=18 deaths) was 82% at 1 year and 79% at 10 years, with independent risk factors including left ventricular hypoplasia ($P<0.001$) and atrial septal defect ($P<0.003$). Freedom from surgical mitral valvotomy (n=11 patients) was 95% at age 6 months and 80% at 10 years, with independent risk factors including the absence of aortic coarctation ($P<0.02$) and the presence of subaortic stenosis ($P<0.04$). There was no significant increase in mean gradient of the PMV over time, but higher gradient was independently associated with the presence of supravalvular mitral stenosis ($P<0.001$), absence of atrial septal defect ($P<0.04$), presence of ventricular septal defect ($P<0.02$), and subsequent mitral valvotomy ($P<0.01$).

Conclusions.—Outcomes for patients with PMV are dependent on the spectrum of associated cardiac lesions. The degree of mitral valve obstruction remains stable, and the majority will not require valvotomy.

▶ An entity that requires almost 25 years to accumulate a series of 84 patients is, by definition, uncommon. Furthermore, when I attempted to do a MEDLINE search with the wording "parachute mitral valve," the only article to emerge is this study from Schaverien et al. I did learn that PMV is defined as a unifocal attachment of the mitral valve chordae to a single or dominant papillary muscle and may cause subvalvar obstruction. It is commonly associated with other cardiac malformations but, from this series, the degree of mitral valve obstruction appears to remain stable and the majority did not require valvotomy. As more and more cardiac disorders are amenable to less-invasive therapeutic procedures, the cardiac catheter becomes a surgical as well as a diagnostic instrument. We can predict that ultimately fewer and fewer neonates will require open thoracotomy operative interventions.

A. A. Fanaroff, MD

Central Venous Lines in Neonates: A Study of 2186 Catheters

Cartwright DW (Royal Brisbane and Women's Hosp, Queensland, Australia)
Arch Dis Child Fetal Neonatal Ed 89:F504-F508, 2004   6–7

Introduction.—At the Grantley Stable Neonatal Unit, Royal Brisbane and Women's Hospital (Queensland, Australia), percutaneously inserted silicone central venous lines (CVLs) have been used since 1978; the goal has always been for the catheter tip to be in the middle of the right atrium. A computerized database exists of all infants admitted since May 1, 1983, and includes information concerning basic and clinical data, diagnoses, and management. Described is the use of CVLs at this institution, with an emphasis on the occurrence of pleural and pericardial effusions, septicemia, and reasons for line removal.

Methods.—The data for all infants admitted between January 1, 1984, through December 31, 2002, in whom a CVL line was placed were reviewed in the neonatal database and patient medical records. Autopsy reports of all infants who died were reviewed.

Results.—Of a total of 18,761 admissions, 2186 catheters were placed in 1862 infants for a total of 35,159 days (median, 14 days; range, 1-99 days). The tip was positioned in the right atrium in 1282 (58.6%) catheters. A total of 142 infants (7.6%) died with a CVL in place; 89 (4.8%) had the catheter tip in the right atrium. Thirty-two of these 89 infant underwent autopsy. No autopsies showed tension in the pericardium or milky fluid resembling intralipid. One case (0.05% of catheters) of nonlethal pericardial effusion was observed in an infant whose catheter was inappropriately left coiled in the right atrium. There were no cases of pleural effusion associated with CVL use. Most catheters (1523 [69.7%]) were removed electively. Septicemia occurred in 116 catheters (5.3%; Table 3).

Conclusion.—This is the largest reported series of percutaneously placed CVLs. These findings endorse the safety of placing catheter tips in the right atrium (Table 4) with contrast injection localization and illustrate the value of keeping records of all CVLs. Strict insertion and management principles may enhance the safety of CVLs.

TABLE 3.—Organisms that Caused Septicemia (n = 116)

CoNS	28	*Acinetobacter* sp	3
MRSA	15	GBS	3
Klebsiella sp	11	*Bacillus* sp	3
Pseudomonas sp	12	*Serratia* sp	3
Enterococcus faecalis	10	*Micrococcus*	2
Staphylococcus aureus	7	*Citrobacter* sp	2
Escherichia coli	5	*Morganella* sp	1
Candida sp	5	*Aeromonas* sp	1
Enterobacter sp	4	*Enterococcus faecium*	1

Abbreviations: CoNS, Coagulase-negative *Staphylococcus; MRSA,* methicillin-resistant *S. aureus; GBS,* Group B *Streptococcus.*

(Courtesy of Cartwright DW: Central venous lines in neonates: A study of 2186 catheters. *Arch Dis Child Fetal Neonatal Ed* 89:F504-F508, 2004, with permission from the BMJ Publishing Group.)

TABLE 4.—Insertion and Management Principles

1. Inserted by experienced staff (consultant or senior registrar)
2. Aim to insert too far and pull back away from vessel walls
3. Never leave a catheter where it does not easily and repeatedly withdraw blood during the insertion procedure
4. ALWAYS inject with radio-opaque contrast for *x* ray examination (if you don't inject it, you don't know where the tip is)
5. Be actively injecting during x ray examination to see contrast coming from the end of the catheter
6. Sterile technique for insertion, and for line changes (three times/week)
7. No drug injections—catheter used for parenteral nutrition only
8. Antifungal prophylaxis of oral and topical nystatin
9. Cover insertion site with bio-occlusive dressing and leave undisturbed. No coils of catheter under dressing

(Courtesy of Cartwright DW: Central venous lines in neonates: A study of 2186 catheters. *Arch Dis Child Fetal Neonatal Ed* 89:F504-F508, 2004, with permission from the BMJ Publishing Group.)

▶ Dr Cartwright reports the experience with percutaneously placed silicone CVLs over an 18-year period (1984-2002). From January 1, 1996, the author prospectively collected data that included dates of insertion and removal, insertion site, catheter tip location, reason for removal, and tip culture results. The autopsy reports of all babies who died with a catheter in place were reviewed, and data from 2186 catheters were compiled and evaluated. This is the largest series of percutaneously inserted silicone CVLs reported. Although serious, sometimes fatal complications are associated with CVLs (usually related to infection or migration of the catheter tip into body cavities with subsequent accumulation of fluid), this report documents a remarkably low rate of complications. The risk of catheter-related sepsis was 5.3%, with reported rates ranging from 0 to 46%. There was only 1 case of nonfatal pericardial effusion found and no cases of pleural effusion.

Unique to this study was the insertion of the catheter tip into the right atrium in 59% of the cases. Placement was always confirmed by injecting radiopaque contrast. Further, to ensure proper localization in a large vessel, blood was readily and repeatedly withdrawn from the catheter before fixing with a bio-occlusive dressing. Percutaneously placed CVLs are essential in providing nutrition to the smallest neonates. Nevertheless, the conclusion that it is safe to place catheter tips in the right atrium must be tempered with some caution. The meticulous protocol adopted and followed for inserting and managing CVLs is by no means universal. Anyone using central lines in infants should have a similar protocol in place to ensure proper placement and management of these lines. It is also extremely important to keep unit-specific statistics so that complication rates can be identified and evaluated.

C. J. E. Pryce, MD

Does Radio-opaque Contrast Improve Radiographic Localisation of Percutaneous Central Venous Lines?

Odd DE, Page B, Battin MR, et al (Natl Women's Hosp, Auckland, New Zealand)
Arch Dis Child Fetal Neonatal Ed 89:F41-F43, 2004   6–8

Background.—Percutaneous central venous lines (long lines) are commonly used in neonatal practice. The position of these lines is important, because incorrect placement may be associated with complications.

Aims.—To determine whether the addition of radio-opaque contrast material improves the localisation of long line tips over plain radiography.

Methods.—Radiographs taken to identify long line position were identified in two periods; 106 radiographs without contrast taken between October 1999 and August 2000, and 96 radiographs with contrast between September 2001 and July 2002. Two observers independently reviewed each radiograph to identify the position of the line tip. The formal radiology report was recorded as a third observer.

Results.—The use of contrast increased the proportion of radiographs in which all observers reported they could see the long line tip (53 (55%) *v* 41 (39%)). It also increased the proportion where they agreed on anatomical position (57 (59%) *v* 39 (37%)) and there was a higher kappa coefficient for agreement (0.56 *v* 0.33).

Conclusions.—The use of contrast while taking radiographs for the localisation of long line position improves the likelihood that an observer can see a long line tip and reduces inter-observer variability. Even using contrast, precise localisation of a long line tip can be difficult.

▶ In this study, the authors retrospectively evaluated whether the use of contrast material would improve practitioners' agreement in radiologic identification of line position (tip of catheter) in newborn infants. Although at first glance a not-so-exciting proposition, this publication has significant merit in that practitioners of all levels often struggle to ascertain catheter position in plane radiographs. Placement of percutaneous IV central lines is a very common practice in the neonatal ICU. To minimize the possibility of catastrophic complications, proper placement is crucially important. Their results are clearly encouraging in that a significantly higher percentage of positive identification by all observers, as well as a significantly higher degree of agreement in assessment of anatomic position, were noted. The authors concluded that when evaluating line position radiographically, contrast material should be administered routinely. I certainly cannot subscribe to that policy. Even though line placement sometimes may be difficult to ascertain, for the most part those cases are the exception to the rule in our clinical experience. Based on the results of this study, for example, you would have to give contrast to about 7 or 8 babies to increase the ability of all observers to identify 1 more line tip or to improve agreement in anatomic localization. Furthermore, when all 3 observers could see the tip of the line, addition of contrast did not improve agreement. Simply expressed, I cannot justify the exposure of every infant to contrast material if line identification is not a problem after a plain film. Also in support of my contention is the fact that the safety of this practice has not been extensively evaluated. The authors did not comment on whether the practice they propose has any significant addition of cost to an already expensive system. The findings of this report reinforce my practice of tailoring care to the needs of the patient and the clinical circumstances.

R. J. Rodriguez, MD

7 Respiratory Disorders

Foxa2 Is Required for Transition to Air Breathing at Birth
Wan H, Xu Y, Ikegami M, et al (Univ of Cincinnati, Ohio; Vanderbilt Univ, Nashville, Tenn; Univ of Pennsylvania, Philadelphia; et al)
Proc Natl Acad Sci U S A 101:14449-14454, 2004   7–1

Toward the end of gestation in mammals, the fetal lung undergoes a process of differentiation that is required for transition to air breathing at birth. Respiratory epithelial cells synthesize the surfactant proteins and lipids that together form the pulmonary surfactant complex necessary for lung function. Failure of this process causes respiratory distress syndrome, a leading cause of perinatal death and morbidity in newborn infants. Here we demonstrate that expression of the forkhead gene *Foxa2* in respiratory epithelial cells of the peripheral lung controls pulmonary maturation at birth. Newborn mice lacking *Foxa2* expression in the lung develop severe pulmonary disease on the first day of life, with all of the morphological, molecular, and biochemical features of respiratory distress syndrome in preterm infants, including atelectasis, hyaline membranes, and the lack of pulmonary surfactant lipids and proteins. RNA microarray analysis at embryonic day 18.5 demonstrated that *Foxa2*-regulated expression of a group of genes mediating surfactant protein and lipid synthesis, host defense, and antioxidant production. *Foxa2* regulates a complex pulmonary program of epithelial cell maturation required for transition to air breathing at birth.

▶ This is a fascinating report by an interesting group of authors. Mildred Stahlman, a true pioneer and leader in the field of neonatal-perinatal medicine, was among the first to not only advocate for more aggressive treatment, but to actually do it. She led the charge in the placement of invasive umbilical catheters and using mechanical ventilation for infants with severe respiratory distress syndrome. It must be extremely gratifying for her to participate in this study, which has elucidated the mechanism by which the lung is prepared for air breathing. Jeff Whitsett's laboratory in Cincinnati has relentlessly pursued the study of surfactant and its various proteins, together with the disorders that result from genetic mutations of these proteins, adding considerably to our knowledge of neonatal respiratory disorders. Machiko Ikegami, in collaboration with Alan Jobe first at UCLA but now at Cincinnati University, has also contributed extensively to the study and elucidation of neonatal pulmonary disorders and, more recently, the role of chorioamnionitis and corticosteroids.

Most mortals merely marvel at the manner in which newly born infants smoothly undergo the transition from life underwater to air breathing at birth. The complex cardiovascular and respiratory changes do not happen by accident, but for years investigators had, at best, a superficial understanding of the important processes that determine this transition. There is much preparation and behind-the-scenes work necessary, and we learn in this great collaborative report that a forkhead gene, *Foxa2*, present in the respiratory epithelial cells of the peripheral lung, controls pulmonary maturation at birth. Not only is the surfactant system readied but so, too, is the antioxidant protection as the newborn infant will face considerable oxidative stress.

Our knowledge of the surfactant proteins and their role in disease is enhanced by the report from Shulenin et al,[1] together with the editorial by Mikko Hallman[2] on the *ABCA3* gene mutations in newborns with fatal surfactant deficiency. *ABCA3* is critical for the proper formation of lamellar bodies and surfactant function and may also be important for lung function in other pulmonary diseases. The state-of-the-art report by Whitsett and Weaver[3] and Haataja and Hallman[4] in 2002 will bring any readers up to speed on this fascinating group of disorders.

A. A. Fanaroff, MD

References

1. Shulenin S, Nogee LM, Annilo T, et al: *ABCA3* gene mutations in newborns with fatal surfactant deficiency. *N Engl J Med* 350:1296-1303, 2004.
2. Hallman M: Lung surfactant, respiratory failure, and genes. *N Engl J Med* 350:1278-1280, 2004.
3. Whitsett JA, Weaver TE: Hydrophobic surfactant proteins in lung function and disease. *N Engl J Med* 347:2141-2148, 2002.
4. Haataja R, Hallman M: Surfactant proteins as genetic determinants of multifactorial pulmonary diseases. *Ann Med* 34:324-333, 2002.

Development of Ventilatory Response to Transient Hypercapnia and Hypercapnic Hypoxia in Term Infants

Søvik S, Lossius K (Univ of Oslo, Norway; Rikshospitalet, Oslo, Norway)
Pediatr Res 55:302-309, 2004   7–2

Background.—After birth, infants' peripheral chemoreceptor oxygen sensitivity markedly increases, but studies have not shown a similar increase in the ventilatory responses to carbon dioxide. Because many of these studies used long-term hypercapnic challenges, central chemoreceptors rather than peripheral chemoreceptors were dominant. Whether term infants exhibit a postnatal change in the immediate ventilatory responses to step changes in inspired carbon dioxide and oxygen was investigated.

Methods.—Ventilatory responses were tested in 26 healthy term infants during natural sleep 2 days and 8 weeks after birth. A pneumotachometer recorded the infants' ventilatory responses to a randomized sequence of 15 seconds of hypercapnia, hypoxia, and hypercapnic hypoxia on a breath-by-breath basis. Analysis included the response rate, the stimulus-response time, and the magnitude of the response.

Results.—All 26 infants had successful recordings at 2 days, and 20 had successful recordings at 8 weeks. With age, the mean minute ventilation, mean tidal volume, and heart rate increased, but the respiratory rate decreased. The response rate to hypercapnia increased 30%, the response rate to hypoxia increased 318%, and the response rate to hypercapnic hypoxia increased 302%. A purely additive effect on the minute ventilation rate was noted at 2 days for the hypercapnic hypoxia condition, but at week 8, the rate during hypercapnic hypoxia was greater than the sum of the rates with each single stimulus, which evidenced a more-than-additive interaction between the effects of hypercapnia and hypoxia. The stimulus-response time of infants during hypercapnia on the second day of life was 2.3 seconds longer than during hypercapnic hypoxia or hypoxia, but at the 8-week measurement, the stimulus response time had declined by 3.4 seconds for both hypercapnic conditions and was unchanged for hypoxia. The interaction between age and test gas type was noted to be independently responsible for about two thirds of the decrease in stimulus-response time.

Conclusions.—For these healthy term infants, a more-than-additive interaction between hypercapnic–hypoxic effects and ventilatory response rate emerged by 8 weeks of age. Infants also showed a marked decline in stimulus-response time during hypercapnic stimuli but not during hypoxic stimuli with increasing age. A maturing of the peripheral carbon dioxide chemoreceptor mechanism appears to occur in this time frame. Developing a prompt response to transient hypercapnia may be a necessary component of respiratory stability for infants.

▶ In this article, the authors attempt to show the development of the peripheral chemoreceptor response to carbon dioxide from birth to 2 months of age in 26 sleeping, healthy, full-term infants. The quantitative ventilatory responses were measured with a sophisticated mask valve pneumotachograph system that they have developed, using steady-state gas presentation. Briefly, they showed that the response to carbon dioxide was the same at both ages but that the response time was less, that is, faster at 2 months. The magnitude of the response to a hypoxic stimulus was greater at 2 months. A more-than-additive response to hypoxic hypercapnia was not present until 2 months, the cause of which was interpreted as a maturation of the peripheral chemoreceptor carbon dioxide drive. That no increase occurred in the ventilatory response to carbon dioxide at 2 months detracts from the conclusion about the increased peripheral chemoreceptor drive. Because a 100% oxygen challenge would have physiologically eliminated the carbon dioxide peripheral chemoreceptor drive, it would have been interesting to see whether this test supported their interpretation for the strength of the peripheral chemoreceptor carbon dioxide effect being greater at 2 months. Because the respiratory pattern and drive vary with the sleep state, it would also be important to control for the sleep state in future investigations.

R. L. Ariagno, MD

Effect of Sighs on Breathing Memory and Dynamics in Healthy Infants
Baldwin DN, Suki B, Pillow JJ, et al (Univ Children's Hosp, Bern, Switzerland;
Boston Univ; Univ of Western Australia, Perth)
J Appl Physiol 97:1830-1839, 2004   7–3

Deep inspirations (sighs) play a significant role in altering lung mechanical and airway wall function; however, their role in respiratory control remains unclear. We examined whether sighs act via a resetting mechanism to improve control of the respiratory regulatory system. Effects of sighs on system variability, short- and long-range memory, and stability were assessed in 25 healthy full-term infants at 1 mo of age [mean 36 (range 28-57) days] during quiet sleep. Variability was examined using moving-window coefficient of variation, short-range memory using autocorrelation function, and long-range memory using detrended fluctuation analysis. Stability was examined by studying the behavior of the attractor with use of phase-space plots. Variability of tidal volume (VT) and minute ventilation (VE) increased during the initial 15 breaths after a sigh. Short-range memory of VT decreased during the 50 breaths preceding a sigh, becoming uncorrelated (random) during the 10-breath presigh window. Short-range memory increased after a sigh for the entire 50 breaths compared with the randomized data set and for 20 breaths compared with the presigh window. Similar, but shorter duration, changes were noted in VE. No change in long-range memory was seen after a sigh. Coefficient of variation and range of points located within a defined attractor segment increased after a sigh. Thus control of breathing in healthy infants shows long-range stability and improvement in short-range memory and variability after a sigh. These results add new evidence that the role of sighs is not purely mechanical.

▶ In brief, this is an engineer's view of the effect of the "sigh" on breathing and potentially on neurorespiratory control resetting. The study uses a compliant silicone mask technique covering the mouth and nose of 25 healthy term (3 were near term) subjects assessed during quiet, nonsedated sleep (Prechtl behavioral criteria) at a mean age of 36 days old (maximum, almost 2 months). End tidal carbon dioxide and oxygen and flow measurement were performed by an ultrasonic flowmeter to obtain volume and flow plus timing of respiration event, that is, inspiratory and expiratory time. Data were analyzed for 10-minute time series. They hypothesized that sighs may play a crucial role for lung mechanics and as a resetting mechanism for the negative-feedback control system. They wanted to see if term infants demonstrated alterations in regulation of breathing after sighs during quiet sleep. The effect of sighs on tidal breathing indexes was determined in terms of respiratory variability, short- and long-term memory, and stability. In summary they found that there was increased variability of tidal breathing after a sigh. Sighs usually occurred every 50 to 100 breaths. Short-range breath-to-breath memory of the neurorespiratory control system decreased just before the sigh. After the sigh there was a decrease in tidal volume and inspiratory time and the ratio of inspiratory time over total time. They concluded that the sigh was an important perturbation for maintaining lung volume and airway tone as well as resetting neurorespiratory control. An aside is that some investigators believe that the sigh is an important part of arousal, which also would affect the input to the respiratory control center. In this article behavioral assessment of sleep would not allow assessment of subcortical arousals. Furthermore, during the age studied the majority of sleep would be active or random eye movement, during which vagal tone is inhibited and the physiology is likely to be different than that found during quiet sleep. Also, the 1-month-old infant is still a neonate, but the outliers in this study may represent another physiology, which introduces some heterogeneity in the group studied. Nevertheless, this will be a stimulating report for the engineering and mathematically oriented reader and a difficult or challenging read for all others.

What significance does the study have for clinical neonatology? In brief, variability in the respiratory and cardiac signal is healthy and desirable and represents the most adaptable physiology. Clinically, we are still in the linear mode of analysis and prefer that the infant's vital signs are metronomically stable. In the next era our management strategies will be focused on promoting physiologic signal variability, which should provide the most robust physiologic adaptation and health for our infant patients.

R. L. Ariagno, MD

Changing Incidence and Outcome of Infants With Respiratory Distress Syndrome in the 1990s: A Population-Based Survey
Koivisto M, Marttila R, Kurkinen-Räty M, et al (Univ of Oulu, Finland; Seinäjoki Central Hosp, Finland; Päijät-Häme Central Hosp, Lahti, Finland)
Acta Paediatr 93:177-184, 2004   7–4

Background.—Respiratory distress syndrome (RDS) remains a problem regarding preterm infants. Examined were the overall and gestational age-specific and birth weight–specific incidence of RDS in the 1990s in a neonatal center managing all cases of RDS in northern Finland.

Study Design.—The study group consisted of 58,990 infants born in the region served by Oulu University Hospital from 1990 through 1999. There were 31 infants who died within the first 2 hours after birth. Clinical characteristics, diagnoses, and length of stay were recorded. For all infants born before 33 weeks, records were reviewed for RDS and associated morbidity. After release from the hospital, patients were followed up for up to 1 year of corrected age. Two periods were compared: 1990 to 1995 and 1996 to 1999.

Findings.—Although the overall incidence of RDS did not change between these 2 periods, the gestational age–adjusted incidence decreased. There was a trend toward increased live birth at less than 28 weeks' gestational age. RDS-related mortality (15%) decreased in parallel with overall neonatal mortality. The duration of oxygen therapy decreased and the incidence of pneumothorax increased between these 2 periods. The rate of chronic lung disease at 36 weeks and at 1 year remained unchanged. Neurosensory morbidity also remained unchanged over this time.

Conclusion.—There was a significant decrease in RDS specific to gestational age between the early 1990s and the late 1990s. The therapies introduced did not decrease the overall incidence of RDS, however, as the number of extremely preterm infants increased over this period. RDS-related mortality decreased in parallel with overall neonatal mortality. The course of RDS shortened and acute complications decreased, although long-term morbidity did not change over this time.

▶ Few, if any, studies of the incidence, clinical course, and outcome of neonatal RDS can claim, as this study does, to include all cases of RDS drawn from a regional population that in a decade accounted for almost 60,000 births, with a 98% 1-year follow-up evaluation for infants that had RDS. This comprehensive assessment of data gathered on 488 newborn infants with RDS at a single university hospital (Oulu) in northern Finland between 1990 and 2000 offers insight regarding outcome in the postsurfactant era, before and after the major change in obstetrical practices related to antenatal steroid therapy (which increased from 15% in the 1990-1995 period to 51% in the 1996-1999 epoch) and liberalized use of antibiotics (which may have contributed to the reduced rate of clinical chorioamnionitis from 11% in 1990 to 1995 to 4% in 1996 to 1999).

Despite these developments, however, the overall incidence of RDS did not change significantly (0.87% in 1990-1995, 0.76% in 1996-1999), though the proportion of RDS that occurred in infants born at less than 28 weeks of gestation increased from 19% in 1990 to 1995 to 31% in 1996 to 1999. Death from RDS remained constant at 6%, accounting for about 15% of the overall neonatal mortality during the decade of this study. At 1-year follow-up, it is notable that the incidence of delayed motor development fell from 8% for infants with RDS who were born in the 1990 to 1995 epoch compared to 2% for infants with RDS who were born in the 1996 to 1999 epoch.

Use of these data as a reference point for outcome analysis at neonatal centers outside of the Nordic nations is problematic on several counts, including homogeneity of the population that was studied, universality of comprehensive prenatal care in Finland, tight control of high-risk maternal care within the region, treatment of all infants with RDS at a single neonatal center, and an impressive 98% participation in the 1-year follow-up program. Nevertheless, these data set a lofty standard worth striving for, an outcome that reflects well on a society that embraces universal access to high-quality health care. In the final analysis, however, the quantum leap in neonatal outcome awaits a major decline in the rate of premature birth, which so far has eluded even the Finns.

R. D. Bland, MD

Early Surfactant for Neonates With Mild to Moderate Respiratory Distress Syndrome: A Multicenter, Randomized Trial

Gunkel JH, for the Texas Neonatal Research Group (Univ of Texas, Dallas; et al)
J Pediatr 144:804-808, 2004   7–5

Objective.—We studied the efficacy and safety of electively providing surfactant to preterm infants with mild to moderate respiratory distress syndrome (RDS) not requiring mechanical ventilation.

Study Design.—A 5-center, randomized clinical trial was performed on 132 infants with RDS, birth weight ≥1250 grams, gestational age ≤36 weeks, postnatal age 4 to 24 hours, FIO_2 ≥40% for ≥1 hour, and no immediate need for intubation. Infants were randomly assigned to intubation, surfactant (Survanta, Ross Laboratories, Columbus, Ohio) administration, and expedited extubation (n = 65) or expectant management (n = 67) with subsequent intubation and surfactant treatment as clinically indicated. The primary outcome was duration of mechanical ventilation.

Results.—Infants in the surfactant group had a median duration of mechanical ventilation of 2.2 hours compared with 0.0 hours for control infants, since only 29 of 67 control infants required mechanical ventilation ($P = .001$). Surfactant-treated infants were less likely to require subsequent mechanical ventilation for worsening respiratory disease (26% vs 43%, relative risk = 0.60; 95% CI, 0.37, 0.99). There were no differences in secondary outcomes (duration of nasal continuous positive airway pressure, oxygen therapy, hospital stay, or adverse outcomes).

Conclusions.—Routine elective intubation for administration of surfactant to preterm infants ≥1250 grams with mild to moderate RDS is not recommended.

▶ There are few who doubt that the introduction of surfactant therapy had a major role in reducing morbidity and mortality in preterm infants. Indeed, the careful evaluation and rigorous clinical trials carried out before surfactant was approved provides a wonderful benchmark that other new products should emulate before they are allowed to be introduced into the neonatal clinical arena.

The past 20 years have seen a proliferation of networks, and we are able to see the fruits of labor from the Texas Neonatal Research Group. I was fascinated to read that 4 infants enrolled at a center were all excluded from the analysis because of a protocol violation consisting of the wrong assignment to study intervention in all 4 infants. "This center did not participate further in the study and did not enroll any additional patients." Very appropriate!

The question was simple, the results unequivocal, and the conclusions therefore unambiguous. The results of their study do not support the routine use of intubation solely to administer surfactant in neonates (≥1250 g; gestational age ≤36 weeks; postnatal age 4 to 24 hours; FIO_2 ≥40% for ≥1 hour with respiratory distress syndrome [RDS] and no immediate need for intubation). Mercifully they accepted their findings and omitted the usual call for further, larger, prospective randomized controlled trials. So we can lay to rest the concept of routine elective intubation for administration of surfactant to bigger preterm infants with mild to moderate RDS.

A. A. Fanaroff, MD

Surfactant Does Not Improve Survival Rate in Preterm Infants With Congenital Diaphragmatic Hernia
Lally KP, for the Congenital Diaphragmatic Hernia Study Group (Univ of Texas, Houston; et al)
J Pediatr Surg 39:829-833, 2004   7–6

Background.—Respiratory failure is the principal cause of death in infants with congenital diaphragmatic hernias (CDHs), and hospital mortality rates range from 25% to 40%. An animal model of CDH has been found to be surfactant deficient, and the administration of exogenous surfactant improved the respiratory condition. No consistent data link human infant surfactant production and functioning with CDH, but the use of exogenous surfactant for infants with CDHs has been linked to some benefit. The CDH Study Group Registry database supplied information to compare outcomes for infants less than 37 weeks' gestation who were or were not given exogenous surfactant.

Methods.—The data were obtained prospectively for the CDH registry, and the timing of surfactant use and outcomes were retrospectively analyzed. Survival to discharge was the outcome sought. Patients given a prenatal diagnosis were assessed, as well as those whose cases were determined postnatally.

Results.—The overall survival rate for all patients in the registry was 67%. Surfactant use and outcome data were available for 424 patients, 209 of whom had received surfactant at some time. Both a low 5-minute Apgar score and an earlier gestational age were found more often in infants who received surfactant than in those who did not. Of 182 patients for whom the timing of the first dose was known, 87 received surfactant within 1 hour of birth, 69 received surfactant within 1 to 6 hours, and 26 received surfactant more than 6 hours after birth. Sixty-five percent received 1 dose, 19% received 2 doses, and 29 patients received 3 or more doses. The odds of death were significantly greater for infants receiving surfactant at any time than for infants who did not receive surfactant. In infants with a prenatal diagnosis of CDH, a nonsignificant higher odds ratio of dying was linked to surfactant use. The use of surfactant within 1 hour did not change the odds ratio for patients compared with those not receiving surfactant; even infants with immediate distress who received surfactant had greater odds of death than did those who did not receive surfactant.

Conclusions.—No benefit was achieved with the use of surfactant in infants with CDHs, regardless of when the dose was administered. Preterm infants with CDHs had a lower survival rate when surfactant was given than when it was not.

▶ This article examines the survival rates in preterm infants (<37 weeks' gestation) with CDH to determine whether surfactant use by 1 hour of age results in an improved chance of survival. The laboratory and clinical data regarding surfactant deficiency in the CDH infant is inconclusive. Data on 424 infants reported to the CDH Registry were analyzed; the mean gestational age was 33.7 weeks for the group who received surfactant and 34.9 weeks for the group who did not receive surfactant. This difference in gestational age was significant ($P < .001$). After adjustment for Apgar score and gestational age, the infants who did not receive surfactant had a higher survival rate (76% vs 48%, $P = .05$). The authors conclude that surfactant use is associated with a lower survival rate in preterm infants with CDH. They acknowledge that if surfactant use was reserved for the sickest patients, its use may be a marker for the severity of illness. Nonetheless, even after adjustment for the severity of illness, no benefit was seen.

As the incidence of respiratory distress syndrome and the need for surfactant replacement varies with gestational age and only about 50% of infants born at 30 weeks need surfactant, it may be difficult to demonstrate whether surfactant is beneficial in this cohort of infants of this mean gestational age. It may have been interesting to look at the same analysis in a cohort of infants younger than 30 weeks' with CDH.

K. P. Van Meurs, MD

Timing of Initial Surfactant Treatment for Infants 23 to 29 Weeks' Gestation: Is Routine Practice Evidence Based?

Horbar JD, for the members of the Vermont Oxford Network (Univ of Vermont, Burlington; et al)
Pediatrics 113:1593-1602, 2004   7–7

Objective.—To describe the timing of initial surfactant treatment for high-risk preterm infants in routine practice and compare these findings with evidence from randomized trials and published guidelines.

Methods.—Data from the Vermont Oxford Network Database for infants who were born from 1998 to 2000 and had birth weights 401 to 1500 g and gestational ages of 23 to 29 weeks were analyzed to determine the time after birth at which the initial dose of surfactant was administered. Multivariate models adjusting for clustering of cases within hospitals identified factors associated with surfactant administration and its timing. Evidence on surfactant timing from systematic reviews of randomized trials and from published guidelines was reviewed.

Results.—A total of 47 608 eligible infants were cared for at 341 hospitals in North America that participated in the Vermont Oxford Network Database from 1998 to 2000. Seventy-nine percent of infants received surfactant treatment (77.6% in 1998, 79.4% in 1999, and 79.6% in 2000). Factors that increased the likelihood of surfactant treatment were outborn birth, lower gestational age, lower 1-minute Apgar score, male gender, white race, cesarean delivery, multiple birth, or birth later in the study period. The first dose of surfactant was administered at a median time after birth of 50 minutes (60 minutes in 1998, 51 minutes in 1999, and 42 minutes in 2000). Over the 3-year study period, inborn infants received their initial dose of surfactant earlier than outborn infants (median time: 43 minutes vs 79 minutes). Other factors associated with earlier administration of the initial surfactant dose were gestational age, lower 1-minute Apgar score, cesarean delivery, antenatal steroid treatment, multiple birth, and small size for gestational age. In 2000, 27% of infants received surfactant in the delivery room. There was wide variation among hospitals in the proportion of infants who received surfactant treatment in the delivery room (interquartile range: 0%–75%), in the median time of the initial surfactant dose (interquartile range: 20-90 minutes), and in the proportion of infants who received the first dose >2 hours after birth (interquartile range: 7%–34%). Six systematic reviews of randomized trials of surfactant timing were identified. No national guidelines addressing the timing of surfactant therapy were found.

Conclusion.—Although the time after birth at which the first dose of surfactant is administered to infants 23 to 29 weeks' gestation decreased from 1998 to 2000, in 2000 many infants still received delayed treatment, and delivery room surfactant administration was not routinely practiced at most units. We conclude that there is a gap between evidence from randomized controlled trials that supports prophylactic or early surfactant administration and what is actually done in routine practice at many units.

▶ This study addresses the issues of evidence-based medicine in a nontraditional manner. The authors examined the changes in the timing of surfactant administration within the ever-expanding multinational Vermont Oxford Network over a 3-year period. They compared practice within the Network with the available evidence base (many systematic reviews of randomized trials of surfactant timing, but no national guidelines). Whereas they found reluctance on the part of most units to administer surfactant prophylactically in the delivery room (as evidence suggests for infants ≤29 weeks), the trend over time was to administer the surfactant earlier (median, 60 minutes in 1998 and 42 minutes in 2000).

The authors carefully documented the changes over time but were reluctant to pass judgment or make firm recommendations. They did, however, remind the readers that most of the surfactant trials were completed in an era characterized by low utilization of antenatal corticosteroids (somewhere in the order of 20%), whereas today between 80% and 90% of the extremely low birth weight infants are the beneficiaries of these agents. Should the parameters for surfactant administrations be the same?

The answer is unclear! The authors emphatically state "We do not claim there is a single correct policy or guideline. We do suggest that there is a gap between what the evidence suggests should be done and what is actually done in routine practice at many units. It is the responsibility of each unit to review and modify its own practices in light of its interpretation of the evidence and how it applies in its unit." That is a very reasonable approach.

A. A. Fanaroff, MD

Prophylactic Nasal Continuous Positive Airways Pressure in Newborns of 28–31 Weeks Gestation: Multicentre Randomised Controlled Clinical Trial

Sandri F, for the Pneumology Study Group of the Italian Society of Neonatology (Univ of Bologna, Italy; et al)
Arch Dis Child Fetal Neonatal Ed 89:F394-F398, 2004   7–8

Background.—The role of nasal continuous positive airways pressure (nCPAP) in the management of respiratory distress syndrome in preterm infants is not completely defined.

Objective.—To evaluate the benefits and risks of prophylactic nCPAP in infants of 28–31 weeks gestation.

Design.—Multicentre randomised controlled clinical trial.

Setting.—Seventeen Italian neonatal intensive care units.

Patients.—A total of 230 newborns of 28–31 weeks gestation, not intubated in the delivery room and without major malformations, were randomly assigned to prophylactic or rescue nCPAP.

Interventions.—Prophylactic nCPAP was started within 30 minutes of birth, irrespective of oxygen requirement and clinical status. Rescue nCPAP was started when FIO_2 requirement was > 0.4, for more than 30 minutes, to maintain transcutaneous oxygen saturation between 93% and 96%. Exogenous surfactant was given when FIO_2 requirement was > 0.4 in nCPAP in the presence of radiological signs of respiratory distress syndrome.

Main Outcome Measures.—Primary end point: need for exogenous surfactant. Secondary end points: need for mechanical ventilation and incidence of air leaks.

Results.—Surfactant was needed by 22.6% in the prophylaxis group and 21.7% in the rescue group. Mechanical ventilation was required by 12.2% in both the prophylaxis and rescue group. The incidence of air leaks was 2.6% in both groups. More than 80% of both groups had received prenatal steroids.

Conclusions.—In newborns of 28–31 weeks gestation, there is no greater benefit in giving prophylactic nCPAP than in starting nCPAP when the oxygen requirement increases to a FIO_2 > 0.4.

Randomized Study of Nasal Continuous Positive Airway Pressure in the Preterm Infant With Respiratory Distress Syndrome

Tooley J, Dyke M (Norfolk and Norwich Univ, England)
Acta Paediatr 92:1170-1174, 2003   7–9

Aim.—To evaluate whether very preterm babies can be extubated successfully to nasal continuous positive airway pressure (nCPAP) within one hour of birth after receiving one dose of surfactant in the treatment of respiratory distress syndrome (RDS).

Methods.—Forty-two infants of 25 to 28^{+6} wk of gestation were intubated at birth and given one dose of surfactant. They were then randomized within one hour of birth to either continue with conventional ventilation or to be extubated to nCPAP.

Results.—Eight out of 21 (38%) babies randomized to nCPAP did not require subsequent reventilation. (Ventilation rates of 62% vs 100%, $p = 0.0034$). The smallest baby successfully extubated weighed 745 g. There were also significantly fewer infants intubated in the nCPAP group at 72 h of age (47% vs 81%, $p = 0.025$). There was no significant difference between the two groups in the number of babies that died, developed chronic lung disease or severe intraventricular haemorrhage.

Conclusion.—A significant number of very preterm babies with RDS can be extubated to nCPAP after receiving one dose of surfactant. nCPAP is a potentially useful modality of respiratory support even in very premature infants.

▶ Some 35 years after its introduction into the neonatal arena the role of nCPAP in the management of RDS in preterm infants is not completely defined. In part this has been due to the changed landscape as a result of widespread use of antenatal corticosteroids and the availability of surfactant therapy. As very few infants now die, the end points in trials become need for mechanical ventilation and, in the Sandri et al trial, need for surfactant therapy. Sandri et al reported that in infants with gestational ages between 28 and 31 weeks, prophylactic nCPAP was not superior to starting nCPAP when the oxygen requirement exceeded an Fio_2 of 0.4 as determined by need for surfactant or mechanical ventilation. In both groups approximately 22% of the infants received surfactant. Tooley and Dyke documented that infants intubated for surfactant, but rapidly extubated (by 1 hour), were less likely to need prolonged ventilation. These were both small trials, and larger trials with similar principles but different end points are underway. The proof of the pudding remains in the eating—the unit at Columbia that preferentially uses nCPAP has continued to report the lowest rates of bronchopulmonary dysplasia among hundreds of neonatal ICUs within the Vermont Oxford Network.

A. A. Fanaroff, MD

How Safe Is Intermittent Positive Pressure Ventilation in Preterm Babies Ventilated From Delivery to Newborn Intensive Care Unit?
Tracy M, Downe L, Holberton (Sydney Univ)
Arch Dis Child Fetal Neonatal Ed 89:F84-F87, 2004   7–10

Objectives.—To examine whether clinically determined ventilator settings will produce acceptable arterial blood gas values on arrival, in preterm infants ventilated from delivery to the newborn intensive care unit (NICU). Further, to examine the usefulness of tidal volume and minute ventilation measurements at this time.

Design.—A prospective observational cohort study in a tertiary level 3 NICU.

Patients.—Twenty six preterm infants requiring intubation and mechanical ventilation at the point of delivery to the NICU.

Setting.—Infants who required mechanical ventilation were monitored with a blinded Ventrak 1550 dynamic lung function monitor from the point of delivery to the NICU. A Drager Babylog 2000 transport ventilator was set up to achieve adequate chest wall movement, and FIO(2) was adjusted to achieve preductal SaO_2 of 90-98%. Dynamic lung function monitoring data were recorded and related to the arterial blood gas taken on arrival.

Results.—Mean gestation was 28 weeks (range 23-34) and mean birth weight was 1180 g (range 480-4200). A quarter (26% (95% confidence interval (CI) 12% to 48%)) were hypocarbic, with 20% (95% CI 7% to 39%) below 25 mm Hg, and 38% (95% CI 20% to 60%) had hyperoxia. Some (20% (95% CI 7% to 39%)) were both hypocarbic and hyperoxic. Total minute ventilation per kilogram correlated significantly with the inverse of $PaCO_2$ (p < 0.001).

Conclusions.—Clinically determining appropriate mechanical ventilation settings from the point of delivery to the NICU is difficult, and inadvertent overventilation may be common. Severe hyperoxia can occur in spite of adjustment of the FIO_2 concentration to achieve an SaO_2 range of 90-98%. Limiting minute ventilation during resuscitation may prevent hypocarbia.

▶ These investigators looked at infants who required assisted ventilation from the time of delivery until they reached the neonatal ICU. They used predetermined intermittent positive pressure ventilation settings of 18/5 cm H_2O, inspiratory time of 0.3 seconds, and a rate of 60/min. The inspiratory and expiratory pressures were increased or decreased to achieve acceptable chest wall excursion and oxygenation. They then adjusted the FIO_2 based on pulse oximeter readings and measured arterial blood gases when the baby arrived in the neonatal ICU. The results were not encouraging. A quarter of the babies were hypocarbic, and 1 in 5 had PCO_2 levels below 25 mm Hg. Thirty-eight percent of the infants were hyperoxic, and 20% were both hypocarbic and hyperoxic. A disturbing finding was the observation that in the presence of hypocarbia, pulse oximetry appeared to underestimate the oxygen saturation so that hyperoxia was a significant risk in these infants.

These observations are sobering, and it is certain that we don't do any better (and probably a lot worse) with manual bag ventilation. These investigators have performed a very useful service by providing us with data suggesting that we need to pay more attention to the manner in which we provide assisted ventilation between the delivery room and arrival in the neonatal ICU.

M. J. Maisels, MB, BCh

Predicting Extubation Outcome in Preterm Newborns: A Comparison of Neural Networks With Clinical Experience and Statistical Modeling
Mueller M, Wagner CL, Annibale DJ, et al (Med Univ of South Carolina, Charleston)
Pediatr Res 56:11-18, 2004   7–11

Even though ventilator technology and monitoring of premature infants has improved immensely over the past decades, there are still no standards for weaning and determining optimal extubation time for those infants. Approximately 30% of intubated preterm infants will fail attempted extubation, requiring reintubation and resuming of mechanical ventilation. A machine-learning approach using artificial neural networks (ANNs) to aid in extubation decision making is hereby proposed. Using expert opinion, 51 variables were identified as being relevant for the decision of whether to extubate an infant who is on mechanical ventilation. The data on 183 premature infants, born between 1999 and 2002, were collected by review of medical charts. The ANN extubation model was compared with alternative statistical modeling using multivariate logistic regression and also with the clinician's own predictive insight using sensitivity analysis and receiver operating characteristic curves. The optimal ANN model used 13 parameters and achieved an area under the receiver operating characteristic curve of 0.87 (out-of-sample validation), comparing favorably with multivariate logistic regression. It also compared well with the clinician's expertise, which raises the possibility of being useful as an automated alert tool. Because an ANN learns directly from previous data obtained in the institution where it is to be used, this makes it particularly amenable for application to evidence-based medicine. Given the variety of practices and equipment being used in different hospitals, this may be particularly relevant in the context of caring for preterm newborns who are on mechanical ventilation.

▶ Extubation failure is a common problem, occurring in nearly 40% of extremely low birth weight infants. Mueller et al have adopted a novel machine-learning approach using ANNs to aid in extubation decision. Starting with 51 variables and after applying them to 183 preterm infants, they boiled them down to 13 parameters. They were able to achieve an area under the receiver operating characteristic curve of 0.87, which compared well with the clinician's expertise. The model is institution specific and will require validation but is an intriguing approach to a common problem that has not had a satisfactory evidence-based approach.

Henry Halliday,[1] from Ireland, searched the Cochrane Library for systematic reviews of randomized controlled trials of interventions to facilitate extubation and reduce postextubation atelectasis. Not shy to come up with recommendations, he concluded that "nasal CPAP (NCPAP), nasal intermittent positive pressure ventilation (NIPPV) and methylxanthines are evidence-based treatments to facilitate weaning and extubation of preterm infants but only the first 2 can be recommended for routine use." Impressively, with these modalities the number needed to treat to see a benefit are 6 for NCPAP, 3 for NIPPV, and

4 for methylxanthines. He went on to say "chest physiotherapy and dexamethasone may be effective but should not be used routinely because of serious adverse effects." Most units would accept some of these recommendations but would continue to use methylxanthines. This is reinforced by recent data from a randomized trial in Australia. Steer et al[2] compared 2 doses of caffeine citrate to facilitate extubation. There was greater success with a dosing regimen of 20 mg/kg per day for preterm infants less than 30 weeks' gestation. Importantly, there was no evidence of harm in the first year of life. The Steer et al trial will no doubt please fellow Australians Henderson-Smart and Davis,[3] who, on the basis of a Cochrane review, concluded that methylxanthines increase the chances of successful extubation of preterm infants within 1 week. They had further recommended caffeine as the xanthine of choice, with stratification by gestational age rather than birth weight (a good idea) and neurodevelopmental status to be included as an outcome.

A. A. Fanaroff, MD

References

1. Halliday HL: What interventions facilitate weaning from the ventilator? A review of the evidence from systematic reviews. *Paediatr Respir Rev* 5(suppl A):S347-S352, 2004.
2. Steer P, Flenady V, Shearman A, et al: Caffeine Collaborative Study Group Steering Group. High dose caffeine citrate for extubation of preterm infants: A randomised controlled trial. *Arch Dis Child Fetal Neonatal Ed* 89:F499-F503, 2004.
3. Henderson-Smart DJ, Davis PG: Prophylactic methylxanthines for extubation in preterm infants. *Cochrane Database Syst Rev* 1:CD000139, 2003.

A Randomized Trial of Early Versus Standard Inhaled Nitric Oxide Therapy in Term and Near-Term Newborn Infants With Hypoxic Respiratory Failure

Konduri GG, for the Neonatal Inhaled Nitric Oxide Study Group (Med College of Wisconsin, Milwaukee; Case Western Reserve Univ, Cleveland, Ohio; Univ of Texas, Dallas; et al)
Pediatrics 113:559-564, 2004   7–12

Introduction.—Inhaled nitric oxide (iNO) decreases the rate of extracorporeal membrane oxygenation (ECMO) use and mortality in term and near-term neonates with severe hypoxic respiratory failure. Term and near-term infants were evaluated in a prospective, randomized, double-masked, multicenter trial to determine whether early administration of iNO in neonatal respiratory failure results in additional decreases in the incidence of ECMO use and mortality.

Methods.—Neonates born at 34 weeks' gestation or more were enrolled when they needed assisted ventilation and had an oxygenation index (OI) of at least 15 but less than 25 on any 2 measurements during a 12-hour interval. Infants were randomly assigned to treatment with either early iNO or stimulated initiation of iNO (control subjects). Infants with an OI increased to 25 or more received iNO as standard therapy.

TABLE 4.—Oxygenation Responses to Initial Administration of Study Gas

Variable	Early iNO Group	Control Group	P Value
Response to 5 ppm, n (%)			
No. of infants	145	147	
Complete	84 (58)	36 (24)	.001*
Partial	12 (8)	13 (9)	
None	49 (34)	98 (67)	
Change in Pao$_2$ (mm Hg)†	44 (6 to 111)	8.5 (−8 to 54)	<.0001
Change in OI†	−6.1 (−12 to −1)	−2.2 (−8 to 3)	.0001
Response to 20 ppm, n (%)‡			
No. of infants	50	105	
Complete	18 (36)	19 (18)	.002*
Partial	12 (24)	15 (14)	
None	20 (40)	71 (68)	
Change in Pao$_2$ (mm Hg)†	11 (−3 to 39)	4 (−16 to 28)	.17
Change in OI†	−2.7 (−7 to 1)	−1.6 (−5 to 7)	.17

*Composite P value for each dose by Cochrane-Armitage test for categorical factors with ordered variables.
†Data are medians with first to third quartile ranges shown in parentheses.
‡Infants who had a ≤20 mm Hg increase in Pao$_2$ in response to 5 ppm of study gas (61 early iNO/111 control infants) were eligible to receive the 20-ppm dose. However, 50 early iNO and 105 control infants actually received the 20-ppm dose. Eight of 11 infants in the early iNO group and 5 of 6 infants in the control group who did not receive a trial of 20 ppm of study gas were exited from study gas to standard iNO therapy for rapid deterioration in clinical status. Three of 11 infants in the early iNO and 1 of 6 infants in the control group had discontinuation of study gas for a period of time because of acute deterioration and were later treated with standard iNO.
Abbreviations: iNO, Inhaled nitric oxide; OI, oxygenation index.
(Reproduced by permission of *Pediatrics*, courtesy of Konduri GG, for the Neonatal Inhaled Nitric Oxide Study Group: A randomized trial of early versus standard inhaled nitric oxide therapy in term and near-term newborn infants with hypoxic respiratory failure. *Pediatrics* 113:559-564, 2004.)

Results.—Trial enrollment was ceased after 75% of the target sample size was achieved because of reduced availability of eligible patients. The 150 infants who received early iNO and 149 control infants had similar baseline characteristics. Arterial oxygen tension rose by more than 20 mm Hg in 73% of the early iNO group and in 37% of control subjects after study gas initiation (Table 4). Control subjects received standard iNO and had their OI deteriorate to more than 40 more often than did infants who received early iNO (Table 5). Both groups were similar in the incidence of death (early iNO, 6.7% vs control, 9.4%), ECMO (10.7% vs 12.1%), and their combined incidence (16.7% vs 19.5%).

TABLE 5.—Secondary Outcomes of the Study

Variable	Early iNO Group (N = 150)	Control Group (N = 149)	P Value
Duration of study gas administration, h*	57 ± 48	39 ± 38	<.003
Initiation of standard iNO therapy, n (%)*	61 (41)	81 (54)	<.02
Duration of standard iNO therapy, h†	121 (41-175)	100 (56-158)	.52
Progression to OI >40, n (%)	11 (7)	21 (14)	.056

*Data are mean ± SD.
†Data are shown as medians with first to third quartile ranges in parentheses.
Abbreviations: iNO, Inhaled nitric oxide; OI, oxygenation index.
(Reproduced by permission of *Pediatrics*, courtesy of Konduri GG, for the Neonatal Inhaled Nitric Oxide Study Group: A randomized trial of early versus standard inhaled nitric oxide therapy in term and near-term newborn infants with hypoxic respiratory failure. *Pediatrics* 113:559-564, 2004.)

Conclusion.—Inhaled NO improves oxygenation yet does not decrease the incidence of ECMO and mortality when initiated at an OI of 15 to 25 versus initiation at greater than 25 in term and near-term neonates with respiratory failure.

▶ I am not quite sure what to take away from this study. It seems that the earlier use of iNO, as defined by the OI at entry, resulted in a trend toward fewer babies exceeding an OI of 40 but did not decrease the primary study end points of death or the need for ECMO. In addition, the number of days of mechanical ventilation, duration of oxygen therapy, and length of the hospital stay were no different between the iNO and control groups. The study had some unique features, such as the entry criterion of "hypoxic respiratory failure" and not persistent pulmonary hypertension of the newborn (PPHN), and the use of a lower than usual dose of iNO to try to establish a dose–response relationship.

Is the OI a reasonable way to assess the effectiveness of iNO? One might argue that, because PPHN was not an entry criterion, some measure of improved oxygenation was a reasonable surrogate. However, for changes in the OI to be interpreted, information regarding the mean airway pressure and the fraction of inspired oxygen also need to be provided. Are we comfortable with the comparability of mean airway pressure measurements during conventional and high-frequency oscillatory ventilation?

I presume that most, if not all, the infants had postductal arterial blood gas monitoring through an umbilical artery catheter. The significant rise in PaO_2 in the early iNO group suggests that it could be directly related to reduced pulmonary vascular resistance, improved pulmonary blood flow, and decreased right-to-left shunting. It would have been nice to have had echocardiographic data to see whether stratification of responders and nonresponders was, in fact, related to the degree of PPHN present at study entry.

The authors should be commended for not making specific recommendations until the 18- to 24-month follow-up data are available. Even so, I am not sufficiently convinced after reading this article to alter my conclusion about this population.

S. M. Donn, MD

Impact of a Physiologic Definition on Bronchopulmonary Dysplasia Rates
Walsh MC, for the National Institute of Child Health and Human Development Neonatal Research Network (Case Western Reserve Univ, Cleveland, Ohio; et al)
Pediatrics 114:1305-1311, 2004   7–13

Introduction.—Bronchopulmonary dysplasia (BPD) is the end point for many intervention trials in neonatology. Yet, outcome measures based solely on oxygen administration may be confounded by varying criteria for oxygen administration among physicians. Reported is the use of a physiologic definition of BPD based on oxygen-saturation monitoring in selected infants in low oxygen to determine if the use of the physiologic definition would reduce the variation in observed BPD rates among various neonatal centers.

Methods.—A total of 1598 consecutive inborn premature infants (501-1249 g birth weight) from 17 centers who remained hospitalized at 36 weeks' postmenstrual age were prospectively evaluated and assigned an outcome by using both a clinical and physiologic definition of BPD. The clinical definition of BPD (Fig 1) was oxygen supplementation at exactly 36 weeks' postmenstrual age; the physiologic definition was assigned at 36 weeks' postmenstrual age and included 2 distinct subpopulations. Neonates on positive pressure support or receiving more than 30% supplemental oxygen with saturations between 90% and 96% were assigned to outcome BPD and were evaluated no further. Neonates receiving 30% or less oxygen or effective oxygen more than 30% with saturations of more than 96% underwent a room-air challenge that involved continuous observation and oxygen-saturation monitoring. The outcomes of the room-air challenge were either

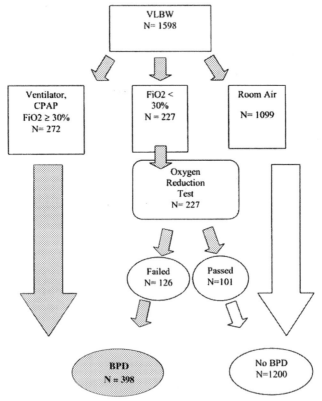

FIGURE 1.—Respiratory outcomes of the physiologic definition of BPD at 36 weeks' postmenstrual age. *Abbreviations: CPAP*, Continuous positive airway pressure; *VLBW*, very low birth weight. (Courtesy of Walsh MC, for the National Institute of Child Health and Human Development Neonatal Research Network. Impact of a physiologic definition on bronchopulmonary dysplasia rates. *Pediatrics* 114:1305-1311, 2004. Reproduced by permission of *Pediatrics*.)

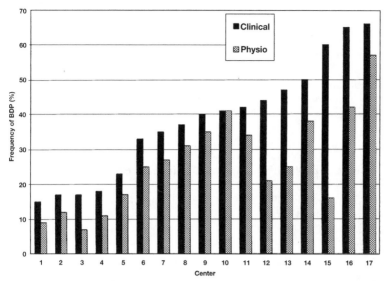

FIGURE 2.—Comparison of BPD rate by the clinical definition and physiologic definition of BPD at each center. The overall reduction in mean BPD rate (*P* < .0001) and the reduction in variation (*P* < .01) between centers are both significant. (Courtesy of Walsh MC, for the National Institute of Child Health and Human Development Neonatal Research Network. Impact of a physiologic definition on bronchopulmonary dysplasia rates. *Pediatrics* 114:1305-1311, 2004. Reproduced by permission of *Pediatrics*.)

"no BPD" (saturations ≥90% during weaning and in room air for 30 minutes) or "BPD" (saturation <90%). At completion of the room-air challenge, all neonates were returned to their baseline oxygen levels. Safety (apnea, bradycardia, increased oxygen use) and outcomes of the physiologic definition versus clinical definition were evaluated.

Results.—A total of 560 (35.0%) neonates were diagnosed with BPD by the clinical definition and 298 (25.5%) were diagnosed by the physiologic definition. All neonates were evaluated safely. There were substantial differences in the impact of the definition on BPD rates among centers (mean reduction, 10%; range, 0.44%). Sixteen centers had a reduction in their BPD rate and 1 had no change (Fig 2).

Conclusion.—The use of the physiologic definition of BPD decreased the overall rate of BPD and decreased the variation among centers. Significant differences were observed among centers in the impact of the physiologic definition; differences remained when using this standardized definition. The magnitude of the change in BPD rate was comparable to that of the magnitude of treatment effects observed in some clinical trials of BPD. The physiologic definition of BPD facilitates the measurement of BPD as an outcome in clinical trials, along with the comparison between and within centers over time.

▶ When one considers the controversy among neonatologists regarding the parameters for supplemental oxygen therapy, it is not surprising that the current clinical definition of BPD is so imprecise. The demonstration that a physiology-based definition decreases both the incidence of BPD diagnosis and diminishes interhospital variations is especially troubling because of its implications for previously published and subsequently influential treatment studies, such as those involving the use of pharmacologic dosages of vitamin A.

The authors have provided a very valuable study. By developing a standard physiologic diagnosis of BPD, they are supplying an essential tool for meaningful interpretation of future prevention and treatment studies.

D. B. DeWitte, MD

Increased Lung Water and Tissue Damage in Bronchopulmonary Dysplasia

Adams EW, Harrison MC, Counsell SJ, et al (Imperial College, London; Queen Mary's Univ Hosp, London)

J Pediatr 145:503-507, 2004   7–14

Introduction.—The incidence of bronchopulmonary dysplasia (BPD) is increasing with improvement in the survival of extremely preterm infants. MRI was used to determine whether water content is increased and unevenly distributed in preterm infants with BPD and whether lesions are distributed homogeneously within the lung.

Methods.—Thirty-five preterm infants (23-35 weeks' gestation) were scanned at or after 28 days postnatal age. Of these, 7 had evidence of respiratory distress syndrome at birth. They were self-ventilating in air at 28 days. Thirteen infants had mild BPD, were oxygen dependent at 28 days, and were self-ventilating in air at 40 weeks' gestational age. Fifteen infants had severe BPD, were oxygen dependent at 40 weeks, or died. Twenty infants underwent MRI to evaluate lung water content; MRI was used in all 35 infants to assess tissue injury. Relative proton density provided an index of water content and distribution and was compared among the 3 groups of infants, between dependent and nondependent lungs, and between rostral and caudal lungs. The location and degree of focal densities and cystlike appearances indicating lung damage were defined.

Results.—Proton density was significantly greater in dependent lung regions. The average proton density, proton density gradient, and severity of lung damage were greater among infants with severe BPD. Indicators of damage were highest in the dorsal lung regions. Bronchopulmonary dysplasia was correlated with higher lung water burden and gravity-dependent atelectasis or alveolar flooding. Lesions occurred more frequently in the dorsal lung regions in infants with severe lung damage.

Conclusion.—Infants with BPD have increased lung water. They are susceptible to gravity-induced collapse and alveolar flooding in the dependent lung. It appears that focal tissue damage is distributed nonhomogeneously.

▶ This brief report presents evidence by MRI, performed within the neonatal ICU of the Hammersmith Hospital in London, that infants with severe BPD have pulmonary edema, most apparent in dependent regions of the lung, with associated focal, nonuniform tissue damage. It's a pity that such a nifty technologic tool as MR could not tell us why these conditions develop.

It's no surprise that pulmonary edema is a prominent feature of the pathology of BPD. It has been well described in patients who have died with the disease as well as in relevant animal models. Nor is it surprising that fluid accumulates mostly in dependent portions of the lung, a finding that has been well documented in experimentally induced pulmonary edema. Less clear are the mechanisms responsible for abnormal fluid accumulation in the lungs of infants with severe BPD. Physiologic studies conducted in the cardiac catheterization lab, as well as in animal models of BPD, indicate that high filtration pressure in the pulmonary circulation contributes to interstitial edema in this disease. When infection sets in, as it often does, lung vascular and epithelial protein permeability likely increase, allowing protein-rich fluid to enter the air spaces. There is considerable experimental evidence, too, that severe hypoxemia and prolonged exposure to high inspired oxygen, which are common in severe BPD, may impair lung epithelial sodium transport and thereby contribute to liquid flooding of air spaces.

Unfortunately, this report of MR studies performed in a group of infants with BPD offers no new information to help sort out the cause of pulmonary edema in this disease, nor does it provide assurance that the images can distinguish between interstitial and alveolar fluid, or that the fluid is a transudate of plasma rather than pus or simply collapsed air spaces. MR is a fantastic method for defining noninvasively and with exquisite precision structural abnormalities of many organ systems, including the lung. But helping diagnose or define the severity of distribution of pulmonary edema is not yet on the list of MR breakthroughs. For now, all we can do is hope.

R. D. Bland, MD

Plasma 8-Isoprostane Is Increased in Preterm Infants Who Develop Bronchopulmonary Dysplasia or Periventricular Leukomalacia
Ahola T, Fellman V, Kjellmer I, et al (Helsinki Univ, Finland; Göteborg Univ, Gothenburg, Sweden; Lund Univ, Sweden)
Pediatr Res 56:88-93, 2004   7–15

Our aim was to assess the plasma free 8-epi-prostaglandin $F_{2\alpha}$ (8-isoprostane) and ascorbyl radical as risk indicators for oxidative damage in extremely low birth weight infants (ELBWIs) and the effect of N-acetylcysteine (NAC) on these markers. Plasma samples were collected on days 3 and 7 of life from infants who were enrolled in a randomized, controlled trial in which i.v. NAC or placebo was administered to ELBWIs during the first week of life, with the aim of preventing bronchopulmonary dysplasia (BPD). Plasma 8-isoprostane was analyzed in 83 infants using an enzyme immunoassay kit. Ascorbyl radical concentration was measured in 61 infants with electron spin resonance spectroscopy. The 8-isoprostane concentrations were similar in the NAC and placebo groups. In infants who later developed BPD or died ($n = 29$), the median (range) 8-isoprostane concentration was significantly higher ($p = 0.001$) on day 3 and day 7 [50.0 pg/mL (19-360) and 57.0 pg/mL (14-460), respectively] than in survivors without BPD [$n = 54$; 34.5 pg/mL (5-240) and 39.5 pg/mL (7-400), respectively]. The 8-isoprostane levels increased significantly more ($p < 0.05$) in infants who later developed periventricular leukomalacia. NAC treatment or the later development of BPD was not related to the ascorbyl radical levels. The ascorbyl radical level decreased significantly in all groups from day 3 to day 7, but the difference between the groups was not significant. The mean (SD) ascorbyl radical level on day 3 was significantly higher ($p < 0.01$) in infants who later developed periventricular leukomalacia [287 (124) versus 194 (90)]. These data suggest that plasma 8-isoprostane could serve as a marker in assessing the risk for BPD development in ELBWIs.

▶ Oxidative stress is implicated in the pathogenesis of several complications of prematurity. The glutathione cycle is one of the most important intracellular antioxidant systems. The synthesis of glutathione may not be adequate in preterm neonates because of the low levels of cysteine available. Therefore, Ahola et al[1] evaluated whether NAC infusion during the first week of life reduces the risk of death or BPD in ELBWIs. In a randomized, double-blind study in Finland, 391 infants requiring mechanical ventilation, with birth weights between 500 and 999 g, were randomly assigned by age 36 hours to receive NAC 16 to 32 mg/kg per day (n = 194) or placebo (n = 197) IV for 6 days. The primary end points were death or BPD, defined as supplementary oxygen requirement at 36 weeks' gestational age. There were no differences in the major outcomes, so we can chalk up another negative but well-intentioned neonatal randomized trial. Nevertheless, getting the most out of the trial, the authors took the opportunity to assess 8-isoprostane and ascorbyl radical as risk indicators for oxidative damage in the study patients and observe the effect of NAC on these markers. The 8-isoprostane levels rose markedly in the infants who had BPD develop or who died as well as in those who had periventricular leukomalacia develop. It takes little imagination to therefore conclude that 8-isoprostane could join the queue of cytokines and inflammatory mediators that serve as markers in assessing the risk for BPD development in ELBWIs.

A. A. Fanaroff, MD

Reference

1. Ahola T, Lapatto R, Raivio KO, et al: N-acetylcysteine does not prevent bronchopulmonary dysplasia in immature infants: A randomized controlled trial. *J Pediatr* 143:713-719, 2003.

Apoptosis and Proliferation in Lungs of Ventilated and Oxygen-Treated Preterm Infants

May M, Ströbel P, Preisshofen T, et al (Univ of Würzburg, Germany)
Eur Respir J 23:113-121, 2004   7–16

Background.—Preterm infants and neonates with respiratory distress syndrome (RDS) require oxygen therapy and exogenous surfactant therapy. However, the effect of these therapies on apoptosis and proliferation of cells in the lung has not been well studied. Apoptosis and proliferation were examined in the lungs of stillborn human fetuses and lung tissue from preterm infants with RDS exposed to mechanical ventilation and to surfactants. The involvement of caspases-3, -8, or -9 in apoptosis was also investigated.

Study Design.—The study group consisted of 29 stillborn fetuses and 27 preterm infants with RDS who received ventilator support with supplemental oxygen. Of the 27 preterm infants, 16 had surfactant therapy and 11 served as control subjects. Lung tissue sections were analyzed for the apoptotic index (AI), calculated as the percentage of nuclei that were terminal deoxynucleotidyltransferase-mediated deoxyuridine triphosphate nick end-labeling (TUNEL)-positive. The proliferation index (PI) was calculated as the percentage of cells that immunostained for Ki-67. Cleaved caspases were also detected by immunohistochemistry.

Findings.—The lung tissue of preterm infants with RDS treated by ventilation with oxygen therapy had significantly increased AI and PI compared to lung tissue from stillborn fetuses. AI and PI increased with ventilation duration. Apoptosis was primarily detected in alveolar epithelial cells, whereas epithelial, endothelial, and smooth muscle cells all had increased PI. Surfactant therapy had no significant effect on either AI or PI. Caspase-3 appeared to be involved in the pathway to apoptosis.

Conclusion.—The number of cells undergoing apoptosis and proliferation increases in the lungs of preterm infants with RDS who are treated with mechanical ventilation. Surfactant treatment was not associated with a significant effect on either AI or PI.

▶ The delicate balance between regulated cell proliferation and programmed cell death is a critical determinant of lung growth during development and the structural remodeling that occurs in response to lung injury. This report by May et al indicates that both cell proliferation and apoptosis are more prevalent in lungs of preterm infants who have died after a period of mechanical ventilation with O_2-rich gas than in stillborn fetuses delivered at roughly the same gestation (28 ± 1 weeks).

Immunolabelling studies suggested that the increased apoptosis associated with lung injury was in epithelial cells, whereas proliferation was not localized to a specific cell type. Treatment with surfactant had no apparent effect on either cell proliferation or apoptosis. These interesting observations are consistent with previous reports of increased lung epithelial cell apoptosis associated with hyperoxia, but they differ from previous reports of decreased proliferation of epithelial cells, fibroblasts, and airway smooth muscle cells exposed to hyperoxia in culture.

The important caveat here is the source of the tissues from which these studies were undertaken. One must be cautious about interpreting data acquired from postmortem histologic studies done on tissues obtained from stillborn fetuses and preterm infants who died several hours or days after birth. The cause and duration of fetal death is unknown in most stillborns, and both of these variables can influence histologic indexes of lung cell multiplication and death.

The lungs of babies who die with respiratory failure after a period of mechanical ventilation with O_2-rich gas have experienced much more than hyperoxia and different degrees of inflation. Most have been exposed to inflammation, often with associated infection, limited supply of nutrients, a variety of drugs, and severe acidosis, all of which may impact both cell proliferation and cell death. The specific impact of surfactant on these processes may be difficult to discern when death occurs several hours or days after surfactant has been given and after a host of intervening events. These concerns aside, the authors deserve a pat on the back for attempting to define important cellular processes that may go awry at a critical stage of lung development and perhaps contribute to failed formation of alveoli and pulmonary capillaries and a disordered extracellular matrix.

R. D. Bland, MD

Survival Rate in Congenital Diaphragmatic Hernia: The Experience of The Canadian Neonatal Network
Javid PJ, Jaksic T, Skarsgard ED, et al (Harvard Med School, Boston; Univ of British Columbia, Vancouver, Canada)
J Pediatr Surg 39:657-660, 2004   7–17

Background.—Congenital diaphragmatic hernias (CDHs) have continued to be associated with a significant mortality rate, despite advances in neonatal intensive care and ventilatory management. Most multicenter studies have reported a survival rate of approximately 65% for infants with CDHs. However, recent single-institution series have reported an improvement in the overall survival rate of infants with CDHs approaching 90%. This improvement has been attributed to several alterations in clinical CDH care, including gentle ventilatory management and improved nutritional support. However, no prospective multicenter data exist to validate these hypotheses. The Canadian Neonatal Network prospectively collects data from 17 pediatric hospitals accounting for 75% of all neonatal ICU beds in Canada. With the use of this database, actual survival rates of neonates with CDHs were compared with predicted outcomes, and whether the institutional CDH volume was associated with improved survival rates was assessed.

Methods.—The actual survival rates for patients with CDHs born during a 22-month period were determined from the registry. Predicted survival

TABLE 1.—Predicted and Actual CDH Survival Rates as
Stratified by Mortality Risk

Risk Category	No.	Predicted Survival Rate (%)	Actual Survival Rate (%)*
Low	46	83	95
Moderate	30	49	77
High	12	18	50

*$P < .05$.
Abbreviation: CDH, Congenital diaphragmatic hernia.
(Courtesy of Javid PJ, Jaksic T, Skarsgard ED, et al: Survival rate in congenital diaphragmatic hernia: The experience of The Canadian Neonatal Network. *J Pediatr Surg* 39:657-660, 2004.)

rates were calculated using the CDH Study Group logistical regression equation, and the actual survival rate was compared with the predicted survival rate with the use of χ^2 analysis. Survival rates were stratified by institutional CDH volume and compared with the use of binomial analysis. A *P* value of less than .05 was considered to be statistically significant.

Results.—Of the approximately 20,500 neonatal admissions in the database, 88 cases of CDH were recorded. Of the 88 neonates with CDHs, 73 (88%) survived to discharge, but the predicted survival rate was 62% (Table 1). Three centers were considered "high-volume" centers and had at least 12 CDH diagnoses; 11 centers were considered "low-volume" centers. The actual CDH survival rate was significantly greater at high-volume versus low-volume centers (90% vs 77%).

Conclusions.—These prospective data showed that the survival rates of Canadian neonates with CDHs are significantly better than those predicted by the CDH Study Group equation. Neonates at high-volume centers in Canada were also shown to have a significantly higher CDH survival rate than those at low-volume centers.

▶ This article compares CDH outcomes in the Canadian Neonatal Network to those predicted with the use of logistic regression equations developed by the CDH Study Group. These equations include birth weight and 5-minute Apgar score. The survival rate in this series of 88 infants with CDH born in a 22-month period (1996-1997) is higher than that predicted (83% vs 62%, *P* < .001). In addition, the authors noted that the survival rate at high-volume centers (>12 patients with CDH; range, 12-15) was higher than that at low-volume centers (<12 patients with CDH; range, 1-9). The authors recognize that the Canadian Neonatal Network dataset does not include infants with CDH admitted to nonneonatal ICU settings or the cohort of infants dying before admission, termed *hidden mortality*. Examination of the clinical practices at high-volume neonatal ICUs may help to determine which clinical practices are responsible for the higher survival rates seen at high-volume centers. Collaborative data collection, analysis, and clinical research are likely to benefit relatively rare conditions such as CDH by identifying the strategies responsible for improved survival rates and by creating an environment in which randomized controlled trials can occur.

K. P. Van Meurs, MD

Is Surfactant Therapy Beneficial in the Treatment of the Term Newborn Infant With Congenital Diaphragmatic Hernia?

Van Meurs K, for the Congenital Diaphragmatic Hernia Study Group (Stanford Univ, Palo Alto, Calif; et al)
J Pediatr 145:312-316, 2004   7–18

Objectives.—To determine the impact of surfactant replacement on survival, need for extracorporeal membrane oxygenation (ECMO), and chronic lung disease in term infants with prenatally diagnosed congenital diaphragmatic hernia (CDH).

Study Design.—Prenatally diagnosed infants born at ≥37 weeks' gestation with immediate distress at delivery and no other major congenital anomalies, who were enrolled in the CDH Registry, were analyzed. For univariate analysis, χ^2 tests were used for categoric variables and unpaired t tests for nominal variables. Multiple logistic regression was used to calculate adjusted odds ratios.

Results.—Eligible infants (n = 522) were identified. Demographic variables were similar between the surfactant-treated (n = 192) and nonsurfactant-treated (n = 330) groups, with the exception of race (white, 88.0% vs 71.2%; P = .0007). The use of ECMO and incidence of chronic lung disease were higher (59.8 vs 50.6, P = .04; 59.9 vs 47.6, P = .0066) and survival lower in the surfactant-treated cohort (57.3 vs 70.0, P = .0033). Adjusted logistic regression for use of ECMO, survival, and chronic lung disease resulted in odds ratios inconsistent with an improved outcome associated with surfactant use.

Conclusions.—This analysis shows no benefit associated with surfactant therapy for term infants with a prenatal diagnosis of isolated CDH.

▶ CDH remains a challenging diagnosis for neonatologists and pediatric surgeons who care for these critically ill newborns. There is little agreement on treatment protocols, underscoring the fact that many questions remain to be answered.

In the absence of randomized controlled trials, the Congenital Diaphragmatic Hernia Study Group provides valuable aggregate data on this relatively infrequent condition. In this observational study that used the CDH Study Group Registry data, the authors conclude that there is no evidence that surfactant replacement benefits term infants with prenatally diagnosed CDH with immediate respiratory distress and no other major anomalies. By univariate analysis, the use of ECMO and incidence of CLD was higher and survival lower in the surfactant-treated cohort.

The authors selected the prenatally diagnosed newborn with immediate respiratory distress to identify a population of similar severity of illness. The inclusion of all CDH infants has hampered meaningful conclusions in many CDH studies, as severity of illness may be the major factor affecting outcome, overshadowing any other factor under investigation. While there were no significant differences in the demographic variables except for race, there were significant differences in use of vasopressors, inhaled vasodilators, sedation, paralysis, alkalinization, and postnatal steroids. This suggests that the surfactant-treated group may have been more severely ill. Multivariate analysis of the risk factors for ECMO and CLD found that surfactant use was not associated with an increase in ECMO or CLD. The authors properly state that the data do not allow them to conclude that surfactant causes worse outcomes but that surfactant therapy provides no benefit.

K. P. Van Meurs, MD

How Low Can You Go? Effectiveness and Safety of Extracorporeal Membrane Oxygenation in Low-Birth-Weight Neonates

Rozmiarek AJ, Qureshi FG, Cassidy L, et al (Univ of Pittsburgh, Pa; Univ of Michigan, Ann Arbor)

J Pediatr Surg 39:845-847, 2004   7–19

Background.—Extracorporeal membrane oxygenation (ECMO) has been shown to be a life-saving therapy in patients with respiratory failure. The experience with ECMO in neonates is extensive, but controversy continues regarding the criteria for infants of low birth weight who may benefit from ECMO. Current guidelines suggest that ECMO should not be used in infants less than 2.0 kg because of a perceived high risk of intracranial hemorrhaging (ICH). However, the concept of a weight threshold for bleeding has been challenged in recent studies. Whether ECMO is a safe and therapeutic intervention for infants weighing less than 2 kg was investigated. The outcomes and survival rates of these infants were also examined.

Methods.—The study group was composed of all patients younger than 30 days old in the Extracorporeal Life Support Organization (ELSO) registry (14,305 patients). These patients were divided into those less than 2 kg (663 patients) and those more than 2 kg (13,462 patients). Multiple regres-

TABLE 3.—Statistically Significant ($P < .05$) Univariate Variables Related to Survival in LBW (≤2.0 kg) and HBW (>2.0 kg) Neonates on ECMO

Factor	LBW Survive	LBW Not Survive	HBW Survive	HBW Not Survive
Variable				
Age (d)	3.1 ± 4.3	4.1 ± 5.8	2.0 ± 4.7	2.7 ± 4.5
Hours on ECMO	161 ± 101	202 ± 177	145.3 ± 86.7	212.8 ± 167
APGAR at 5min	6.9 ± 2.0	6.6 ± 2.2	7.0 ± 2.1	6.6 ± 2.4
Initial pco$_2$	42.6 ± 21.4	51.7 ± 26.2	40.3 ± 18.7	48.4 ± 25.7
Overall Survival Rate	53%		77%*	

Note: Data are mean ± SD.
*$P < .05$.
Abbreviations: LBW, Low birth weight; *HBW*, high birth weight; *ECMO*, extracorporeal membrane oxygenation.
(Courtesy of Rozmiarek AJ, Qureshi FG, Cassidy L, et al: How low can you go? Effectiveness and safety of extracorporeal membrane oxygenation in low-birth-weight neonates. *J Pediatr Surg* 39:845-847, 2004.)

sion analysis was used to determine factors that were predictive of survival and the lowest safe weight for ECMO.

Results.—The overall survival rate was 76%, but this rate was lower in infants less than 2 kg. The survival rate was significantly lower for patients with diaphragmatic hernias, bleeding, and ICH, as determined by regression analysis. The incidence of ICH in infants less than 2.0 kg was 6% versus 4% in those more than 2.0 kg. Regression analysis indicated that the lowest weight at which a survival rate of 40% could be obtained was 1.6 kg (Table 3).

Conclusions.—Cannulation for ECMO may be safe and effective in infants weighing less than 2.0 kg and may be potentially safe and effective in infants weighing as little as 1.6 kg. Bleeding, which occurred in a minority of patients in this study, may be limited by the careful use of anticoagulation therapy.

▶ Rozmiarek et al review the international experience with ECMO in infants weighing less than 2 kg using the ELSO Registry data from 1991 to 2002. They report that the survival rate in the cohort weighing less than 2 kg when compared with that in the cohort weighing more than 2 kg is lower (53% vs 77%, $P < .0001$) and that ICH rates are higher (6% vs 4%, $P < .05$). They note that the ELSO data show a survival rate of 40% in infants with a birth weight of 1.6 kg or more, and they conclude that ECMO cannulation may be relatively safe and effective in babies weighing less than 2 kg. Hirschl et al,[1] using ELSO Registry data in a prior study, have also found that a birth weight of less than 2 kg significantly decreases the probability of survival when compared with a birth weight of more than 2 kg (65% vs 83%, $P < .001$). Two issues are critical: oxygenation index criteria used for ECMO eligibility no longer identify a cohort with an 80% mortality because of improvements in neonatal intensive care, and birth weight may not accurately predict the risk of ICH and mortality because of the inclusion of small-for-gestational-age infants in the ELSO Registry. A review of the ELSO data regarding survival and ICH risk demonstrates that mortality and ICH rates are more tightly correlated with gestational age than they are with birth weight. Decisions regarding the utilization of ECMO in low birth weight infants should include a consideration of gestational age and the risk of death with continued intensive care in a specific infant, even though this may be difficult to predict.

K. P. Van Meurs, MD

Reference

1. Hirschl RB, Schumacher RE, Snedecor SN, et al: The efficacy of extracorporeal life support in premature and low birth weight newborns. *J Pediatr Surg* 28:1336-1340, 1993.

Congenital Diaphragmatic Hernia Repair on Extracorporeal Life Support: A Decade of Lessons Learned

Austin MT, Lovvorn HN III; Feurer ID, et al (Vanderbilt Univ, Nashville, Tenn)
Am Surg 70:389-395, 2004   7–20

Background.—A congenital diaphragmatic hernia (CDH) is still a highly dangerous condition, despite numerous advances in prenatal and neonatal care in recent years. Mortality rates have remained near 50% in babies with CDHs who require extracorporeal membrane oxygenation (ECMO) because of the difficulties in controlling pulmonary hypertension, a result of pulmonary hyperplasia and its associated reduced alveolar surface area and increased pulmonary vascular resistance. The use of ECMO and delayed repair of CDH has dramatically improved survival rates in many series; however, controversy continues regarding the optimal timing of repair for babies who require ECMO and the use of either a venovenous (VV) or a venoarterial (VA) bypass. Both modalities have been shown to be efficacious, but no clear survival advantage has been shown for either modality. The outcomes of infants who underwent repair of CDHs while receiving ECMO were assessed at one institution.

Methods.—A retrospective review was conducted of all infants (n = 30) treated with CDH repair while receiving ECMO at one center between 1992 and 2003.

Results.—Of these patients, 18 were supported by VV and 12 were supported by VA bypass. Transfusion requirements while receiving ECMO were increased 2-fold postoperatively (15-33 mL/kg per day) and then were significantly decreased after decannulation (1.5 mL/kg per day). Nonintracranial hemorrhaging occurred in 7 infants (23%), and intracranial hemorrhaging occurred in 3 (10%). There were 12 deaths (40%), including 1 infant receiving ECMO secondary to refractory pulmonary hypertension. The mean length of stay for the 18 infants who survived (60%) was 48 days.

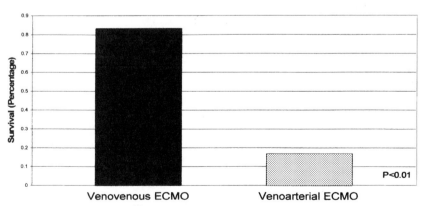

FIGURE 2.—Survival rate was significantly increased in patients receiving venovenous bypass (*P* < .01). *Abbreviation: ECMO*, Extracorporeal membrane oxygenation. (Courtesy of Austin MT, Lovvorn HN III, Feurer ID, et al: Congenital diaphragmatic hernia repair on extracorporeal life support: A decade of lessons learned. *Am Surg* 70:389-395, 2004.)

Comparisons between survivors and nonsurvivors showed a significantly increased mortality rate for infants who were supported by VA bypass (Fig 2). However, no other variable was predictive of survival.

Conclusions.—Repair of CDHs while infants are receiving ECMO is technically feasible. The survival rate in this study was similar to that of the Extracorporeal Life Support Organization (ELSO) registry, and CDH repair in infants who require ECMO was associated with few bleeding complications.

▶ Austin et al describe the practice of repairing CDH in infants on ECMO at a single center with 30 cases over a 10-year period and attempt to determine which clinical factors and practices influence survival. They report that transfusion requirements of infants on ECMO double after repair, patients with a VA bypass have a higher mortality rate, and patients with a VV bypass have higher transfusion requirements. They conclude that CDH repair in infants on ECMO is relatively safe because the survival rate seen for their patients is above the average reported to the ELSO Registry. The authors believe that the favorable results reported with delayed repair in several articles are possibly secondary to selection bias. The interpretation of data in this article suffers from a lack of randomization as well as a small sample size, which makes it difficult to come to any conclusion regarding their practices. The severity of pulmonary hypoplasia is probably the chief determinant of survival in CDH infants, and unfortunately, this variable is not easily measured. Data analysis on the utility of various treatments in CDH infants is flawed unless it compares infants whose conditions are of equivalent severity.

K. P. Van Meurs, MD

Cost Effectiveness Analysis of Neonatal Extracorporeal Membrane Oxygenation Based on Four Year Results From the UK Collaborative ECMO Trial

Petrou S, Edwards L (Univ of Oxford, England)
Arch Dis Child Fetal Neonatal Ed 89:F263-F268, 2004   7–21

Objective.—To assess the cost effectiveness of extracorporeal membrane oxygenation (ECMO) for mature newborn infants with severe respiratory failure over a four year time span.

Design.—Cost effectiveness analysis based on a randomised controlled trial in which infants were individually allocated to ECMO (intervention) or conventional management (control) and then followed up to 4 years of age.

Setting.—Infants were recruited from 55 approved recruiting hospitals throughout the United Kingdom. Infants allocated to ECMO were transferred to one of five specialist regional centres. Follow up of surviving infants was performed in the community.

Subjects.—A total of 185 mature (gestational age at birth ≥ 35 weeks, birth weight ≥2000 g) newborn infants with severe respiratory failure (oxygenation index ≥40).

Main Outcome Measures.—Incremental cost per additional life year gained; incremental cost per additional disability-free life year gained.

Results.—Over four years, the policy of neonatal ECMO was effective at reducing known death or severe disability (relative risk = 0.64; 95% confidence interval 0.47 to 0.86; p = 0.004). After adjustment for censoring and discounting at 6%, the mean additional health service cost of neonatal ECMO was £17367 (95% confidence interval £12072 to £22224) per infant (£UK, 2001 prices). Over four years, the incremental cost of neonatal ECMO was £16707 (£9828 to £37924) per life year gained and £24775 (£13106 to £69690) per disability-free life year gained. These results remained robust after variations in the values of key variables performed as part of a sensitivity analysis.

Conclusions.—The study provides rigorous evidence of the cost effectiveness of ECMO at four years for mature infants with severe respiratory failure.

▶ This study follows previous studies of the randomized, controlled trial of ECMO conducted in the United Kingdom in 1993. Four-year follow-up demonstrated impressive decreases in mortality rate (33% in the ECMO vs 59% in the conventional group) and increases in disability-free survival (50% vs 37%). This study explores the question of whether the additional expense required to achieve these improved outcomes was worth it. The key here is not the tabulation of costs, an essential analytical step that was exquisitely accomplished by these researchers, but rather coming to grips with the notion of worth. Their approach was to determine the cost of each additional year of life gained and also the cost of each disability-free year of life gained from ECMO and then plot these against willingness-to-pay thresholds. In England a new technology is considered cost effective if the cost of each of these outcomes is less than £30,000. For ECMO, each year gained cost well under this threshold (£16,700 per additional year and £24,800 per additional disability-free year). In reflecting on this study, the quandary for U.S. neonatologists is not how to translate pounds into dollars, but rather deciding how much we should be willing to spend on a new technology to gain an additional disability-free year of life.

J. B. Gould, MD, MPH

The Pediatric Investigators Collaborative Network on Infections in Canada Study of Predictors of Hospitalization for Respiratory Syncytial Virus Infection for Infants Born at 33 Through 35 Completed Weeks of Gestation

Law BJ, Langley JM, Allen U, et al (Univ of Manitoba, Winnipeg, Canada; Dalhousie Univ, Halifax, Canada; Hosp for Sick Children, Toronto; et al)
Pediatr Infect Dis J 23:806-814, 2004   7–22

Introduction.—Infants born at 33 through 35 weeks' gestation are at increased risk for severe respiratory syncytial virus (RSV) infection. The risk for hospitalization for RSV infection can be lowered by as much as 80% with palivizumab prophylaxis. Approximately 3% to 5% of annual births are among infants who are 33 to 35 weeks' gestation. The American Academy of Pediatrics guidelines recommend restricting prophylaxis to infants with 2 or more risk factors, including child-care attendance, preschool-aged siblings, exposure to environmental air pollutants, congenital abnormalities of the airways, or severe neuromuscular disease. Independent risk factors for hospitalization for RSV infection were assessed in a multicenter, prospective, observational cohort investigation of 33 to 35 weeks' gestation infants followed through their first RSV season (2001-2002 or 2002-2003).

Methods.—Baseline data were obtained during parent interview and review of medical records. Respiratory tract illnesses were documented at the time of monthly follow-up calls. Medical records were reviewed for emergency department visits or hospitalizations.

Results.—Of 1860 enrolled infants, 1832 (98.5%) were followed up for at least 1 month; 1760 (94.6%) completed all follow-ups. Of 140 (7.6%) who were hospitalized for respiratory tract illnesses, 66 had proven RSV infection. Independent predictors for hospitalization for RSV infection included day-care attendance (odds ratio [OR], 12.32; 95% confidence interval [CI], 2.56-59.34); November through January birth (OR, 4.89; 95% CI, 2.57-9.29); preschool-aged sibling(s) (OR, 2.76; 95% CI, 1.51-5.03); birth weight less than tenth percentile (OR, 2.19; 95% CI, 1.14-4.22); male sex (OR, 1.91; 95% CI, 1.10-3.31); 2 or more smokers in the home (OR, 1.87; 95% CI, 1.0703.26); and households with more than 5 people, including the research subject (OR, 1.79; 95% CI, 1.02-3.16). Family history of eczema (OR, 0.42; 95% CI, 0.18-0.996) was a protective factor.

Conclusion.—Specific host/environmental factors may be used to identify which infants aged 33 to 35 weeks' gestation are at highest risk for hospitalization for RSV infection and likely to benefit from prophylaxis with palivizumab.

▶ Every year we go through the cycle of RSV infection in our pediatric units. The majority of infants who require admission with RSV are healthy, term newborns but, although much smaller in number, it is the preterm newborns who are at the greatest risk. Prophylaxis with palivizumab significantly reduces the risk of hospitalization with RSV infection, and the American Academy of Pediatrics recommendations for its use in infants born at 32 weeks of gestation or earlier have been widely adopted. We would also like to give palivizumab to infants of 33 to 35 weeks of gestation, but the numbers make the cost prohibitive. Thus, the American Academy of Pediatrics recommends that prophylaxis be restricted to infants who have risk factors such as child-care attendance, school-aged siblings, exposure to environmental air pollutants, congenital anomalies of the airways, or severe neuromuscular disease. Although these risks are considered to be additive,[1] there is, currently, no evidence to support this belief.

In an attempt to better define the risks for RSV infection in infants born at 33 to 35 weeks of gestation, the Canadian investigators undertook a multicenter study to identify independent risk factors for hospitalization with RSV infection. They collected data prospectively from 16 pediatric centers across Canada during 2 winter respiratory seasons. In a German study,[2] the risk of hospitalization varied from a low of 0.4% for premature infants with no other risk factors to a high of 55.9% for male premature infants with chronic lung disease discharged between October and December to a home with 1 or more siblings attending day care.

We now need to prospectively evaluate a population of infants before discharge for the risk factors noted in this article. We could assign a risk score based on the odds ratios and then document the actual incidence of admission with RSV disease. In this way we can better define the risk of hospitalization for RSV infection and provide improved guidelines for the use of palivizumab prophylaxis in infants of 33 to 35 weeks of gestation.

M. J. Maisels, MD

C. J. E. Pryce, MD

References

1. American Academy of Pediatrics Committee on Infectious Diseases and Committee on Fetus and Newborn: Revised indications for the use of palivizumab and respiratory syncytial virus immune globulin intravenous for the prevention of respiratory syncytial virus infection. *Pediatrics* 112:1442-1446, 2003.
2. Liese JG, Grill E, Fischer B, et al: Incidence and risk factors of respiratory syncytial virus-related hospitalizations in premature infants in Germany. *Eur J Pediatr* 162:230-236, 2003.

8 Central Nervous System and Special Senses

General Neurology

The Scottish Perinatal Neuropathology Study: Clinicopathological Correlation in Early Neonatal Deaths

Becher JC, Bell JE, Keeling JW, et al (Univ of Edinburgh, Scotland; Royal Hosp for Sick Children, Edinburgh, Scotland)
Arch Dis Child Fetal Neonatal Ed 89:F399-F407, 2004   8–1

Background.—Lethal malformations, prematurity, and birth asphyxia are the 3 major causes of neonatal death. The first 2 may be considered by the public to be unavoidable circumstances, but birth asphyxia implies a lack of care during labor. However, a proportion of neonatal deaths from asphyxia have been shown in other studies to be associated with pre-existing brain injuries. In the current study, epidemiologic characteristics of infants displaying signs of birth asphyxia were compared with those not showing signs; the neuropathologic features of birth asphyxia were also determined and, if possible, the timing of the brain insult was compared between those infants who had and had not asphyxiated. In addition, the clinical features of infants who had died of birth asphyxia with and without prelabor damage were compared.

Methods.—This study was conducted among 22 Scottish delivery units over a 2-year period. Clinical details were collected on early neonatal deaths. Requests for postmortem examinations included separate requests for detailed neuropathologic examinations of the brain. The infants included in the study were classified into 2 groups—those who had died of birth asphyxia and those who had died of other causes (Fig 1). Clinicopathologic correlation was used to determine the time of the brain insult.

Results.—Detailed clinical data were available for 137 of 174 early neonatal deaths that met the criteria for inclusion. From this group, 70 of 88 parents who had agreed to postmortem examination consented to a detailed examination of additional samples from the brain. In 53 of these cases, the

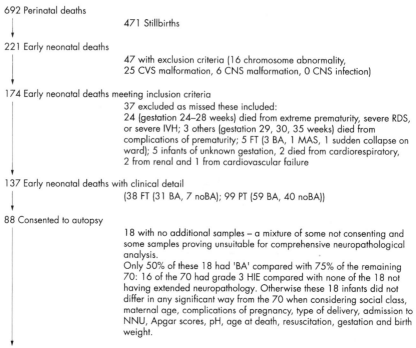

692 Perinatal deaths

    471 Stillbirths

221 Early neonatal deaths

    47 with exclusion criteria (16 chromosome abnormality,
    25 CVS malformation, 6 CNS malformation, 0 CNS infection)

174 Early neonatal deaths meeting inclusion criteria

    37 excluded as missed these included:
    24 (gestation 24–28 weeks) died from extreme prematurity, severe RDS,
    or severe IVH; 3 others (gestation 29, 30, 35 weeks) died from
    complications of prematurity; 5 FT (3 BA, 1 MAS, 1 sudden collapse on
    ward); 5 infants of unknown gestation, 2 died from cardiorespiratory,
    2 from renal and 1 from cardiovascular failure

137 Early neonatal deaths with clinical detail

    (38 FT (31 BA, 7 noBA); 99 PT (59 BA, 40 noBA))

88 Consented to autopsy

    18 with no additional samples – a mixture of some not consenting and
    some samples proving unsuitable for comprehensive neuropathological
    analysis.
    Only 50% of these 18 had 'BA' compared with 75% of the remaining
    70: 16 of the 70 had grade 3 HIE compared with none of the 18 not
    having extended neuropathology. Otherwise these 18 infants did not
    differ in any significant way from the 70 when considering social class,
    maternal age, complications of pregnancy, type of delivery, admission to
    NNU, Apgar scores, pH, age at death, resuscitation, gestation and birth
    weight.

70 Consented to additional study samples

    53 BA   17 noBA

23 FT   30 PT   3 FT   14 PT

           Died ≤ 3 days

21 FT   25 PT   2 FT   11 PT

PND noPND   PND noPND   PND noPND   PND noPND
13 (62%) 8 (38%)   13 (52%) 12 (48%)   1   1   0   11

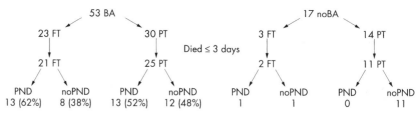

FIGURE 1.—The Scottish perinatal deaths cohort. *Abbreviations: FT*, Full term; *RDS*, respiratory distress syndrome; *PT*, preterm < 37 weeks; *IVH*, intraventricular hemorrhage; *BA*, birth asphyxia; *MAS*, meconium aspiration syndrome; *noBA*, no birth asphyxia; *HIE*, hypoxic–ischemic encephalopathy; *PND*, prenatal brain damage; *NNU*, neonatal unit; *noPND*, no prenatal brain damage; *CVS*, cardiovascular system. (Courtesy of Becher JC, Bell JE, Keeling JW, et al: The Scottish perinatal neuropathology study: Clinicopathological correlation in early neonatal deaths. *Arch Dis Child Fetal Neonatal Ed* 89:F399-F407, 2004, with permission from the BMJ Publishing Group.)

infant was born in an asphyxiated condition. Damage consistent with the onset of asphyxia before the start of labor was present in all the asphyxiated infants, in 38% of the mature and in 52% of the preterm infants with features of birth asphyxia but without encephalopathy, and in only 1 of 12 infants without any signs of birth asphyxia (Tables 1 and 2).

Conclusions.—Brain injury was found to predate the onset of labor in a large proportion of neonatal deaths. Prelabor brain injuries are more common in infants born in an asphyxiated condition.

TABLE 1.—Timing of Injury to the Central Nervous System After Cerebral Insult

Pathological Feature	Timing of Onset After Injury	References
Neuronal eosinophilia	6-24 hours	60-62
Neuronal karyorrhexis	12-48 hours	61, 63-65
Infarcts—necrosis	3-8 hours	60, 65, 66
Infarcts—cavitation	14-42 days	65-68
White matter gliosis	3-11 days	31, 32, 58, 60, 61, 65, 67, 69, 70
Grey matter gliosis	3-5 days	30, 63, 68, 71
Microglial upregulation	3 hours-3 days	60, 61, 66, 67, 71
Macrophage infiltration	3-7 days	63, 65-68
Fresh haemorrhage	Minutes	67
Haemosiderin deposits	2-3 days	27, 67, 72
Mineralisation	3-14 days	58, 60, 65, 67

(Courtesy of Becher JC, Bell JE, Keeling JW, et al: The Scottish perinatal neuropathology study: Clinicopathological correlation in early neonatal deaths. *Arch Dis Child Fetal Neonatal Ed* 89:F399-F407, 2004, with permission from the BMJ Publishing Group.)

▶ This review of a 2-year period of all 22 Scottish delivery units is a useful benchmark for determining the cause of neonatal deaths associated with asphyxia. The bottom line is that many of these neonatal asphyxial deaths are associated with pre-existing brain injuries. A weakness of the study is that only half (51%) of 137 eligible infants had detailed neuropathologic investigations. A major assumption is that focal or diffuse astrocytic hyperplasia and parenchymal macrophage accumulation represent cellular reactions that require 3 days to become established. If this were assumed, then most of the infants

TABLE 2.—Clinical Features of Birth Asphyxia in 137 Early Neonatal Deaths

Features of Asphyxia	Full Term	Preterm
Total number of infants	38	99
Single feature only		
Apgar ≤ 5 at 5 min	9	35
Cord pH < 7.1	0	1
1st pH < 7.1	1	8
NNE	1	0
Two features		
Low Apgar and low pH	7	9
Low Apgar and NNE	2	1
Low pH and NNE	0	1
Three features		
Low pH, low Apgar, and NNE	11	4
Total with some indication of asphyxia	31 (82%)	59 (60%)

Note: All infants had a 5-minute Apgar score. Only 12 full-term infants and 11 preterm infants had cord pH measured. An additional 22 full-term infants and 35 preterm infants had the pH measured on arrival in the local neonatal unit. Sixteen full-term infants at 12 hours of age were not paralyzed, and 14 of these had features of an encephalopathy. Nineteen preterm infants remained alive and nonparalyzed at 12 hours; 6 had an encephalopathy.

Abbreviation: NNE, Neonatal encephalopathy.

(Courtesy of Becher JC, Bell JE, Keeling JW, et al: The Scottish perinatal neuropathology study: Clinicopathological correlation in early neonatal deaths. *Arch Dis Child Fetal Neonatal Ed* 89:F399-F407, 2004, with permission from the BMJ Publishing Group.)

with features of birth asphyxia must have sustained brain damage prenatally, including all 8 in the full-term encephalopathic group. The implications for surviving infants are also uncertain. Because many asphyxiated infants have no evidence of pre-existing brain damage and infants who are not asphyxiated at birth often display only recent postnatal damage, the hope is that some individuals might be "rescued" by such therapies as hypothermia. Nonetheless, others are clearly beyond rescue when they present. The importance of the Scottish findings is that they suggest that the "asphyxiated" encephalopathic infant may not necessarily represent mismanagement of labor or lack of vigilance in the pregnancy.

D. K. Stevenson, MD

Early Experience Alters Brain Function and Structure
Als H, Duffy FH, McAnulty GB, et al (Harvard Med School, Boston; Univ of Geneva; Brigham and Women's Hosp, Boston)
Pediatrics 113:846-857, 2004   8–2

Introduction.—There is increasing evidence that features of brain structure and function are different between medically healthy preterm infants and their term counterparts when evaluated at comparable age points. Although some differences may be explained by the cumulative effect of minor medical complications linked with premature birth, the infant's sensory experience in the newborn ICU environment—including exposure to bright lights, high sound levels, and frequent noxious interventions—may have deleterious effects on the immature brain and alter its subsequent development.

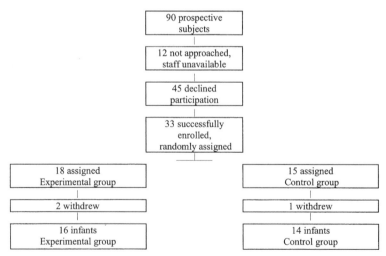

FIGURE 1.—Subject-selection process. (Reproduced by permission of *Pediatrics* courtesy of Als H, Duffy FH, McAnulty GB, et al: Early experience alters brain function and structure. *Pediatrics* 113:846-857, 2004.)

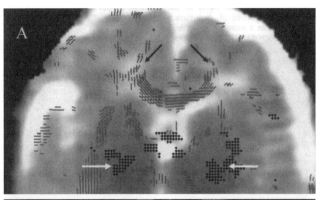

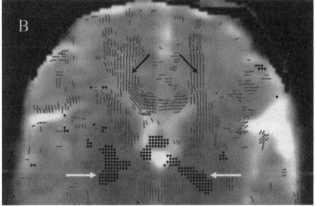

FIGURE 3.—MRI diffusion tensor imaging: Comparison of control and experimental group infants at 2 weeks' corrected age. Shown are examples of diffusion tensor maps from identical axial slices through the frontal lobes of a representative control group (**A**) and an experimental group (**B**) infant obtained at 2 weeks' corrected age. In each example, the principal eigenvectors (shown in *gray* and *black*) overlie the apparent diffusion coefficient map to show anisotropy in white matter. The *gray lines* denote eigenvectors located within the plane of the image, and the *black dots* indicate eigenvectors oriented mostly perpendicular to the image plane. The ratio of E1//E3 has been used as a threshold to show only eigenvectors at those voxels where E1/E3 exceeds a threshold value of 1.3 in both images. Note the greater anisotropy of white matter found in the experimental infant (**B**) as compared with the control infant (**A**) at the posterior limbs of the internal capsule (*white arrows*) and the frontal white matter adjacent to the corpus callosum (*black arrows*). The greater anisotropy found in the experimental infant (**B**) suggests more advanced white matter development in these regions as compared with white matter found in the control infant (**A**). (Reproduced by permission of *Pediatrics* courtesy of Als H, Duffy FH, McAnulty GB, et al: Early experience alters brain function and structure. *Pediatrics* 113:846-857, 2004.)

The effects of early experience on brain function and structure were examined in a randomized, clinical trial.

Methods.—The neurodevelopmental effectiveness of the Newborn Individualized Developmental Care and Assessment Program (NIDCAP) was examined in 30 preterm infants, 28 to 33 weeks' gestational age at birth, who were free of known developmental risk factors (Fig 1). The NIDCAP was started within 72 hours of ICU admission and continued to age 2 weeks, corrected for prematurity.

TABLE 3.—Assessment of Preterm Infants' Behavior System and
Prechtl Scores at 2 Weeks' Corrected Age

Variable	Control (n = 14)	Experimental (n = 16)	P
APIB system scores			
Autonomic system	5.56 (1.41)	4.59 (1.26)	.06
Motor system	6.29 (1.01)	4.70 (1.23)	.001‡
State system	5.22 (1.34)	4.62 (0.90)	.12
Attention system	6.91 (1.83)	6.54 (1.69)	.58
Self-regulation system	6.11 (1.26)	4.94 (1.07)	.01†
Examiner facilitation	6.89 (1.76)	5.74 (1.67)	.08
Prechtl scores			
Trunk and limb posture (0-6)	2.21 (1.31)	0.81 (1.05)	.004*
Motility (0-2)	1.07 (0.48)	0.50 (0.73)	.02
Pathological movements (0-11)	3.79 (1.48)	1.50 (1.46)	.002*
Motor system tone (0-2)	1.00 (0.00)	0.63 (0.62)	—
Intensity of responses (0-2)	0.85 (0.36)	0.25 (0.45)	.0004†
Threshold of responses (0-1)	0.85 (0.36)	0.44 (0.51)	.02
Moro response (0-2)	1.47 (0.75)	0.38 (0.62)	.002*
State stability (0-1)	0.86 (0.63)	0.38 (0.50)	.005*
Crying (0-2)	0.93 (0.48)	0.69 (0.48)	.18
Hemisyndrome (0-14)	2.32 (2.27)	1.50 (2.56)	.36
Syndromes abnormal reactivity (0-2)	1.16 (0.62)	0.56 (0.73)	.03
Total Prechtl (percent abnormal)	38.30 (9.55)	17.33 (15.52)	.0001†

Note: Shown are Assessment of Preterm Infants Behavior (*APIB*) system scores at 2 weeks' corrected age (range, 1-9; lower scores denote more appropriate responses) and Prechtl scores (ranges shown in *parentheses*; lower scores denote more appropriate responses). Multivariate analysis of variance (*MANOVA*) for the APIB: F = 3.19; df = 6,23; P = .02; MANOVA for the Prechtl: F = 3.35; df = 12,17; P = .01. Data shown are means (standard deviation). Probabilities in **bold type** indicate significant differences (Holm's correction).
*P < .05.
†P < .01.
‡P < .001.
(Reproduced by permission of *Pediatrics* courtesy of Als H, Duffy FH, McAnulty GB, et al: Early experience alters brain function and structure. *Pediatrics* 113:846-857, 2004.)

Fourteen control subjects and 16 infants in the experimental group were evaluated at 2 weeks' and 9 months' corrected age in measures of health status, growth, and neurobehavior (the Assessment of Preterm Infants' Behavior and the Prechtl Neurologic Examination of the Fullterm Newborn Infant). At 2 weeks' corrected age, they underwent electroencelographic spectral coherence, MR diffusion tensor imaging (Fig 3), and measurements of transverse relaxation time.

Results.—The groups were medically and demographically comparable before and after treatment. The experimental group demonstrated significantly better neurobehavioral functioning (Table 3), increased coherence between frontal and a broad spectrum of mainly occipital brain regions, and higher relative anisotropy in the left internal capsule, with a trend for right internal capsule and frontal white matter (Table 5). Transverse relaxation time did not differ between groups.

Behavioral function was improved at 9 months' corrected age (Table 4). The association among the 3 neurodevelopmental domains was significant. Consistently better function and more mature fiber function was observed for infants in the experimental versus the control group.

TABLE 5.—Magnetic Resonance Diffusion Tensor
Imaging at 2 Weeks' Corrected Age

Variable	Control ($n = 8$)	Experimental ($n = 15$)	P
RA			
Frontal white matter	12.03 (2.76)	14.66 (4.52)	.10
Right internal capsule	35.20 (6.98)	41.54 (7.14)	.06
Left internal capsule	35.18 (4.30)	40.19 (5.31)	.03
Corpus callosum	40.43 (11.79)	40.23 (12.69)	.97
Ratio of E1/E3			
Frontal white matter	1.27 (0.08)	1.35 (0.13)	.09
Right internal capsule	1.98 (0.25)	2.25 (0.34)	.05
Left internal capsule	1.96 (0.13)	2.17 (0.21)	**.008***
Corpus callosum	2.18 (0.55)	2.17 (0.52)	.99

Note: Higher scores represent more mature fiber tract development. Multivariant analysis of variance (*MANOVA*) for RA: F = 2.85 (2-tailed); df = 4.18; $P = .05$; MANOVA for the ratio of E1/E3: F = 2.88 (2-tailed); df = 4,18; $P = .05$. Data shown are means (standard deviation). Probabilities in *bold type* indicate significant differences (Holm's correction).
*$P < .05$.
†$P < .01$.
‡$P < .001$.
(Reproduced by permission of *Pediatrics* courtesy of Als H, Duffy FH, McAnulty GB, et al: Early experience alters brain function and structure. *Pediatrics* 113:846-857, 2004.)

TABLE 4.—Bayley II at 9 Months' Corrected Age

Variable	Control ($n = 13$)	Experimental ($n = 11$)	P
Mental scale			
MDI	94.85 (9.22)	109.55 (7.23)	.0002‡
MDI < 100/≥ 100, percentile	69/31	9/91	.003†
Percentile	39 (20)	72 (15)	.0002‡
Age equivalent, mo	8.39 (1.19)	10.27 (0.79)	.0001‡
Motor scale			
PDI	89.23 (14.88)	107.00 (9.28)	.002†
PDI < 100/ ≥ 100, percentile	77/23	9/91	.003†
Percentile	31 (21)	67 (20)	.0004†
Age equivalent, mo	8.00 (1.53)	9.91 (0.70)	.0009†
BRS, percentile			
Orient/engagement	57 (28)	71 (22)	.19
Emotional regulation	39 (27)	67 (23)	.01*
Motor quality	23 (22)	57 (32)	.007*
Total score	39 (23)	73 (16)	.0004†

Note: Multivariate analysis of variance (*MANOVA*) of mental developmental index (*MDI*), psychomotor developmental index (*PDI*), and 4 Behavior Rating Scale (*BRS*); F = 3.59 (2-tailed); df = 6,17; $P = .027$. Data shown are means (standard deviation). Probabilities shown in *bold type* indicate significant differences (Holm's correction). MDI and PDI: mean = 100; standard deviation = 15.
*$P < .05$.
†$P < .01$.
‡$P < .001$.
(From Als H, Duffy FH, McAnulty GB, et al: Early experience alters brain function and structure. *Pediatrics* 113:846-857, 2004. Courtesy of Bayley N: *Bayley Scales of Infant Development*, ed 2. San Antonio, Tex, Psychological Corporation, 1993.)

Conclusion.—This is the first in vivo evidence of enhanced brain function and structure via the NIDCAP. The quality of experience before term may significantly impact brain development.

▶ NIDCAP has had a debated impact on developmental and behavioral outcomes. This study is also challenged because of its sample size and the fact that the experiment is necessarily unmasked. Nonetheless, the findings are provocative and consistent with our understanding of how early behavioral interventions might impact the developing nervous system, not only in terms of its function but its actual structure. In fact, structure and function are always inextricably intertwined in development, and that there is an observable change in structure associated with a change in a function is not surprising.

What is supported by the observations is that the impact of complex behavioral programs can be consequential and measurable in terms of function and structure. Thus, all interventions that we undertake, as well as the unintended influences of the environments we create for our patients, need to be carefully considered, perhaps even systematically studied, as important contributors to long-term neurodevelopmental outcome.

D. K. Stevenson, MD

Sounds and Silence: An Optical Topography Study of Language Recognition at Birth
Peña M, Maki A, Kovačić D, Dehaene-Lambertz G, et al (Internatl School for Advanced Studies, Trieste, Italy; Hitachi Advanced Research Lab, Saitama, Japan; École des Hautes Études en Sciences Sociales, Paris; et al)
Proc Natl Acad Sci U S A 100:11702-11705, 2003   8–3

Does the neonate's brain have left hemisphere (LH) dominance for speech? Twelve full-term neonates participated in an optical topography study designed to assess whether the neonate brain responds specifically to linguistic stimuli. Participants were tested with normal infant-directed speech, with the same utterances played in reverse and without auditory stimulation. We used a 24-channel optical topography device to assess changes in the concentration of total hemoglobin in response to auditory stimulation in 12 areas of the right hemisphere and 12 areas of the LH. We found that LH temporal areas showed significantly more activation when infants were exposed to normal speech than to backward speech or silence. We conclude that neonates are born with an LH superiority to process specific properties of speech.

▶ The work of Peña et al, published in one of the most prestigious journals, not only has a catchy title but also deals with sophisticated technology and unequivocally provides the answer to the question "Does the neonate's brain have LH dominance for speech?" The authors are to be complimented on this outstanding report, which demonstrated that, indeed, the LH lights up in response to normal speech. A PubMed search revealed no other similar articles in the neonate. I guess this becomes a landmark publication.

De Regnier et al[1] at Northwestern University evaluated the effects of post-conceptional age and postnatal experience on the development of neonatal auditory recognition memory in a group of preterm infants tested at 35 to 38 weeks' postconceptional age and less than 1 week old and 2 groups of term infants, the first less than a week old and the second group aged 8 to 30 days. They observed that the development of recognition of the maternal voice correlated with postconceptual age, but there were qualitative effects of postnatal experience. These near-term infants at least recognized their mothers' voices.

Therien et al[2] evaluated the effects of extreme prematurity on the neural pathway for auditory recognition memory by using event-related potentials. Because infants must be able to detect and discriminate sounds before recognizing them, 2 paradigms were used to assess these functions. The first evaluated the detection and discrimination of speech sounds. The second tested recognition of the mother's voice compared with a stranger's. Infants with no evidence of major imaging abnormalities were used, but despite this the preterm infants demonstrated no evidence of maternal voice recognition and significant other differences from the term infants. They commented that "No specific patterns of auditory detection or discrimination were associated with patterns of recognition memory, suggesting that the function of multiple neural pathways may have been altered in this group of preterm infants. These results provide a functional corroboration of magnetic resonance imaging studies showing effects of prematurity on early brain development, even among preterm infants with normal cranial ultrasonography." The facts speak for themselves, but the findings are nonetheless distressing. One can merely speculate whether these pathways can be induced by more intense input from the mother. Should we be playing recordings of the parents' voices in the isolette rather than the current lullabies or rock music?

A. A. Fanaroff, MD

References

1. deRegnier RA, Wewerka S, Georgieff MK, et al: Influences of postconceptional age and postnatal experience on the development of auditory recognition memory in the newborn infant. *Dev Psychobiol* 41:216-225, 2002.
2. Therien JM, Worwa CT, Mattia FR, et al: Altered pathways for auditory discrimination and recognition memory in preterm infants. *Dev Med Child Neurol* 46:816-824, 2004.

Frequency and Natural History of Subdural Haemorrhages in Babies and Relation to Obstetric Factors

Whitby EH, Griffiths PD, Rutter S, et al (Univ of Sheffield, England; Univ of Hull, England; Central Sheffield Teachings Hosps, England)
Lancet 363:846-851, 2004   8–4

Background.—Subdural haematomas are thought to be uncommon in babies born at term. This view is mainly based on findings in symptomatic neonates and babies in whom subdural haemorrhages are detected fortuitously. We aimed to establish the frequency of subdural haemorrhages in asymptomatic term neonates; to study the natural history of such subdural haematomas; and to ascertain which obstetric factors, if any, are associated with presence of subdural haematoma.

Methods.—We did a prospective study in babies who were born in the Jessop wing of the Central Sheffield University Hospitals between March, 2001, and November, 2002. We scanned neonates with a 0.2 T magnetic resonance machine.

Findings.—111 babies underwent MRI in this study. 49 were born by normal vertex delivery without instrumentation, 25 by caesarean section, four with forceps, 13 ventouse, 18 failed ventouse leading to forceps, one failed ventouse leading to caesarean section, and one failed forceps leading to caesarean section. Nine babies had subdural haemorrhages: three were normal vaginal deliveries (risk 6.1%), five were delivered by forceps after an attempted ventouse delivery (27.8%) (Fig 2), and one had a traumatic ventouse delivery (7.7%). All babies with subdural haemorrhage were assessed clinically but no intervention was needed. All were rescanned at 4 weeks and haematomas had completely resolved.

Interpretation.—Presence of unilateral and bilateral subdural haemorrhage is not necessarily indicative of excessive birth trauma.

▶ Traumatic injury to the neonatal brain is now much less common than in previous decades. Surprisingly, subdural hemorrhage occurs more frequently than intraventricular or subarachnoid hemorrhage often associated with instrumental and assisted deliveries (forceps or vacuum) but, as noted by the authors, relatively most commonly with spontaneous vaginal delivery. Breysen et al[1] documented 4 cases in which blunt abdominal trauma during pregnancy caused fetal cranial injury, including 1 subdural hemorrhage. Haase et al[2] added a case in which subdural hemorrhage followed a traumatic delivery by cesarean section.

The report from Whitby et al, based on MRI scanning, documents many more cases of subdural hemorrhage than would have been recognized clinically. Selection bias includes the fact that many parents refused the study because they had to wait 48 hours for the neonatal MRI. And some parents may have consented because of a perception that their labor was difficult and therefore something may be wrong with the baby. Furthermore, the high proportion of babies delivered by forceps after failed vacuum may create bias toward a higher incidence of subdural hemorrhages in the cohort. Reassuringly,

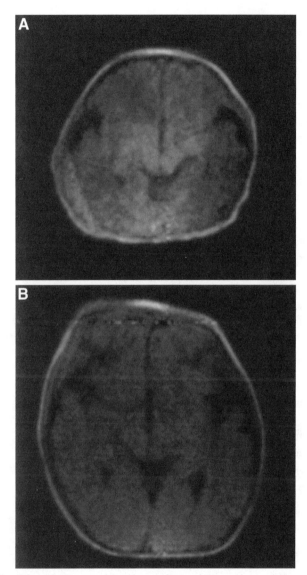

FIGURE 2.—Baby with (**A**) acute subdural haemorrhage and (**B**) complete resolution at 4 weeks. This neonate was delivered by forceps after an attempted ventouse delivery. (Courtesy of Whitby EH, Griffiths PD, Rutter S, et al: Frequency and natural history of subdural haemorrhages in babies and relation to obstetric factors. *Lancet* 363:846-851, 2004. Reprinted with permission from Elsevier.)

none of the babies needed intervention and the hemorrhages had resolved when rescanned at age 4 weeks, and all the babies were clinically normal at 2 years of age. This reinforces the notion that subdural hemorrhage rarely causes significant long-term damage. This MRI exercise also provides evidence to support their conclusion that "the presence of unilateral and bilateral subdural hemorrhage is not necessarily indicative of excessive birth trauma." Now let's make the plaintiff lawyers aware of this concept.

A. A. Fanaroff, MD

References

1. Breysen L, Cossey V, Mussen E, et al: Fetal trauma: Brain imaging in four neonates. *Eur Radiol* 14:1609-1614, 2004.
2. Haase R, Kursawe I, Nagel F, et al: Acute subdural hematoma after caesarean section: A case report. *Pediatr Crit Care Med* 4:246-248, 2003.

Placental Fetal Thrombotic Vasculopathy Is Associated With Neonatal Encephalopathy

McDonald DGM, Kelehan P, McMenamin JB, et al (Royal College of Surgeons in Ireland, Dublin; Univ College, Dublin; Natl Maternity Hosp, Dublin, Ireland)

Hum Pathol 35:875-880, 2004   8–5

Neonatal encephalopathy (NE) remains an important cause of morbidity and mortality in the term infant, and many cases have an antepartum, rather than an intrapartum, etiology. Chronic processes such as thrombosis result in changes in the placenta. We sought to determine whether histopathological examination of the placenta in cases of NE, focusing on these changes, could identify significant antenatal processes that are not recognized by clin-

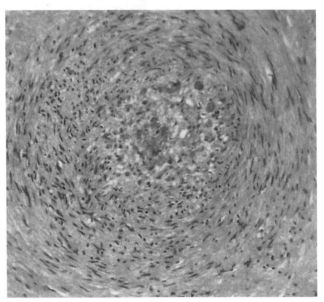

FIGURE 2.—A fetal stem artery shows hemorrhagic endovasculitis, with fibrosis of the lumen, red cell fragmentation, and partial recanalization. (Courtesy of McDonald DGM, Kelehan P, McMenamin JB, et al: Placental fetal thrombotic vasculopathy is associated with neonatal encephalopathy. *Hum Pathol* 35:875-880, 2004.)

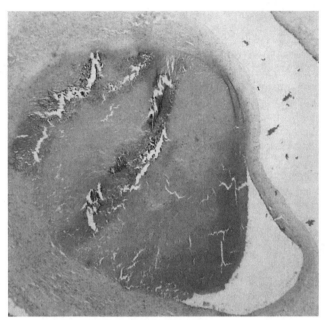

FIGURE 4.—A chorionic plate vessel shows almost total occlusion by a partly calcified thrombus. (Courtesy of McDonald DGM, Kelehan P, McMenamin JB, et al: Placental fetal thrombotic vasculopathy is associated with neonatal encephalopathy. *Hum Pathol* 35:875-880, 2004.)

ical assessment alone. Infants born at term with NE were identified retrospectively over a 12-year period. Placental tissue from deliveries during the study period was available for reexamination (Figs 2 and 4). Controls were selected from a cohort of 1000 consecutive deliveries on which clinical and pathological data were collected as part of an earlier study. Bivariate and multivariate analyses of clinical and pathological factors for cases and controls were used to test for an independent association with NE. Clinical and placental data was collected on 93 cases of NE and 387 controls. The placental features of fetal thrombotic vasculopathy (FTV), funisitis (signifying a fetal response to infection), and accelerated villous maturation were independently associated with NE. Of the clinical factors studied, meconium-stained liquor and abnormal cardiotocograph were independently associated. There were no independently associated clinical antenatal factors. Placental features of infection, thrombosis, and disturbed uteroplacental flow are significant independent factors in the etiology of NE in this study. Acute and chronic features suggest that NE may result from acute stress in an already compromised infant. The absence of significant clinical antenatal factors supports the value of placental examination in the investigation of infants with NE.

▶ The placenta is often the forgotten evidence that may provide definitive and ultimate clues to the etiology of NE. Not only may it explain the course of events, but it could also save millions of dollars in lawsuits. As a large proportion of the cases of severe NE will land in law offices and many in the courts, it is prudent to ensure that the placental examination becomes an integral part of the medical record. This examination should be performed by an EXPERIENCED PLACENTAL PATHOLOGIST. The findings must be incorporated into the medical record and the discharge diagnosis reflect these observations. In this manner many cases will be deflected from the legal system.

McDonald et al reviewed the placental pathology on 93 cases of NE and matched them with 387 controls. Meconium-stained amniotic fluid and an abnormal fetal heart rate tracing were the clinical features associated with NE, but otherwise the antenatal history was noninformative.

There were distinctive placental pathologic features (including fetal thrombotic vasculopathy, funisitis, and accelerated villous maturation) independently associated with NE. fetal thrombotic vasculopathy signifies a chronic thrombotic process within the fetal vasculature, and I liked the analogy that the placental vessels are as much a part of the fetal circulation as the deep leg veins are of an adult. The placental pathology was consistent with the findings of Redline and O'Riordan[1] from our own institution. Having an expert placental pathologist such as Redline is an invaluable asset for the maternal-fetal, neonatal-perinatal team. It is the equivalent of having an exclusive with Sherlock Holmes. He adds breadth and depth to the interpretation of the placenta and will either directly make the diagnosis or point the clinicians in the right direction.

A. A. Fanaroff, MD

Reference

1. Redline R, O'Riordan MA: Placental lesions associated with cerebral palsy and neurologic impairment following term birth. *Arch Pathol Lab Med* 124:1785-1791, 2000.

Neonatal Cerebral White Matter Injury in Preterm Infants Is Associated With Culture Positive Infections and Only Rarely With Metabolic Acidosis
Graham EM, Holcroft CJ, Rai KK, et al (Johns Hopkins Univ, Baltimore, Md; Ross Med School, Dominica, West Indies)
Am J Obstet Gynecol 191:1305-1310, 2004   8–6

Background.—Neonatal cerebral white matter injury, characterized by periventricular leukomalacia and ventricular dilatation, is a common precursor of neurologic impairment and cerebral palsy. The risk factors associated with the development of neonatal cerebral white matter injury were examined in this retrospective case-control study.

Study Design.—The study group consisted of 150 cases of white matter injury at a single institution between May 1994 and September 2001. Each case was matched to a control subject by using the next delivery of the same gestational age at that institution. Cases and controls were compared to determine risks for white matter injury.

Findings.—There were no differences between the 2 groups in number of cesarean births or umbilical arterial pH (metabolic acidosis). Case patients had a significant increase in positive blood, CSF, and tracheal cultures during the neonatal period. Conditional logistic regression indicated a significant association between multiple gestations, intraventricular hemorrhage, positive tracheal cultures, and cerebral white matter injury.

Conclusion.—Although intrapartum hypoxia-ischemia, chorioamionitis, and funisitis were not associated with cerebral white matter injury in this study, neonatal infection was.

▶ Well, there is good news and bad news in our attempts to predict and prevent CNS injury in preterm infants. The good news for obstetricians is that in this study, intrapartum hypoxia was not related to the development of white matter injury. The incidence of white matter injury was similar in patients with and without metabolic acidosis.

The bad news is that the current popular belief that chorioamnionitis is a major contributing factor to neonatal white matter injury in preterm infants was not confirmed by this study, again leading to confusion about the causal relationship between infection and brain injury. Although the link between chorioamnionitis and subsequent development of cerebral palsy was first described in term infants, there have been a number of other studies linking this obstetric complication to neonatal brain injury at all gestational ages.

This study again proves that the pathogenesis of neonatal brain injury—and, in this case, cerebral white matter injury—is not a simple matter. It is intriguing to note that intrapartum infection and hypoxic ischemia were not related but that neonatal culture-proven sepsis was related. This suggests that perhaps the intrauterine environment is protective against infection until the baby is delivered.

Current interest in the pro-inflammatory cytokines and their relationship to neonatal brain injury makes this finding particularly important. Overwhelming evidence points to the fact that chorioamnionitis in both the preterm and term infants has some relationship to brain injury by way of the pro-inflammatory cytokine mechanism.

These observations raise the question whether or not neonatal brain injury requires a "double hit," ie, both intrapartum and postdelivery release of cytokines, which may be of different classes. The final common pathway of the production of reactive oxygen species and subsequent damage to the CNS cells is always an important consideration.

M. L. Druzin, MD

Cerebellar Vermian Atrophy After Neonatal Hypoxic-Ischemic Encephalopathy

Sargent MA, Poskitt KJ, Roland EH, et al (British Columbia's Children's Hosp, Vancouver, Canada)

AJNR Am J Neuroradiol 25:1008-1015, 2004   8–7

Background.—Pathologic evidence of cerebellar injury caused by asphyxia at birth has been well documented, but neuroimaging evidence is sparse. The early and late imaging findings in the cerebellum of infants who had neonatal hypoxic-ischemic encephalopathy with thalamic edema shown by neonatal CT were evaluated retrospectively.

Study Design.—The study group consisted of 55 newborns with hypoxic-ischemic encephalopathy and CT-verified thalamic edema. Twenty-six newborns had follow-up neuroimaging. All images were reviewed for hemorrhage, edema, atrophy, and CT attenuation or MR signal intensity abnormalities. Neonatal autopsy findings were available for 4 cases.

Findings.—All 55 infants had thalamic edema, and half also had diffuse cerebral cortical edema. The cerebellar vermis appeared normal on all neonatal images. However, atrophy of the cerebral vermis was detected in 46% of patients on follow-up studies. One patient had cerebellar hemispheric atrophy. Cerebellar vermian atrophy was more common among those without cortical edema.

Conclusions.—Cerebellar vermian atrophy appears to be common during follow-up in many patients who had neonatal hypoxic-ischemic encephalopathy with CT evidence of thalamic edema.

▶ Radiologic markers that distinguish acute profound asphyxia from prolonged partial asphyxia are useful diagnostic tools. Early evidence of thalamic edema correlates with acute near-total intrauterine asphyxia. This report suggests that superior vermian atrophy may be a late sign of acute profound asphyxia in these term newborns. A retrospective review of 55 patients with radiologic evidence of thalamic edema was done, 26 of whom had follow-up imaging. At 3 days of age, all infants had thalamic edema, with or without cortical edema, and no evidence of cerebellar damage. Evaluation of follow-up imaging performed after the neonatal period confirmed thalamic damage in the vast majority of these patients and demonstrated cerebellar vermian atrophy in approximately half of them. The etiology of the cerebellar atrophy is unclear. It may be due to apoptosis or necrosis, resulting either directly from hypoxia or secondarily from loss of cerebellar inputs. In addition, whether patients with cortical edema, but not thalamic edema, have any late cerebellar changes has not yet been addressed, so the specific link with thalamic edema remains unclear. However, this report is significant because it shows that radiologic evidence of cerebellar damage after neonatal hypoxic-ischemic encephalopathy is relatively common, not relatively rare, as previously thought. Indeed, given the improvements in neuroimaging and the fact that this study included images obtained over more than a decade, this report may underestimate the extent of cerebellar damage in such patients. This report should stimulate further examination of the extent of cerebellar damage seen after neonatal hypoxic-ischemic encephalopathy, both radiologically and functionally.

A. Penn, MD, PhD

Multiorgan Dysfunction in Infants With Post-asphyxial Hypoxic-Ischaemic Encephalopathy

Shah P, Riphagen S, Beyene J, et al (Univ of Toronto)
Arch Dis Child Fetal Neonatal Ed 89:F152-F155, 2004   8–8

Background.—Multiorgan dysfunction (MOD) is one of four consensus based criteria for the diagnosis of intrapartum asphyxia. The theoretical concept behind MOD is the diving reflex (conservation of blood flow to vital organs at the cost of non-vital organs).

Objectives.—To assess the patterns of involvement of each major organ/system and combinations of involvement in infants with post-asphyxial hypoxic-ischaemic encephalopathy (HIE), and to describe this in relation to long term outcome.

Design.—Retrospective cohort study.

Setting.—Regional tertiary neonatal intensive care unit at the Hospital for Sick Children, Toronto, Canada.

Patients.—Term neonates with post-intrapartal asphyxial HIE assessed for kidney, cardiovascular system, lung, and liver function.

Outcome.—Death and presence or absence of severe neurodevelopmental disability.

Results.—Out of 130 of 144 eligible infants with outcome data, 80 (62%) had severe adverse outcome and 50 (38%) had good outcome. All infants had evidence of MOD (at least one organ dysfunction in addition to HIE). Renal, cardiovascular, pulmonary, and hepatic dysfunction was present in 58-88% of infants with good outcome and 64-86% of infants with adverse outcome.

Conclusions.—MOD was present in all the infants with severe post-asphyxial HIE. However, there was no association between MOD and outcome in these infants. No relation between individual or combinations of organ involvements and long term outcomes was observed.

▶ One of the requirements for the definition of significant intrapartum asphyxia is the presence of MOD. In this retrospective cohort study, the investigators reviewed the clinical data of infants with documented HIE. They found that all infants who had severe postasphyxial HIE had evidence of dysfunction of at least 1 organ/system in addition to the CNS. This observation confirms the criteria established by the American College of Obstetrics and Gynecology for the definition of significant HIE. They did not, however, find any relationship between the presence or absence of MOD and death or severe disability.

M. J. Maisels, MB, BCh

Prognostic Significance of Amplitude-Integrated EEG During the First 72 Hours After Birth in Severely Asphyxiated Neonates

Ter Horst HJ, Sommer C, Bergman KA, et al (Univ Hosp, Groningen, The Netherlands)
Pediatr Res 55:1026-1033, 2004   8–9

Background.—Birth asphyxia is responsible for approximately 20% to 30% of all cases of cerebral palsy and is a major cause of perinatally acquired brain injury in full-term infants. In the first few hours after birth, continuous amplitude-integrated electroencephalography (aEEG) recorded with a cerebral function monitor is one of the most accurate bedside methods for establishing a neurologic prognosis for asphyxiated infants. The prognostic accuracy of aEEG very soon after perinatal asphyxia has made it the best method for identification of groups eligible for potentially neuroprotective treatments. The natural course of aEEG patterns during the first 72 hours of life was determined in relation to neurologic outcomes in a group of severely asphyxiated term infants.

Methods.—A retrospective study was conducted of 30 infants admitted to a neonatal ICU from October 1998 to February 2001. aEEG traces obtained during the first 72 hours after birth were assessed by pattern recognition: continuous normal voltage (CNV), discontinuous normal voltage (DNV), burst suppression (BS), continuous low voltage (CLV), and flat trace (FT). Epileptic activity was also determined. The course of aEEG patterns was examined in relation to neurologic findings at 24 months.

Results.—Initial findings showed that 17 of 30 infants had severely abnormal aEEG patterns (BS or worse), which changed spontaneously to normal voltage patterns (CNV or DNV) in 7 infants within 48 hours. The prognosis was better the sooner the abnormalities on aEEG disappeared. The likelihood ratio of a BS pattern or worse predicting an adverse outcome was 2.7 between 0 and 6 hours and increased to its highest value of 19 between 24 and 36 hours; however, after 48 hours it was not significant. Normal voltage patterns (CNV and DNV) up to 48 hours of life were predictive of normal neurologic outcomes.

Conclusions.—The course of aEEG patterns was found to increase the prognostic value of aEEG monitoring in asphyxiated infants. Spontaneous recovery from severely abnormal aEEG patterns is not an uncommon occurrence.

▶ Continuous aEEG has been used as a bedside method of assessing the neurologic status of high-risk newborns. aEEG has been used to select patients for neuroprotective therapy after perinatal asphyxia because it has been shown to be useful in identifying newborns with more severe encephalopathies and worse outcomes within several hours after birth. In this technique, a single-channel EEG from biparietal electrodes is recorded. The recorded signal is then processed by rectifying and integrating the EEG amplitudes and is then displayed semilogarithmically with the use of a compressed time scale.

This study extends previous studies by analyzing the natural course of aEEG patterns during the first 72 hours after birth in a group of severely asphyxiated term infants. It attempts to correlate the evolution of patterns with neurologic outcomes. The authors evaluated the aEEG of 30 infants who were admitted to their neonatal ICU during a 2.5-year period. The aEEG tracings were assessed by pattern recognition. The patterns included CNV, DNV, BS, CLV, and FT. Epileptic activity and status epilepticus were also determined. The course of aEEG patterns was examined in relation to neurologic findings at 24 months of age.

Initially, 17 of 30 infants had severely abnormal aEEG patterns (BS, CLV, or FT), which changed to normal voltage patterns (CNV or DNV) in 7 within 48 hours. The sooner the severe abnormal patterns on aEEG changed to a normal voltage one, the better was the prognosis. Persistent abnormal aEEG patterns were predictive of severe deficits or death. Normal voltage patterns (CNV and DNV) up to 48 hours of life were predictive of normal neurologic outcomes.

The study findings indicate that the course of aEEG patterns adds to the prognostic value of aEEG monitoring in asphyxiated infants. When aEEG background patterns were normal voltage (CNV or DNV), the prognosis was good. The persistence of severely abnormal patterns (FT, CLV, or BS) after 48 hours was associated with universally poor outcomes. This article is important in showing that spontaneous recovery of severely abnormal aEEG patterns is not uncommon. If the recovery occurs before 24 hours of age, the prognosis can be good. These findings are similar to previous studies that used conventional neonatal EEG.

The study could not differentiate a particular evolution of aEEG patterns that separated infants with normal outcomes from those with mild deficits. Severely abnormal aEEG patterns, if present, tended to improve slightly later in the group of infants with mild deficits, between 24 and 36 hours instead of before 12 hours of age; however, the numbers in the subgroups were too small for statistical significance.

The study also found that 10 of 30 had epileptic activity on aEEG. It appears that 6 of these had status epilepticus, and they all had adverse outcomes.

aEEG is being used more commonly in intensive care nurseries around the world as a method of assessing the neurologic status of high-risk newborns and identifying those that are likely to develop severe neurologic deficits. This technique relies on a limited number of channels, usually a single bipolar derivation from the parietal regions. Newer monitors allow 2-channel recordings (1 from each hemisphere) and have the capability to simultaneously compare with the continuous EEG from the same electrodes. In previous comparative studies of aEEG and standard neonatal EEG, the former was very good at detecting severely abnormal patterns, such as BS, CLV, and FT. The capability to detect seizures was fairly good, although brief seizure discharges could be missed. Focal seizures can be missed because of the limited array of electrodes (as was the case in this study).

The interpretation of various patterns, such as seizures and discontinuous patterns, requires experience and education on the part of the neonatal staff. The authors state that interpretation by pattern recognition can be easily learned by nurses, junior medical staff, and neonatologists after a short period of training. The ability to make frequent correlations with the continuous EEG from more than 1 channel (available in newer monitors) should improve the acceptance of this technique by neurologists and neurophysiologists. As the authors point out, management decisions about hypoxic–ischemic encephalopathy or the treatment of neonatal seizures should not be made solely on the basis of a single test such as the aEEG.

J. S. Hahn, MD

Perinatal Stroke in Term Infants With Neonatal Encephalopathy

Ramaswamy V, Miller SP, Barkovich AJ, et al (Univ of California, San Francisco)
Neurology 62:2088-2091, 2004   8–10

Background.—Perinatal stroke is a serious, under-recognized event; the incidence, clinical presentation, and pathogenesis of perinatal stroke are poorly understood. Most cases are associated with infection and cardiac and blood disorders, but it has been reported that < 5% of perinatal stroke is associated with asphyxia. Although perinatal stroke has a heterogeneous etiology, the most common presentation is reported as seizures without encephalopathy. The risk of neurodevelopmental impairment after neonatal stroke is dependent on the etiology of the stroke. The occurrence, clinical presentation, and outcome of perinatal stroke in term infants presenting with neonatal encephalopathy was determined.

Methods.—A prospective cohort study was conducted of MRI predictors of outcome in 124 term neonates with encephalopathy. Newborns were studied with MRI at a median of 7 days. Strokes were defined as focal parenchymal infarcts, either in an arterial or venous distribution and were identified by a neuroradiologist blinded to the clinical condition. Outcome was determined at 30 months using the Bayley Scales of Infant Development Mental Index (MDI) and an examination done by a neurologist blinded to the neonatal condition and imaging studies.

Results.—Six newborns in the cohort were identified with perinatal strokes (4.8% prevalence). Of these newborns with stroke, the median birthweight was 3518 g, and 5 of the 6 were male. Significant resuscitation was required in all 6 patients. Neurodevelopmental outcome at 30 months was abnormal in all 6 patients and significantly worse than that of the entire cohort.

Conclusions.—Acute focal strokes are an uncommon but serious event in newborns with encephalopathy. These strokes are associated with substantial risk for abnormal neurodevelopmental outcome in the setting of neonatal encephalopathy.

▶ Although Ramaswamy et al only identified 6 infants with evidence of an acute focal stroke amongst 124 encephalopathic term infants, they all had a poor neurologic outcome. They concluded that perinatal strokes were not that common, but had serious consequences.

Golomb[1] reviewed the current thinking about strokes in and around the time of delivery and reported that arterial ischemic stroke around the time of birth is recognized about 1 in 4000 full-term infants. Although the presentation varies with either neurological and/or systemic signs observed in the newborn, seizures are most commonly the clinical finding that triggers assessment. In many children, perinatal stroke is recognized only retrospectively, with emerging hemiparesis or seizures after the early months of life. The known risk factors for perinatal stroke include hereditary or acquired thrombophilias; infection, pre-eclampsia, diabetes, and drug use in the mother; and infection, dehydration, complex congenital heart disease, extracorporeal membrane oxygenation, and catheter placement in the neonate. So be on the alert for this condition and remember that the placenta may yield valuable clues to the underlying cause.

A. A. Fanaroff, MD

Reference

1. Golomb M: The contribution of prothrombotic disorders to peri- and neonatal ischemic stroke. *Semin Thromb Hemost* 29:415-424, 2003.

Neonatal Cerebral Infarction and Neuromotor Outcome at School Age
Mercuri E, Barnett A, Rutherford M (Imperial College School of Medicine, Lond)
Pediatrics 113:95-100, 2004   8–11

Introduction.—Hemiplegia is the most feared and common motor sequela related to neonatal cerebral infarction. Not all infants with these lesions have abnormal motor outcome. Reported is the neuromotor follow-up at early school age of 22 children who had cerebral infarction on neonatal MRI.

Methods.—Twenty-two children with evidence of cerebral infarction on neonatal brain MRI (18, arterial infarction; 4, border-zone lesions) were evaluated at school age via a structured neurologic examination and the Movement Assessment Battery for Children, a battery of tests designed to investigate motor functioning.

Results.—Of 22 children evaluated, 6 (30%) had hemiplegia, and 7 (30%) demonstrated some neuromotor abnormality, including asymmetry on the neurologic examination or poor scores on the neuromotor test without any sign of asymmetry (4 and 3 children, respectively). A normal motor outcome was seen in the remaining 9 children. Hemiplegia occurred only in children with concomitant involvement of hemispheres, the internal capsule, and basal ganglia on brain MRI. Children with involvement of the internal capsule, associated with either basal ganglia or hemispheric lesions, did not manifest hemiplegia; they still had motor difficulties (Table 1).

Conclusion.—Hemiplegia occurs in a relatively small proportion of children with neonatal cerebral infarction, but other signs of neuromotor impairment may be present and may become more obvious at school age, when

TABLE 1.—Details of Clinical and MRI Findings

No.	Age	Infarct	Site	Basal Ganglia/Thalami	Internal Capsule	Neurological Examination	Mov ABC (Percentile)
				Neonatal MRI			
1	12 d	Lenticulostriate b	Normal	L lentiform/caudate	L decreased SI ALIC	Asymmetry	Normal (45)
2	10 d	Lenticulostriate b	Normal	L lentiform/caudate	L decreased SI ALIC	Normal	Abnormal (3)
3	10 d	Cortical b	R F,P	Normal	Normal	Normal	Normal (75)
4	8 d	Cortical b	L F,P	Normal	Normal	Normal	Normal (65)
5	3 d	Cortical b	L P	Normal	Normal	Normal	Normal (79)
6	6 d	Cortical b	L P,T,O	Normal	Normal	Normal	Normal (93)
7	5 d	Cortical b	L P,T,O	Normal	Normal	Normal	Normal (62)
8	4 d	Cortical b	L P,O	L lentiform	Normal	Asymmetry	Normal (79)
9	4 d	Cortical b	L F,P	L lentiform/caudate	Normal	Normal	Normal (72)
10	7 d	Cortical b/contralateral	L P,T	L lentiform R thalamus	Normal	Normal	Normal (72)
11	6 d	Cortical b	L P	Normal	L decreased SI PLIC	Asymmetry	Normal (16)
12	6 d	Cortical b	L F,P	Normal	L decreased SI PLIC	Normal	Abnormal (4)
13	4 d	Cortical b	L P,T,O	L lentiform/thalamus	L decreased SI PLIC	Normal	Abnormal (1)
14	4 d	Cortical b	L P,O	L lentiform/caudate	L loss of SI PLIC	Normal	Normal (18)
15	10 d	Cortical b/contralateral	R P,O; L O	R thalamus	R decreased SI PLIC	R hemi (Mod*)	Abnormal (2)
16	7 d	Main b/contralateral	L F,P,T,O	L lentiform	L decreased SI PLIC	L hemi (Mod*)	Normal (6)
17	5 d	Main b/contralateral	R F,P,T,O	R lentiform/thalamus	R decreased SI PLIC	R hemi (Mod*)	Abnormal (3)
18	5 d	Main b/contralateral	L F,P,T,O	L lentiform/thalamus	Bilat. decreased SI PLIC	L hemi (Mild*)	Abnormal (3)
19	9 d	Border zone	Bilat P,O	Normal	Normal	Normal	Normal (50)
20	6 d	Border zone	L F,P,T,O; R O	Normal	Normal	Normal	Normal (18)
21	5 d	Border zone	Bilat P,O	Normal	Normal	Asymmetry	Normal (28)
22	6 d	Border zone	Bilat. P,O (L>R)	L lentiform R lentiform	Bilat decreased SI PLIC	R hemi (Mild*)	Abnormal (3)

*Classification according to Claeys et al.

Abbreviations: b, Branch; *Bilat,* bilateral; *SI,* signal intensity; *F,* frontal; *P,* parietal; *T,* temporal; *O,* occipital; *L,* left; *R,* right; *Mod,* moderate; *ALIC,* anterior limb of the internal capsule; *PLIC,* posterior limb of the internal capsule.

(Reproduced by permission of *Pediatrics,* courtesy of Mercuri E, Barnett A, Rutherford M: Neonatal cerebral infarction and neuromuscular outcome at school age. *Pediatrics* 113:95-113, 2004.)

a more specific evaluation can be performed. Involvement of the internal capsule on neonatal MRI seems to be predictive of the presence of these abnormalities.

▶ Impressively, fewer than 30% of children with a history of neonatal cerebral infarction will have hemiplegia, but the good news is tempered by the recognition that some children without apparent hemiplegia may have asymmetry on their neurologic examination or poor neuromotor functioning, which indicates that a similar percentage of children (approximately 28%) have neuromotor impairment that could affect their everyday school performance. This latter group of children may not be recognized early because injuries involving the internal capsule, which seems to predict such an outcome, may not become obvious until a later age, when a more detailed assessment can be performed. The recovery of a baby from a stroke is remarkable compared with adults with similar injuries, but a longer term look at neurobehavioral capacities is required before being too reassuring to parents who are obviously hopeful that their baby will be the one that recovers completely. At least for the full-term infant with a symptomatic stroke, a careful MRI evaluation of the internal capsule, including diffusion-weighted imaging, should allow detection of abnormalities within the first week, which will provide some ability to prognosticate. Nonetheless, larger prospective studies are required before statistics such as those described in this cohort can be generalized with confidence. Also, when prematurity is added to the list of factors that can affect the long-term outcome, prognostication must be undertaken with even more circumspection. Combining optimism with realism is not science; rather, it is an art.

D. K. Stevenson, MD

▶ We need good long-term follow up on these infants, and the authors show us that a normal neurologic examination between 18 and 36 months of age in patients with previous neonatal cerebral infarction does not guarantee a normal examination at school age. In fact, 7 out of the 15 children (47%) who were considered normal between 18 and 36 months, showed minor neuromotor difficulties or asymmetries at school age. The authors speculate that the difference was likely related either to the ability to perform a more detailed examination at school age or the development of late onset mild joint contractures causing asymmetry of posture or walking.

The MRI findings were good predictors of neuromotor outcome. All 3 children with main branch MCA infarctions had hemiplegia and all children with internal capsule infarction had either hemiplegia, asymmetry in tone or abnormal motor competence. In contrast, most children with cerebral infarction that spared the internal capsule were normal.

There is also some good news. Most children with neonatal cerebral infarction have normal cognitive development and more than half have a normal neurologic examination and motor competence. We will await further studies from this group on how these children do with regard to their language, memory, behavior, and school performance.

B. Gebara, MD

Intracranial Hemorrhage in Premature Neonates Treated With Extracorporeal Membrane Oxygenation Correlates With Conceptional Age

Hardart GE, Hardart MKM, Arnold JH (Columbia Univ, New York; Harvard Med School, Boston)

J Pediatr 145:184-189, 2004   8–12

Objective.—To determine the effect of patient age on the risk of intracranial hemorrhage (ICH) in premature neonates treated with extracorporeal membrane oxygenation (ECMO).

Study Design.—This was a retrospective cohort study of neonates of <37 weeks' gestation treated with ECMO in the years 1992 through 2000 and reported to the Extracorporeal Life Support Organization Registry (n = 1524). The relation between ICH and patient age, defined as gestational age, postnatal age (PNA), and postconceptional age (PCA), was determined with the use of multiple logistic regression analysis.

Results.—PNA was inversely correlated with ICH in the univariate analysis ($P = .01$) but not in the multivariate analysis ($P = .36$). PCA showed a strong univariate correlation with decreasing ICH: 26% of patients ≤ 32 weeks' PCA developed ICH as compared with 6% of patients with PCA of 38 weeks ($P = .004$). Multiple logistic regression identified as independent predictors of ICH: PCA ($P = .005$), sepsis ($P = .004$), acidosis ($P = .0004$), and treatment with sodium bicarbonate ($P = .002$). Gestational age was correlated with ICH in the multivariate model only when PNA was included.

Conclusions.—Postnatal age is not a strong independent predictor of ICH in premature neonates treated with ECMO. PCA is the best age-related predictor of ECMO-related ICH in premature infants.

▶ This study by Griffin et al began with a reasonable hypothesis but is emblematic of the difficulties inherent in doing clinical research when the event rate is rather low. I commend the investigators for their persistence in adhering to a study protocol for nearly 8 years (and enduring all of those institutional review board renewals), but this unfortunately confounds interpretation of the results. I would argue that a baby with an oxygenation index of more than 40 in 2000 was probably a lot sicker than a baby with an oxygenation index more than 40 in 1993. This time frame encompassed the evolution of so many "modern" therapies, including high-frequency ventilation and inhaled nitric oxide, and it obviously affected patient accrual.

Still another problem that has plagued ECMO research is studying the treatment as if it were the disease. The population in this study is relatively typical of the infants treated with ECMO in the 1990s; it is a group of newborns with very heterogeneous primary lung disorders, each of which is too small to allow stratification. This is evident by what the authors tried to do in removing the infants with congenital diaphragmatic hernia from analysis. Yes, they are a different group. So are those infants with sepsis, especially if inflammatory mediators play a role in the genesis of capillary leak and pulmonary edema.

Although the study was masked, the rather predictable effects of dexamethasone on blood pressure prevent total removal of investigator bias. Additionally, the authors gave a reasonable explanation as to why they chose the dose of dexamethasone used in the study but, given the relatively long half-life, why was such a short interval between doses used?

No information is provided regarding cannulation techniques. It might have been helpful to know if both venoarterial and venovenous ECMO were utilized, and whether there were differences related to the dexamethasone. Since venovenous runs are usually longer, one might expect a larger effect if the treatment worked.

S. M. Donn, MD

Brain Imaging

Magnetic Resonance Imaging and T2 Relaxometry of Cerebral White Matter and Hippocampus in Children Born Preterm

Abernethy LJ, Klafkowski G, Foulder-Hughes L, et al (Royal Liverpool Children's Hosp, England; Univ of Liverpool, England)
Pediatr Res 54:868-874, 2003   8–13

Background.—The improved survival rate of very premature infants over the past 20 years has led to an increased interest in their long-term neurodevelopmental outcomes. Reported series have shown rates of major disability in these infants of 10% to 15%, and most of these are cerebral palsy and hearing and visual disabilities. Most of the remaining children attend normal schools, but it has been reported that one third to one half of these children experience behavioral and specific learning difficulties often associated with minor motor impairment (MMI). This syndrome is often referred to as developmental coordination disorder. Imaging studies have clearly shown lesions associated with major neurodevelopmental disabilities, but this has not been the case with MMI. Compared with term children, preterm infants have been shown to have smaller brains and less cortical complexity and, in many cases, delayed myelination. Quantitative MRI in adolescents who were born preterm has shown significant associations between caudate and hippocampal volumes and intelligence, as well as everyday memory. Whether intelligence and MMI in preterm children without major disabilities are associated with cerebral white matter (CWM) and hippocampal abnormalities on MRI was determined.

Methods.—The study included 103 preterm children who were studied at 7 years of age with MRI brain scans, including a T2-mapping sequence from which T2 relaxation times of the CWM and hippocampal formations were calculated. No major disabilities were present in any of the children, and all attended normal schools and had been assessed for IQ and MMI.

Results.—On MRI, visible lesions, which were associated with a lower IQ and a greater frequency of MMI, were seen in 20 children. The mean (SD) IQ in these patients was 90 (14.1). MMI was identified in 25 children, and this group was shown to have significantly longer T2 relaxation times for CWM but not for the hippocampus compared with children without MMI. These differences persisted even when only children without visible lesions on scans were considered. No significant correlation was observed between IQ and T2 relaxation times.

Conclusions.—Preterm children with no subsequent major disabilities may, in addition to visible lesions on MR images, have a diffuse abnormality of CWM, which is identified as an increased T2 relaxation time. This abnormality closely correlated with MMI but not with full-scale IQ.

▶ Advanced and novel quantitative imaging techniques such as volumetric MRI and diffusion tensor imaging are important in the investigation of brain injury and development in the preterm infant. In this study, Abernethy et al elegantly demonstrate the additional information gained by T2 relaxometry over qualitative MRI alone in delineating the type and location of brain findings associated with MMI. The authors also focus further interest on the differences between brain lesions linked with cognitive deficits and those linked with motor delays. The significant association of a prolonged CWM T2 relaxation time with MMI among children 7 years of age who were born preterm tantalizes the reader to speculate on the mechanism of such a finding. Additional investigation with prospective serial quantitative imaging beginning in the neonatal period may allow us to recognize the antecedent insult or developmental phenomena and, ultimately, intervene before damage is done.

S. R. Hintz, MD

Diffusion-Weighted Magnetic Resonance Imaging in Term Perinatal Brain Injury: A Comparison With Site of Lesion and Time From Birth

Rutherford M, Counsell S, Allsop J, et al (Imperial College, London)
Pediatrics 114:1004-1014, 2004   8–14

Introduction.—MRI provides detailed information concerning the pattern of lesions after perinatal brain injury. It is an excellent predictor of outcome in infants with hypoxic-ischemic encephalopathy. Abnormalities on MRI may take several days to become obvious, a period in which maximal benefit from interventions designed to modify perinatal brain injury may be obtained and in which important clinical decisions may need to be made. Diffusion-weighted MRI (DWI) techniques have been used to evaluate the developing brain and are of value in neonates with perinatal strokes. Abnormalities are most obvious 1 to 4 days after delivery, with the abnormal signal intensity gradually decreasing by the end of the first week as the conventional imaging appearances become more abnormal. The relation between contemporaneous DWI and conventional MRI was examined in 63 symptomatic term infants with early seizures thought to be hypoxic-ischemic in origin and 15 control subjects to establish a more objective method for confirming tissue injury.

Methods.—Apparent diffusion coefficients (ADC) were acquired for multiple regions of the brain. Comparisons were made across lesion groups, along with age at scan; infants were divided into those who were scanned during the first week and those who were scanned after the first week. This division was performed because of the known process of pseudonormalization of ADC values that occurs at approximately 7 days.

Results.—The ADC values in the 15 control subjects were (median [range]): 1 (1-1.15) × 10⁻³/mm² per second in the thalami, 1.1 (1-1.3) × 10⁻³/mm² per second in the lentiform nuclei, 1.5 (1.3-1.7) × 10⁻³/mm² per second in the centrum semiovale, 1.6 (1.46-1.7) × 10⁻³/mm² per second in the anterior white matter (WM), and 1.55 (1.35-1.85) × 10⁻³/mm² per second in the posterior WM. Little variation occurred over time. The ADC values were significantly decreased during the initial week after severe injury to either WM or basal ganglia and thalami (BGT); the values normalized at completion of the first week, then increased during week 2. The ADC values were either normal or increased in moderate BGT and WM lesions compared with control subjects. The ADC values less than 1.1×10^{-3}/mm² per second were always linked with WM infarction and values less than 0.8×10^{-3}/mm² per second were linked with thalamic infarction.

Conclusion.—A decreased ADC soon after delivery permits the presence of tissue infarction to be verified when conventional imaging changes may be subtle. Because both moderate WM and BGT lesions may have normal or increased ADC values, a normal ADC value during the first week of life does not signify normal tissue. The ADC values should always be measured in combination with visual analysis of both conventional MRI and DWI for maximum detection of pathologic tissue, and timing of the scans needs to be considered when interpreting findings.

▶ In related articles, Hunt et al[1] and Rutherford et al[2] discuss the use of DWI in the detection of perinatal brain injury and the prediction of outcome. Both articles point out the earlier detection of tissue damage with DWI compared with more conventional T1 and T2 imaging. Conventional MRI techniques rely on the differences of water relaxation in damaged tissue, whereas DWI is derived from the increased diffusion of water in damaged tissues, which may occur within hours of an injury. Earlier detection can lead to more rapid intervention in the appropriate clinical setting. Neuroimagers have relied on DWI to detect stroke in adult patients since the late '90s.[3] During the past 2 years, several studies have demonstrated the use of DWI in the neonate.[4,5] The studies by Hunt et al and Rutherford et al further establish DWI as a practical and reliable methodology for the early detection of perinatal brain injury and the prediction of long-term outcome.

G. Trock, MD

References

1. Hunt RW, Neil JJ, et al: Apparent diffusion coefficient in the posterior limb of the internal capsule predicts outcome after perinatal brain injury. *Pediatrics* 114:999-1003, 2004.
2. Rutherford M, Counsell SJ, et al: Diffusion weighted magnetic resonance imaging in term perinatal brain injury: A comparison with site of lesion and time from birth. *Pediatrics* 114:1004-1014, 2004.
3. Read SJ, Jackson GD, et al: Experience with diffusion weighted imaging in an adult stroke unit. *Cerebrovasc Dis* 8:135-143, 1998.

4. Counsell SJ, Allsop JM, et al: Diffusion weighted imaging of the brain in preterm infants with focal and diffuse white matter abnormality. *Pediatrics* 112:1-7, 2003.
5. Roelants-Van Run AM, Van Der Grond J, et al: Diffusion weighted imaging in neonates: Relation with histopathology. *Proc Int Soc Magnet Res Med* 9, 2001.

Ultrasound Abnormalities Preceding Cerebral Palsy in High-Risk Preterm Infants

de Vries LS, van Haastert I-LC, Rademaker KJ, et al (Wilhelmina Children's Hosp, Utrecht, The Netherlands)
J Pediatr 144:815-820, 2004   8–15

Background.—Cranial US was considered to be the method of choice for assessment of the brain in high-risk preterm infants after its introduction in the late 1970s. Later, neonatal MRI was found to be superior to US for the detection of subtle white matter lesions. However, neonatal MRI is expensive and time consuming, and patients require transport and, possibly, sedation. Several recently published studies have reported that only 40% to 50% of infants with cerebral palsy (CP) had lesions on neonatal US. There is concern that this information may lead to a decreased use of cranial US during the neonatal period. Performance of only 1 or 2 scans in the first few weeks of life decreases the reliability of cyst detection, and unexpected cases of CP may occur. Sequential high-resolution cranial US was assessed for its capability to predict CP in high-risk preterm infants.

Methods.—A group of 2139 preterm infants was studied, including 1636 who were 32 weeks' gestational age or less (group A) and 503 who were 33 to 36 weeks' gestational age (group B). US was performed with the use of a 7.5-MHz transducer once weekly until the infants were discharged and at 40 weeks' postmenstrual age. Major abnormalities found on US were grade III and IV hemorrhages, cystic periventricular leukomalacia (c-PVL), and focal infarction. A diagnosis of CP was made at a minimum age of 24 months.

Results.—Of the 1460 survivors in group A, 76 (5%) had CP. Abnormalities found on US were present in 70 of 76 infants (92%): major abnormalities were found in 58 of these patients (83%), and minor abnormalities were found in 12 (17%). In 295 of the patients with major abnormalities found on US, cysts were first detected beyond day 28. An additional 6 infants without abnormalities found on US had CP, and 3 of these infants had ataxic CP. Of the 469 survivors in group B, 29 (6%) had CP. Abnormalities found on US were present in 28 of these infants (96%) and were considered major in 25 patients (89%) and minor in 3 (11%). CP also developed in 1 infant who had no abnormalities found at US. Sequential high-resolution cranial US was determined to have a specificity of 95% and 99% and a sensitivity of 76% and 86% for finding major abnormalities in groups A and B, respectively. The positive predictive values were 58% in group A and 83% in group B.

Conclusions.—Seventy-nine percent of patients with CP in this study had major abnormal findings on US. Sequential scans with a 7.5-MHz transducer are required for detection of c-PVL, the most predictive US marker for CP.

▶ The authors provide crucial evidence that, in skilled hands and with the use of high-resolution techniques, serial cranial US can be an extremely powerful diagnostic modality in the preterm population. De Vries et al carefully evaluated findings of weekly in-hospital cranial US studies among preterm survivors with CP diagnosed at 24 months and found that 76% of infants with an estimated gestational age (EGA) of ≤32 weeks and 86% of infants ≥32 weeks' EGA had had "major" abnormal cranial US findings. Not surprisingly, extensive or advanced c-PVL was associated with the worst outcomes at 24 months. Perhaps most importantly, however, of the 70 infants ≤32 weeks' EGA with abnormalities found on US and CP at 24 months, 17 had no detectable abnormalities on US before day 28 Of these late findings, all were major abnormalities. Conversely, 63 of the 121 surviving infants born at ≤32 weeks' gestational age with major abnormalities found on US did not develop CP. Furthermore, approximately 80% of surviving infants ≤32 weeks' EGA with grade III intraventricular hemorrhages and more than half of surviving infants ≤32 weeks' EGA with unilateral parenchymal hemorrhages did not develop CP. The negative predictive value of US for linking major abnormalities with CP at 24 months was outstanding (99%), but the positive predictive value was quite disappointing (48%) among infants ≤32 weeks' EGA.

The challenges to investigators in this area of research are clear. A complete picture of neurodevelopmental findings for all infants ≤32 weeks' gestational age during a given study period, not just those with major abnormalities found on US or those who developed CP specifically, would add greatly to our understanding of the predictive capabilities of high-quality serial cranial US. It will also be extremely important to pursue further studies with the use of both serial US and MRI at near-term to assess the combined power of these diagnostic modalities to predict adverse neurodevelopmental outcomes. Finally, predictive models that include both clinical and radiologic factors may provide a more reliable and integrated basis of understanding for physicians and families.

S. R. Hintz, MD

▶ Linda DeVries has not only been a pioneer in the use of US to detect brain injury in the preterm infant, but she has also been most persistent and productive. Her present study, derived from a huge database and collection of images, illustrates how reliably experienced operators with state-of-the-art equipment can detect major US abnormalities of the brain. The specificity and sensitivity were spectacular and the positive predictive value of 83% in the more mature infants remarkable. US is an effective means of determining abnormalities in the preterm infant. However, the question is whether it is being supplanted by other modalities.

Additional neuroimaging modalities are now readily available and used according to the suspected underlying pathology. Arzoumanian et al[1] have demonstrated that neonatal diffusion tensor imaging may allow earlier detection of specific anatomic findings of microstructural abnormalities in infants at risk for neurologic abnormalities and disability. They concluded that the "combination of conventional MRI and diffusion tensor imaging may increase the predictive value of neonatal MR imaging for later neurologic outcome abnormalities and may become the basis for future interventional clinical studies to improve outcomes." Furthermore, MRI has become an important determinant of diagnosis and management for children with motor delay and varying combinations of spastic diplegia, quadriplegia, hemiplegia, and extrapyramidal movement disorders.[2,3] MRI and diffusion-weighted imaging can also be used effectively in neonatal encephalopathies. For reasons of cost and availability, US remains the most common evaluation for brain injury. MRI is gaining in popularity, and the combination of cystic lesions, ventricular dilatation, cortical atrophy, and thinning of the corpus callosum are all indicators of poor neurodevelopmental outcome. The correlations between more subtle neonatal MRI changes and long-term development are still underway.

A. A. Fanaroff, MD

References

1. Arzoumanian Y, Mirmiran M, Barnes PD, et al: Diffusion tensor brain imaging findings at term-equivalent age may predict neurologic abnormalities in low birth weight preterm infants. *AJNR Am J Neuroradiol* 24:1646-1653, 2003.
2. Serdaroglu G, Tekgul H, Kitis O, et al: Correlative value of magnetic resonance imaging for neurodevelopmental outcome in periventricular leukomalacia. *Dev Med Child Neurol* 46:733-739, 2004.
3. Kwong KL, Wong YC, Fong CM, et al: Magnetic resonance imaging in 122 children with spastic cerebral palsy. *Pediatr Neurol* 31:172-176, 2004.

Sex Differences in Cerebral Volumes of 8-Year-Olds Born Preterm

Reiss AL, Kesler SR, Vohr B, et al (Stanford Univ, Calif; Brown Univ, Providence, RI; Yale Univ, New Haven, Conn)
J Pediatr 145:242-249, 2004   8–16

Introduction.—We investigate sex-associated effects of preterm birth on cerebral gray matter (GM) and white matter (WM) volumes. Preterm chil-

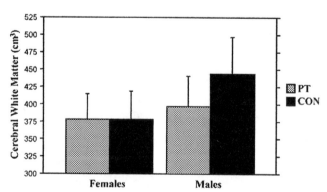

FIGURE 2.—Mean (and SD) of cerebral WM volumes (in cm³) by group and sex. A significant reduction is observed in males within the preterm (PT) group as compared with control (CON) males. The two female groups show comparable means. (Courtesy of Reiss AL, Kesler SR, Vohr B, et al: Sex differences in cerebral volumes of 8-year-olds born premature. *J Pediatr* 145:242-249. Copyright 2004 by Elsevier.)

TABLE 3.—Neuroanatomical Variables by Group (All Values Are in Cm^3)

	Preterm Males (n = 36) Mean (SD)	Preterm Females (n = 29) Mean (SD)	Control Males (n = 14) Mean (SD)	Control Females (n = 17) Mean (SD)
Cerebral GM**[b]	654.6 (49.7)	627.6 (46.6)	694.3 (68.6)	648.0 (54.1)
Cerebral WM**[c]†	396.7 (44.3)	380.8 (33.5)	443.7 (52.7)	378.1 (40.2)
Frontal lobe WM[c]	142.6 (16.5)	135.7 (12.0)	157.2 (22.9)	134.9 (18.1)
Parietal lobe WM*[b]	107.7 (12.5)	104.8 (11.6)	117.2 (12.9)	105.4 (11.6)
Temporal lobe WM**[c]†	62.2 (9.3)	59.1 (7.0)	72.8 (14.0)	58.8 (6.5)
Occipital lobe WM[c]	47.5 (8.3)	45.1 (7.9)	53.4 (10.1)	42.5 (7.4)
Subcortical WM*[a]†	36.7 (3.7)	36.2 (3.4)	43.1 (5.1)	36.5 (4.7)
Cerebral CSF	99.3 (14.4)	104.7 (18.2)	110.7 (17.3)	109.5 (16.0)

Significant group effect (control > preterm; *$P \le .05$, **$P \le .01$).
Significant sex effect (males > females; [a]$P \le .05$, [b]$P \le .01$, [c]$P \le .001$).
†Significant group by sex interaction (preterm males > control males *and* preterm females = control females; $P \le .05$).
(Courtesy of Reiss AL, Kesler SR, Vohr B, et al: Sex differences in cerebral volumes of 8-year-olds born premature. *J Pediatr* 145:242-249. Copyright 2004 by Elsevier.)

dren (n = 65) and 31 healthy, term control children had usable magnetic resonance imaging (MRI) data acquired at 8 years of age. Both GM and WM volumes were significantly reduced in the preterm group compared with controls. However, only males with preterm birth had significantly reduced WM compared with term males (P = .021), whereas WM volumes were equivalent in the female groups. Lower birth weight was associated with reduced WM in both boys and girls with preterm birth, whereas intraventricular hemorrhage (IVH) was associated with reduced GM in girls only. Positive correlations between GM and cognitive outcome were observed in girls with preterm birth but not boys. We conclude that preterm birth has a significant impact on brain development with increased risk for smaller GM and WM cerebral volumes. Males appear particularly vulnerable to adverse effects of preterm birth on WM development (Fig 2). However, girls with preterm birth show stronger correlations between neuro-anatomical variables and both neonatal risk factors and cognitive outcome, compared with boys. These findings indicate that the sex of the very preterm newborn influences the mechanisms by which the developing brain is affected (Table 3).

▶ If you are born some 12 to 16 weeks before term, it is not surprising that some of the processes involved in the growth and proliferation of the cells of the CNS might be affected. Studies have shown an association between lower IQ scores and educational difficulties of preterm children and the reduced size of different areas of the brain.[1] Decreased brain volumes have also been found in adolescents who were born preterm and in adult survivors of very low birth weight.[2,3] These authors show that at 8 years of age, preterm boys have significantly reduced volumes of WM compared with term boys, while in girls, WM volumes were similar in preterm and term infants. Here we have another explanation for why boys consistently demonstrate poorer neurodevelopmental outcome than do girls of similar gestation Whatever your sex, there is no advantage in being born prematurely; but if you have the choice, be a girl.

M. J. Maisels, MB, BCh

References

1. Abraham H, Tornoczky T, Kosztolanyi G, et al: Cell proliferation correlates with postconceptual and not with postnatal age in the hippocampal dentate gyrus, temporal neocortex and cerebellar cortex of preterm infants. *Early Hum Dev* 78:29-43, 2004.
2. Nosarti C, Al-Asady MH, Frangou S, et al: Adolescents who are very preterm have decreased brain volumes. *Brain* 125:1616-1623, 2002.
3. Fearon P, O'Connell P, Frangou S, et al: Brain volumes in adult survivors of very low birth weight: A sibling-controlled study. *Pediatrics* 114:367-371, 2004.

Brain Volumes in Adult Survivors of Very Low Birth Weight: A Sibling-Controlled Study

Fearon P, O'Connell P, Frangou S, et al (Inst of Psychiatry, London; Univ College Hosp, London)
Pediatrics 114:367-371, 2004   8–17

Background.—Very low birth weight (VLBW), defined as less than 1500 g, has been associated with an increased risk of brain injury perinatally and can influence cognition, neurologic status, and behavioral functioning during childhood. Whether brain damage resulting from VLBW persists into adulthood was investigated.

Methods.—The volumes of the whole brain, gray matter, ventricles, bilateral hippocampal areas, and corpus callosum were obtained from structural MRI scans in 33 adults born with VLBW and in 18 of their normal birth weight siblings.

Results.—The VLBW group had a mean birth weight of 1172 g. No difference was found between the VLBW and sibling groups with respect to whole brain volume, cerebral gray matter volume, anterior or middle corpus callosum volume, or bilateral hippocampal volume. Compared with the control subjects, the VLBW adults had a larger ventricular volume and a smaller posterior corpus callosum volume: the ventricular volume was increased by 46%, and the posterior corpus callosum volume declined by 17%.

Conclusions.—Some brain structures differ in volume between adults born with VLBW and their siblings born with normal birth weight. Thus, the structural consequences for the brain of the VLBW infant extend into adulthood. Whether these differences translate into impaired psychological and social functioning was not determined.

▶ This is one of the more recent important studies from this group of investigators. They report brain findings from VLBW preterm infants surviving into adulthood. Of significance, this article provides data on young adult subjects (mean age, 23 years; N = 33) and term normal birth weight sibling controls (N = 18). The main findings were that VLBW individuals had a 46% increase in total ventricular volume and a 17% reduction in posterior callosum volume. Although no other statistically significant differences were found, all the volumes measured were less in the VLBW group. The lack of significance may be due to the sample size and the heterogeneous group of preterm infants (ie, 6% were not actually preterm: they had gestations of 37 weeks). Functional data were not provided, but the neurological status of the subjects was stated to be normal.

Although the authors concede that the functional significance of these brain volume differences is unclear, they do offer a review of the literature and the association of cognition issues with decreases in hippocampal and cerebellar volumes. This is an older cohort of individuals: the question remains whether intensive care has made significant changes to affect this outcome. More studies are needed to investigate the structure–function relationships, the long-term significance of these findings, and whether early intensive care or later interventions will affect these structural, potentially adverse, functional outcomes.

R. L. Ariagno, MD

Special Senses

Flavor Programming During Infancy
Mennella JA, Griffin CE, Beauchamp GK (Monell Chemical Senses Ctr, Philadelphia)
Pediatrics 113:840-845, 2004   8–18

Background.—One of the fundamental mysteries of human behavior involves the source of individual differences in food preferences and habits. Genetic differences may underlie some of these differences, but there is increasing evidence that experience may have important influences on later functioning and preferences. In a previous study, it was reported that clinical observations have shown that early experience with formulas establishes subsequent preferences. The goals of this study were to test the hypothesis that prior exposure to formula with a particular flavor can affect later acceptance of that and other formulas and to determine whether this experimental approach could be used to investigate the existence of sensitive periods in the development of human flavor preferences.

Methods.—Infants whose parents chose to use formula feeding were randomly assigned to one of 4 groups by the second week of life (Fig 1). One group was assigned to be fed a milk-based formula (Enfamil), while another was fed with a particularly unpleasant-tasting protein hydrolysate formula (Nutramigen). The remaining 2 groups were assigned to be fed Nutramigen for 3 months and Enfamil for 4 months.

The timing of exposure differed between the groups. After 7 months of exposure, infants were videotaped on 3 separate days while feeding, in counterbalanced order, Enfamil, Nutramigen, and Alimentum, a novel hydrolysate formula. Interrelated measures of behavior included intake, duration of formula feeding, facial expressions, and mothers' judgment of infant acceptance.

Results.—For each of the 4 interrelated measures of behavior, previous exposure to Nutramigen was found to significantly enhance subsequent accep-

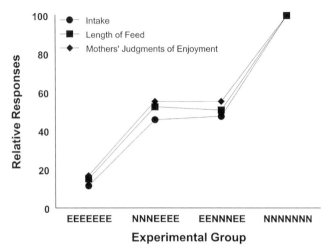

FIGURE 1.—Relative responses of the 4 groups of infants to Nutramigen at the 7.5-month test session. The points (connected by *lines* to enhance visual appreciation only) represent relative response for 4 of the behaviors monitored: the amount of formula consumed (*black circles*), the duration of the feed (*black squares*), and the mother's perception of her infant's enjoyment of the formula (*black diamonds*) at the 7.5-month test sessions. The response of group NNNNNNN was set to 100%. The groups differed in the type of formula the infants were fed during the entire 7 months preceding the test session. One group of infants was assigned to be fed Enfamil (EEEEEEE), another group was fed the protein hydrolysate formula, Nutramigen (NNNNNNN), and the remaining 2 groups were fed Nutramigen for 3 months and Enfamil for 4 months (NNNEEEE and EENNNEE). The timing of exposure differed between the groups. (Reproduced by permission of *Pediatrics* courtesy of Mennella JA, Griffin CE, Beauchamp GK: Flavor programming during infancy. *Pediatrics* 113:840-845, 2004.)

tance of both Nutramigen and Alimentum (Fig 1). Acceptance was greater after 7 months of exposure than after 3 months of exposure.

Conclusion.—These findings have clarified the origins of clinical difficulties in introducing hydrolysate formulas during older infancy. The results of this experiment also demonstrated that variation in formula flavor provided a useful model for investigation of the effects of long-term exposure differences on later acceptance. Such early variation under more species-typical circumstances (eg, exposure to different flavors in amniotic fluid and mothers' milk) may be the source of individual differences in food acceptability throughout the life span.

▶ Neonatologists are becoming familiar with the concept of the fetal origins of adult disease. However, the programming of the biology that makes us who we are, reaches beyond somatic growth and intermediary metabolism. Our tastes are no exception. The authors present convincing data on flavor programming during infancy. I have tasted most of the substances, foods and medicines, we "ask" babies to eat, and many are quite unpleasant or down right nasty with respect to their taste. Although there may be innate "dislikes," perhaps determined by a hard-wiring of preferences that reflect selection pressures on the species, most tastes are probably acquired.

Apparently, there are "critical periods" for such acquisitions, and we may be impacted lifelong with respect to what we like and dislike of the flavors we experience in our foods. I am now beginning to wonder what my mother and others fed me. Somehow Brussels sprouts have never been high on my list of preferences despite my knowledge about their many nutritional benefits.

D. K. Stevenson, MD

Regression of Retinopathy by Squalamine in a Mouse Model
Higgins RD, Yan Y, Geng Y, et al (Georgetown Univ, Washington, DC; Genaera Corp, Plymouth Meeting, Pa)
Pediatr Res 56:144-149, 2004   8–19

The goal of this study was to determine whether an antiangiogenic agent, squalamine, given late during the evolution of oxygen-induced retinopathy (OIR) in the mouse, could improve retinal neovascularization. OIR was induced in neonatal C57BL6 mice and the neonates were treated s.c. with squalamine doses begun at various times after OIR induction. A system of retinal whole mounts and assessment of neovascular nuclei extending beyond the inner limiting membrane from animals reared under room air or OIR conditions and killed periodically from d 12 to 21 were used to assess retinopathy in squalamine-treated and untreated animals. OIR evolved after 75% oxygen exposure in neonatal mice with florid retinal neovascularization developing by d 14. Squalamine (single dose, 25 mg/kg s.c.) given on d 15 or 16, but not d 17, substantially improved retinal neovascularization in the mouse model of OIR. There was improvement seen in the degree of blood vessel tuft formation, blood vessel tortuosity, and central vasoconstriction with squalamine treatment at d 15 or 16. Single-dose squalamine at d 12 was effective at reducing subsequent development of retinal neovascularization at doses as low as 1 mg/kg. Squalamine is a very active inhibitor of OIR in mouse neonates at doses as low as 1 mg/kg given once. Further, squalamine given late in the course of OIR improves retinopathy by inducing regression of retinal neovessels and abrogating invasion of new vessels beyond the inner-limiting membrane of the retina.

► The management of retinopathy of prematurity (ROP), a developmental vascular anomaly occurring in the incompletely vascularized retina of the premature infant, has changed considerably over the last 20 years. Screening and treatment protocols have been established to provide timely therapy to infants at risk, and the classification and reporting have been standardized. Cryotherapy, laser photoablation, vitrectomy, and scleral buckling have proven effective but also have inherent risks of complications. As the pathophysiology of the disorder is clarified, newer options become apparent. There are a number of approaches to inhibit angiogenesis, for example. Higgins et al, in this elegant study, prove that squalamine is a potent inhibitor of OIR and improves retinopathy by inducing regression of retinal neovessels and inhibiting invasion of new vessels beyond the inner-limiting membrane of the retina. In the same mouse model Sharma et al[1] demonstrated that ibuprofen improves OIR when administered concurrently with the injury phase without affecting the normal retinal development of the animals.

It is a huge leap from mice to human beings, but it is encouraging to see the emergence of alternative noninvasive therapies.

While talking of noninvasive approaches, here is something to ponder: Screening for detection of retinopathy currently is limited to indirect ophthalmoscopy, which requires considerable examiner skill and experience. Jokl et al[2] investigated whether conventional 10 MHz B-scan US could document the clinical stages of ROP as accurately as indirect ophthalmoscopy. The ultrasonographer, without use of papillary mydriatics or lid speculum, determined the presence or absence of a ridge or tractional elements, if present on the ridge. US grade did correlate with clinical grade and did not appear to cause harm ($R = .79$, $P < .001$). However, 9 eyes were overdiagnosed by 1 stage and 1 eye, in which a peripheral detachment was mistaken for an artifact, was underdiagnosed. The technology is advancing and has the potential to be used as a screening process, reducing the work load for the ophthalmologists.

A. A. Fanaroff, MD

References

1. Sharma J, Barr SM, Geng Y, et al: Ibuprofen improves oxygen-induced retinopathy in a mouse model. *Curr Eye Res* 27:309-314, 2003.
2. Jokl DH, Silverman RH, Springer AD, et al: Comparison of ultrasonic and ophthalmoscopic evaluation of retinopathy of prematurity. *J Pediatr Ophthalmol Strabismus* 41:345-350, 2004.

Involution of Threshold Retinopathy of Prematurity After Diode Laser Photocoagulation
Coats DK, Miller AM, McCreery KMB, et al (Baylor College of Medicine, Houston)
Ophthalmology 111:1894-1898, 2004   8–20

Objective.—To characterize the process of involution of threshold retinopathy of prematurity after transpupillary diode laser photocoagulation.

Design.—Retrospective case series.

Participants.—Neonates with threshold retinopathy who underwent diode laser photocoagulation of the peripheral avascular retina.

Methods.—A retrospective chart review was done of the weekly examination records of infants treated for threshold disease. Features that were studied included the presence of residual stage 3 neovascularization, plus disease, and development of retinal detachment (RD).

Main Outcome Measures.—Timing of full involution and/or development of an RD.

Results.—Of 262 eyes of 138 infants treated, full involution without RD was seen in 8%, 43%, 64%, 73%, and 86% of eyes at postoperative weeks 1, 2, 3, 4, and 9 ± 3, respectively. Retinal detachments were diagnosed cumulatively in 0%, 1.5%, 4.2%, 6.5%, and 14% of eyes at weeks 1, 2, 3, 4, and 9 ± 3, respectively.

Conclusions.—Full involution of laser-treated threshold retinopathy of prematurity required more than 2 weeks in more than half of treated eyes. Most RDs were not detected until ≥3 weeks after treatment.

▶ With increased survival of less-mature infants the risks of threshold disease requiring intervention have increased. Coats et al[1] looked at the incidence of threshold retinopathy of prematurity (ROP) in infants less than 25 weeks' gestation, including 7 at 23 weeks and 42 at 24 weeks. Initial screenings were at 5 weeks of age and continued until the infants were no longer at risk for serious ROP. ROP developed in all eyes. Thirteen (13%) eyes of 7 (14%) patients developed prethreshold disease and regressed without treatment. Threshold retinopathy was noted in 41% of the infants at a mean postconceptional age of 34 weeks and required treatment.

The results of the transpupillary diode laser photocoagulation are somewhat reassuring. Complete resolution was seen in 86% of the eyes, but retinal detachment still occurred in 14%. Full involution took longer than 2 weeks in more than half the treated eyes and 14% resolved beyond 4 weeks after therapy. Most retinal detachments were noted 3 weeks or more after laser therapy. Concerns have been raised about the risks of cataract after laser therapy, but Paysse et al[2] only noted 1 cataract among 293 eyes treated with transpupillary diode laser photocoagulation. This cataract consisted of peripheral cortical punctate lenticular opacities that were not progressive or visually significant. They commented that transpupillary diode laser photocoagulation may be safer than argon laser photocoagulation for treatment of threshold ROP. Threshold retinopathy remains a formidable problem among the smallest, least mature babies in the neonatal ICU.

A. A. Fanaroff, MD

References

1. Coats DK, Paysse EA, Steinkuller PG: Threshold retinopathy of prematurity in neonates less than 25 weeks' estimated gestational age. *J AAPOS* 4:183-185, 2000.
2. Paysse EA, Miller A, McCreery KM, et al: Acquired cataracts after diode laser photocoagulation for threshold retinopathy of prematurity. *Ophthalmology* 109:1662-1665, 2002.

Trends in the Incidence of Severe Retinopathy of Prematurity in a Geographically Defined Population Over a 10-Year Period

Hameed B, Shyamanur K, Kotecha S, et al (Leicester Royal Infirmary, England; Leicester Univ, England; Univ Med School, Leicester, England)
Pediatrics 113:1653-1657, 2004   8–21

Objective.—To examine trends in the incidence of severe (≥grade 3) retinopathy of prematurity (ROP) in infants with birth weight of ≤1250 g in a geographically defined population over a 10-year period.

1990-1994

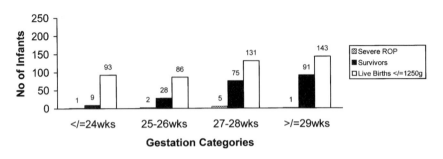

Gestation Categories

1995-1999

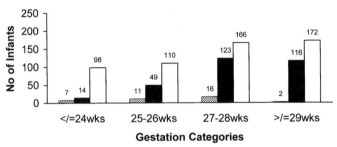

Gestation Categories

FIGURE 2.—Distribution of cases by gestation for the 2 time periods. (Courtesy of Hameed B, Shyamanur K, Kotecha S, et al: Trends in the incidence of severe retinopathy of prematurity in a geographically defined population over a 10-year period. *Pediatrics* 113:1653-1657, 2004. Reprinted by permission of *Pediatrics*.)

Methods.—An observational study was conducted of all infants who had a birth weight ≤1250 g and were born to mothers who were resident in the county of Leicestershire, United Kingdom, during the period January 1, 1990, to December 30, 1999. Cases were identified by the Trent Neonatal Survey. The incidence of severe ROP (≥grade 3) was compared in 2 successive 5-year periods: 1990-1994 and 1995-1999.

Results.—Comparing the first 5-year period (1990-1994) with the second (1995-1999), the total number of live births fell (60 789 vs 56 564). However, there was a significant increase in the number of births with birth weight ≤1250 g (including live and dead; 615 vs 734; live births only: 455 vs 556). Survival to 42 weeks of infants who were born at ≤1250 g was significantly better in the latter time period (203 vs 302; odds ratio [OR] for death: 0.54; 95% confidence interval [CI]: 0.39-0.75) (Fig 2). The number of cases of severe ROP was 4 times higher during the second time period compared with the first (9 vs 36). A significantly increased risk for the development of severe ROP was seen during the second time period (OR: 2.92; 95% CI: 1.37-6.20). Even after allowing for the change in gestation induced by the improved survival during the second time period, the increased risk remained (OR: 2.81; 95% CI: 1.27-6.21).

Conclusions.—There is strong evidence that the incidence of severe ROP among infants with birth weight ≤1250 g increased in the latter half of the last decade. The increased risk seems to be independent of the increase in survival.

▶ In this geographically defined population, the incidence of severe ROP among surviving infants less than 1250 g was 4.4% from 1990 to 1994 versus 11.9% from 1995 to 1999. In the latter time period, there were more survivors at less than or equal to 26 weeks' gestation, but even when this was taken into account, the differences in ROP incidence remained. There is no ready explanation for why this increase in severe ROP has occurred. Because this is a geographically defined, population-based study, it is not susceptible to the vagaries of the changes in incidence of a relatively low frequency event in an individual neonatal ICU. We need additional population-based studies to see if this change is occurring as well in other parts of the world.

M. J. Maisels, MB, BCh

Long-term Ocular Prognosis in 327 Children With Congenital Toxoplasmosis

Wallon M, Kodjikian L, Binquet C, et al (Hôpital de la Croix-Rousse, Lyon, France; Centre Hospitalier Universitaire, Dijon, France; Univ of Bern, Switzerland)
Pediatrics 113:1567-1572, 2004   8–22

Introduction.—Retinochoroiditis is the most common consequence of congenital toxoplasmosis, with ocular lesions reported in as many as 80% of untreated, congenitally infected children. Early diagnosis and treatment may decrease the risk of visual impairment in these children. Reported was

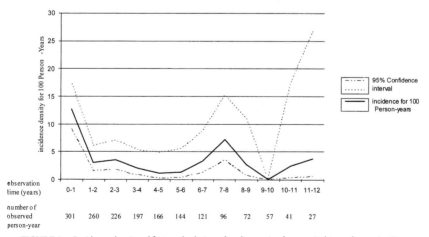

FIGURE 1.—Incidence density of first ocular lesion after diagnosis of congenital toxoplasmosis. (Reproduced by permission of *Pediatrics* courtesy of Wallon M, Kodjikian L, Binquet C, et al: Long-term ocular prognosis in 327 children with congenital toxoplasmosis. *Pediatrics* 113:1567-1572, 2004.)

TABLE 5.—New and Secondary Events Detected After Birth in 327 Children with Congenital Toxoplasmosis

	No. of Children	%
Secondary events	23	29
New ocular lesion	19	24
Reactivation of old lesions	1	1
New and reactivated lesions	3	4
No secondary events	56	71

(Reproduced by permission of *Pediatrics* courtesy of Wallon M, Kodjikian L, Binquet C, et al: Long-term ocular prognosis in 327 children with congenital toxoplasmosis. *Pediatrics* 113:1567-1572, 2004.)

the clinical evolution of ocular lesions and final visual function in a prospective cohort of congenitally infected children identified during monthly maternal prenatal screening.

Methods.—A total of 327 congenitally infected children who were monitored for up to 14 years were included. Data were recorded regarding maternal infection; time and type of therapy; antenatal, neonatal, and postnatal workups; and ocular status.

Results.—All except 52 mothers had been treated. Pyrimethamine and sulfadiazine were administered in utero to 38% of children and after birth to 72% of infants. Fansidar was given for an average of 337 days in all except 2 children. At a median follow-up of 6 years, 79 (24%) children had a minimum of 1 retinochoroidal lesion (Fig 1). In 23 (29%) children, at least 1 new event was diagnosed up to 10 years after identification of the first lesion: reactivation of an existing lesion, new lesion in a previously healthy location, or both in 1, 19, and 3 cases, respectively (Table 5).

Of 55 children with lesions in 1 eye, 45 had final visual acuity data available; 31 (69%) had normal vision. Twenty-four children had lesions in both eyes. Of the 21 for whom final visual acuity data were available, 11 had normal vision in both eyes. None of the children had bilateral visual impairment.

Conclusion.—Clinicians, parents, and elder children with congenital infection need to understand that late-onset retinal lesions and relapse can occur for many years after birth. The overall ocular prognosis of congenital toxoplasmosis is satisfactory in patients for whom the infection is identified early and treated appropriately.

▶ The authors report on the most frequent consequence of congenital toxoplasmosis, retinochoroiditis, which occurred in 24% of congenitally infected children over a median 6-year follow-up in the described cohort. What is important for the neonatologist to recognize is that only 11% of the diagnoses were made in the first month of life and more than half were made after the first year of life.

Unfortunately, follow-up with respect to visual impairment was incomplete for this cohort, and the statistics reported are difficult to interpret, not only because of the incompleteness of follow-up but also because of the early diagnosis and more frequent treatment of infants with congenital toxoplasmosis. Another factor making interpretation difficult is that there is unavoidably imperfect information with respect to the actual date of onset of maternal infection, which may affect ultimate visual acuity. Moreover, even if an effort were made to understand the actual time of onset of the maternal infection, such information would likely still represent a "best guess" in most cases.

Ultimately, the study was not population-based and the authors acknowledge this fact. Even with its limitations, the message is clear that ocular manifestations of congenital toxoplasmosis may be delayed, and clinical counseling should take this into consideration. The good news is that the functional visual outcome is usually not severe impairment.

D. K. Stevenson, MD

Visual Impairment in Children Born Prematurely From 1972 Through 1989
Rudanko S-L, Fellman V, Laatikainen L (Finnish Natl Agency for Welfare and Health, Helsinki; Univ of Helsinki)
Ophthalmology 110:1639-1645, 2003   8–23

Purpose.—To investigate the incidence and causes of visual impairment in children born prematurely in Finland from 1972 through 1989, and to determine what conditions and factors were associated with its occurrence

Design.—Retrospective, cross-sectional study.

Subjects.—All visually impaired individuals from 0 to 17 years of age who had been born at fewer than 37 gestational weeks in Finland from 1972 through 1989 for whom records were available in the Finnish Register of Visual Impairment were eligible for this study.

Methods.—Data in the Finnish Register of Visual Impairment relating to 556 children were supplemented with data from hospital records, and from the Register of Births, the Register of Congenital Malformations, the Finnish Care Register, and the Finnish Cancer Register. Data relating to causes associated with visual impairment in particular were collected. Data relating to the children born prematurely were compared with data relating to children born at full term. The chi-square test (Mantel-Haenszel), the Mann-Whitney *U* test, Fisher exact test, and stepwise logistic regression analysis were used in statistical analysis of the data.

Main Outcome Measures.—Visual acuity, ophthalmologic diagnoses, associated systemic disease, multiple handicap, gestational age, birth weight, 5-minute Apgar scores, and prenatal, perinatal, and infantile or juvenile disorders or disease and treatment.

Results.—One hundred twenty-five of the 556 visually impaired children (23%; 11/100,000 children less than 18 years of age) had been born preterm. Retinopathy of prematurity, optic atrophy, and cerebral amblyopia were the main diagnoses associated with visual impairment (in 46%, 28%, and 12% of cases, respectively). Sixty-six percent of those born prematurely with visual impairment were also affected by other handicaps (mental, motor, auditory), 54% by cerebral palsy and 36% by epilepsy. Eighty-eight of the 125 children (70%) born preterm with visual impairment were blind. Very low birth weight (<1500 g), young gestational age (fewer than 30 weeks), prenatal infection, hyperbilirubinemia, respiratory disorders, asphyxia, and lengthy mechanical ventilation were associated with an increased risk of visual impairment.

Conclusions.—Premature birth was a major risk factor of severe visual impairment and blindness in childhood. The visual impairment often was accompanied by cerebral palsy, epilepsy, and other motor and mental handicaps. Retinopathy of prematurity, optic atrophy, and cerebral amblyopia were the main diagnoses associated with visual impairment. During the 18 years covered by the study, the increasing incidence of survival of infants born weighing fewer than 1500 g was associated with increasing incidence of blindness.

Visual Impairment in Children Born at Full Term From 1972 Through 1989 in Finland
Rudanko S-L, Laatikainen L (Finnish Natl Agency for Welfare and Health, Helsinki; Univ of Helsinki)
Ophthalmology 111:2307-2312, 2004   8–24

Objective.—To investigate the incidence, prevalence, and causes of visual impairment in children born at full term and to determine conditions and factors associated with visual impairment.

Design.—Retrospective, cross-sectional, population-based study.

Participants.—All visually impaired individuals from 0 to 17 years of age who were born at full term from 1972 through 1989 in Finland and recorded in the Finnish Register of Visual Impairment (n = 556) were eligible for this study.

Methods.—Data in the Finnish Register of Visual Impairment relating to 556 subjects were supplemented with data from hospital records and other national registers (Register of Births, Register of Congenital Malformations, Finnish Care Register, and Finnish Cancer Register). Data relating to the children born at full term were compared with Finnish perinatal and vital statistics and with data concerning children born prematurely. The chi-square test (Mantel-Haenszel) and stepwise logistic regression analysis were used in statistical analysis of the data.

Main Outcome Measures.—Visual acuity, time of onset of visual impairment, ophthalmic diagnosis of visual impairment, systemic disease, multiple handicap, 5-minute Apgar score, prenatal disorders, perinatal disorders, disorders arising during infancy and childhood, and treatment.

Results.—Four hundred thirty-one of the 556 individuals with visual impairment (78%) had been born at full term. Visual impairment was predominantly associated with genetic (53%) and prenatal (34%) factors. Ocular malformations (34%), retinal diseases (31%), and neuro-ophthalmologic disorders (26%) were the main ophthalmic diagnoses. Optic nerve atrophy (20%) and congenital cataract (13%) were the most common single diagnoses. The occurrence of blindness, systemic disease, and multiple handicap was 40%, 43%, and 45%, respectively.

Conclusions.—The incidence of visual impairment in children born at full term did not decline during the 2 decades covered by this study. The findings reflected the lack of treatment for genetic eye diseases. The results also confirmed an obvious need for further understanding of mechanisms underlying congenital anomalies of the human visual system.

▶ These 2 articles (Abstract 8–23 and Abstract 8–24) complement each other and provide a comprehensive view of the causes of visual impairment in term and preterm infants over an 18-year period. The data are derived from a retrospective, cross-sectional, population-based study that used the Finnish Register of Visual Impairment supplemented with data from hospital records and other national registers. A total of 556 subjects with visual impairment were identified, including 431 children born at term and 125 preterm infants. Each cohort is reported in a separate article. The prematurity rate in Finland during the period under consideration was less than 5%, yet premature birth accounted for 23% of the visually impaired children and adolescents. Retinopathy of prematurity, optic atrophy, and cerebral amblyopia were the main diagnoses associated with visual impairment. Furthermore, the visual impairment was often accompanied by cerebral palsy, epilepsy, and other motor and mental handicaps. During the 18 years covered by the study, the increasing incidence of survival of infants born weighing less than 1500 g was associated with increasing incidence of blindness. To place these data in perspective, the period 1972 through 1989 is before the landmark Cryotherapy Trial in which cryotherapy reduced the risk of unfavorable ocular outcome from threshold retinopathy of prematurity.[1] Since then screening and treatment protocols have been standardized so that infants are closely monitored and interventions such as cryotherapy, laser photoablation, vitrectomy, and scleral buckling have proven effective. Also, oxygen management protocols have reduced the incidence of retinopathy.[2] The net effect has been a reduction in blindness from retinopathy despite further improvements in survival of extremely low birth weight infants after the introduction of surfactant therapy and widespread use of antenatal corticosteroids.

In the term infant, visual impairment was predominantly associated with genetic and prenatal factors. Not surprisingly, no decline was seen during the second decade, as there are few treatments or cures for genetic diseases of the eye. Ocular malformations, retinal diseases, and neuro-ophthalmologic disorders were the main diagnoses leading to impaired vision. Optic nerve atrophy and congenital cataract were the most common single diagnoses. There was substantial morbidity with blindness (40%), systemic disease (43%), and multiple handicaps (45%). Perinatal asphyxia is a potent cause of cerebral injury that may include the visual cortex. Injuries to the visual cortex, which is essential in visual processing, can produce blindness, referred to as "cortical blindness." In children some degree of visual recovery has been noted, and for that reason the term "cortical visual impairment" has been suggested as a more appropriate diagnosis. Hoyt[3] deemed the term "inaccurate, as a significant number of children with visual loss and neurologic damage have injuries to the noncerebral pathways (for example, optic radiations in children with periventricular leukomalacia)." Mercuri et al[4] monitored 39 children with severe neonatal encephalopathy who had early cerebral imaging. They reported that the presence and severity of visual impairment was related to the severity and site of brain lesions. Furthermore, the assessment of visual function performed in the first year was a reliable indicator of visual function at school age. Moderate or severe basal ganglia lesions and severe white matter changes were always associated with abnormal visual function. Infants with normal MRI, minimal basal ganglia lesions, and minimal or moderate white matter involvement tended to have normal vision.

A. A. Fanaroff, MD

References

1. Multicenter trial of cryotherapy for retinopathy of prematurity. Three-month outcome. Cryotherapy for Retinopathy of Prematurity Cooperative Group. *Arch Ophthalmol* 108:195-204, 1990.
2. Chow LC, Wright KW, Sola A, CSMC Oxygen Administration Study Group: Can changes in clinical practice decrease the incidence of severe retinopathy of prematurity in very low birth weight infants? *Pediatrics* 111:339-345, 2003.
3. Hoyt CS: Visual function in the brain-damaged child. *Eye* 17:369-384, 2003.
4. Mercuri E, Anker S, Guzzetta A, et al: Visual function at school age in children with neonatal encephalopathy and low Apgar scores. *Arch Dis Child Fetal Neonatal Ed* 89:F258-F262, 2004.

Educational and Social Competencies at 8 Years in Children With Threshold Retinopathy of Prematurity in the CRYO-ROP Multicenter Study

Msall ME, for the Cryotherapy for Retinopathy of Prematurity Cooperative Group (Univ of Chicago; et al)

Pediatrics 113:790-799, 2004   8–25

Background.—The increased survival rates of infants with extremely low and very low birth weights have raised concerns about the impact of neurosensory disabilities in long-term survivors. The educational status of children with threshold retinopathy of prematurity (ROP) at 8 years of age was investigated.

Methods.—This prospective cohort study analyzed data on children with birth weights of less than 1251 g and threshold ROP in the Cryotherapy for Retinopathy of Prematurity multicenter trial. Two hundred sixteen of 255 survivors (85%) were evaluated at 5.5 and 8 years. Visual status, functional skills, and social data were evaluated at 5.5 years. At 8 years, a questionnaire was administered to elicit information on the need for special education classes, developmental disabilities, rehabilitation treatments, and academic and social competencies. Visual status was judged to be favorable or unfavorable based on the better eye.

Findings.—When children with unfavorable visual status were compared with those with favorable visual status. Major impairments were found to be significantly more prevalent in those with unfavorable status. Cerebral palsy was documented in 39% and 16%, respectively; developmental disability, 57% versus 22%; autism, 9% versus 1%; and epilepsy, 23% versus 3%. Special education services were reported for 63% of the children with unfavorable visual status, compared with 27% for those with favorable visual status.

Eighty-four percent of the children with an unfavorable status had below–grade-level academic performance, compared with 48% of those with a favorable status. In addition, school-based rehabilitation services were significantly less common for children with favorable visual status.

Factors associated with significantly lower rates of special education placement and below–grade-level academic performance at age 8 were favorable visual status, favorable functional ratings at 5.5 years, markers of higher socioeconomic status, and nonblack race. In a multivariate logistic regression analysis, only favorable visual status and functional status significantly predicted decreasing special education placement.

Conclusion.—Threshold ROP correlates with high rates of developmental, educational, and social challenges in middle childhood. Vision preservation was associated with a clear advantage. More than half of children with favorable visual status performed at grade level.

▶ Extremely low birth weight infants are at high risk for neurosensory disabilities. It is estimated that 50% of very low birth weight survivors need special education support while 10% to 30% of them have severe neurosensory disorders including cerebral palsy, blindness, hearing loss, and neurodevelopmental disabilities. However, these studies did not specifically look at the relationship between visual status and the need for special education services.

In a previous study of infants enrolled in the Cryotherapy for Retinopathy of Prematurity (CRYO-ROP) multicenter trial, the authors reported a strong association between severity of ROP and functional limitations at 5.5 years of age. In this study, they report the educational and social outcomes at 8 years of age in infants with threshold ROP.

Two hundred and sixteen infants with a birth weight of less than 1250 g enrolled in the CRYO-ROP trial were evaluated at 5.5 years and 8 years of age. Visual, functional, and social status was assessed at 5.5 years, and a questionnaire was administered at age 8 years to obtain information about special education, developmental and rehabilitation treatment, and social and academic issues. Visual status was classified as favorable or unfavorable based on assessment of grating acuity by the Teller acuity card procedure. Overall, a much higher proportion of infants with unfavorable visual status had neurodevelopmental, behavioral or learning disorders at 8 years of age compared to infants with a favorable visual status (70% vs 56%).

Similarly, a much higher proportion of infants with an unfavorable visual status required special education (63.4% vs 27.1%) and rehabilitation for speech-language problems, physical therapy, or visual services. A much higher percentage of infants with a favorable visual status showed competency in mathematics (55% vs 20%), reading (50% vs 18%), and handwriting (50% vs 17%) at 8 years of age. Social competency as assessed by unsupervised play (38% vs 80%), peer interaction (39% vs 77%), and practical judgment (32% vs

67%) was worse in children with an unfavorable visual status. After controlling for several variables, it appears that only unfavorable visual status and a low WeeFim score (a measure of functional independence) at age 5.5 years were significant predictors of special education placement at age 8 years.

This study has some limitations in that it only looked at infants with threshold ROP, which includes only a small subset of very low birth weight infants, and bilateral vision impairment was higher in this cohort as 1 eye was not treated with ablative surgery. Also, it is difficult to separate the effect of visual loss from the effect of any underlying undetected neurologic injury on the above outcomes. Nevertheless, the results of this study indicate that infants with threshold ROP, and particularly those with an unfavorable visual status, are at high risk for long term neurodevelopmental problems and should be referred for comprehensive early intervention services.

A. Madan, MD

Nutritional Effects on Auditory Brainstem Maturation in Healthy Term Infants
Ünay B, Sarici SÜ, Ulaş ÜH, et al (Gülhane Military Med Academy, Ankara, Turkey)
Arch Dis Child Fetal Neonatal Ed 89:F177-F179, 2004   8–26

Objective.—To assess the effects of dietary long chain polyunsaturated fatty acid (LCPUFA) supplementation on auditory brainstem maturation of healthy term newborns during the first 16 weeks of life by measuring brainstem auditory evoked potentials (BAEPs).

Design.—Throughout the 16 week study period, infants in the formula A group (n = 28) were assigned to be fed exclusively with the same formula supplemented with DHA, and infants in the formula B group (n = 26) were assigned to receive only a DHA unsupplemented but otherwise similar formula. During the study period, the first 26 consecutive infants to be fed exclusively on their mother's milk for at least the first 16 weeks of life were chosen as the control group. BAEP measurements were performed twice: at the first and 16th week of age.

Results.—There were no significant differences among the study and control groups in the BAEP measurements performed at the study entry. At 16 weeks of age, all absolute wave and interpeak latencies in the study and control groups had significantly decreased. The decreases were significantly greater in the formula A and control groups than in the formula B group.

Conclusions.—Infants fed on human milk or a formula supplemented with LCPUFAs during the first 16 weeks of life show more rapid BAEP maturation than infants fed on a standard formula. Although the clinical importance and long term effects of these findings remain to be determined, routine supplementation of formulas with LCPUFAs should be considered.

▶ If you haven't had a visit from your formula representative extolling the virtues of added LCPUFA to infant formulas, you are probably on an extended sabbatical overseas. Using BAEPs, these Turkish investigators show that infants fed human milk or formula supplemented with LCPUFAs during the first 16 weeks of life have accelerated maturation of the BAEP compared with infants fed standard formulas. These data are consistent with other observations regarding the benefits of supplementing formulas with LCPUFAs in term as well as preterm infants. Of course, all of this only reemphasizes the obvious—the ideal nutrition for both term and preterm infants is human milk. Please read the recent excellent policy statement on breastfeeding from the American Academy of Pediatrics.[1]

M. J. Maisels, MB, BCh

Reference

1. American Academy of Pediatrics, Section on Breastfeeding: Breastfeeding and the use of human milk. *Pediatrics* 115:496-506, 2005.

Salt Wasting and Deafness Resulting From Mutations in Two Chloride Channels

Schlingmann KP, Konrad M, Jeck N, et al (Philipps Univ of Marburg, Germany; Olgahospital Stuttgart, Germany)
N Engl J Med 350:1314-1319, 2004   8–27

Background.—A newly identified phenotype of antenatal Bartter's syndrome has been identified in which both severe renal salt wasting and sensorineural deafness are present. This new phenotype has been designated as antenatal Bartter's syndrome with sensorineural deafness (BSND). The case of a child with renal salt wasting and deafness who had no mutation in the *BSND* gene was presented.

Case Report.—The patient was born to consanguineous parents (first cousins) at 28 weeks' gestation with a birth weight of 1250 g. The baby was at the fortieth percentile for gestational age. Severe maternal polyhydramnios had necessitated repeated amniocenteses during the last 6 weeks of gestation. Within 72 hours after birth the child had polyuria and volume depletion associated with hypokalemia and metabolic alkalosis, which required supplementation with water, sodium, and potassium chloride. Antenatal Bartter's syndrome was diagnosed on the basis of excessive urinary prostaglandin E-M excretion, and treatment with indomethacin was initiated 10 days after birth. Response was unsatisfactory, and the indomethacin was discontinued. Treatment with rofecoxib was initiated and the patient was monitored. However, he required supplementary potassium and sodium for fluid and electrolyte balance. Audiometry at 8 weeks showed bilateral sensorineural deafness at 8 weeks, and genetic analysis was performed for a *BSND* gene defect.

Conclusions.—The patient in this report had a combined ClC-Ka and ClC-Kb chloride channel defect but did not have phenotypic features that would be mirrored by a simple superposition of the 2 monogenic phenotypes. Combined impairment of ClC-Ka and ClC-Kb results in a phenotype that mimics antenatal Bartter's syndrome with deafness through defects in barttin, the beta subunit common to the ClC-K–type chloride channels. These channels are suggested to be regulated by barttin.

▶ In 1962 Bartter et al described a syndrome of hypokalemic, hypochloremic metabolic alkalosis. Other characteristics of the disorder included increased urinary excretion of potassium and prostaglandins, normal or low blood pressure despite increased plasma renin activity, high serum aldosterone concentrations, a relative vascular resistance to the pressor effects of exogenous angiotensin II, and hyperplasia of the juxtaglomerular apparatus. Bartter's syndrome has an autosomal recessive mode of inheritance and is not a single disease, but a set of closely related renal tubular disorders. At least 3 phenotypic subgroups have been identified: an antenatal hypercalciuric variant, also termed hyperprostaglandin E syndrome, which is characterized by polyhydramnios, prematurity, and dehydration (severe volume depletion) at birth; classic Bartter's syndrome, which presents in children, often as failure to thrive; and a hypocalciuric-hypomagnesemic variant known as Gitelman's syndrome, which often presents in adults. This heterogeneity and the diverse array of physiologic derangements long confounded efforts to understand the fundamental defects in these syndromes.[1] However, over the past few years the mysteries have been solved, the mutations for the hypokalemic salt-losing tubulopathies identified, and the inner workings of the tubules demystified. As these authors state, "Molecular genetic analyses of the different forms of Bartter's syndrome have revealed mutations in various genes encoding ion channels and transporters that mediate transepithelial salt reabsorption along distal nephron segments: the sodium-potassium-chloride co-transporter NKCC2, and the potassium channel ROMK in antenatal Bartter's syndrome (genetically defined as Bartter's types I and II, respectively); the chloride channel ClC-Kb in classic Bartter's syndrome (Bartter's type III), and the sodium-chloride co-transporter (NCCT) in Gitelman's variant."

In 1995 Landau et al[2] identified a phenotype of antenatal Bartter's syndrome, with both severe renal salt wasting and sensorineural deafness; it is called antenatal Bartter's syndrome with sensorineural deafness (BSND, or Bartter's type IV). In contrast to the other Bartter variants, the underlying genetic defect does not affect a bona fide ion-transport protein. Rather, mutations in the *BSND* gene product, a protein called barttin, indirectly interfere with epithelial salt transport by impairing the barttin-dependent insertion in the plasma membrane of ClC-Kb and the closely related chloride channel ClC-Ka, both of which associate with barttin in the epithelial cells of the kidney and the inner ear. Schlingmann et al add their case of a child born of consanguineous parents with the syndrome yet a normal *BSND* gene. The child had mutations in each of 2 genes encoding the chloride transporters ClC-Ka and ClC-Kb. The data provide strong evidence that barttin regulates ClC-K–type chloride channels, and thus provide new insight into renal salt handling. The case report is fascinating and reads like a Sherlock Holmes short story Under usual circumstances a single case report does not warrant publication in the *New England Journal of Medicine*, accompanied by a commentary/editorial. However, this is a unique case reported by Schlingmann and associates, whc have been at the forefront of the studies on the variants of Bartter's syndrome. The accompanying exquisitely illustrated commentary by Bichet and Fujiwara[3] provides deep insight into renal tubular function and salt and water metabolism.

A. A. Fanaroff, MD

References

1. Guay-Woodford LM: Bartter syndrome: Unraveling the pathophysiologic enigma. *Am J Med* 105:151-161, 1998.
2. Landau D, Shalev H, Ohaly M, et al: Infantile variant of Bartter syndrome and sensorineural deafness: A new autosomal recessive disorder. *Am J Med Genet* 59:454-459, 1995.
3. Bichet DG, Fujiwara TM: Reabsorption of sodium chloride—Lessons from the chloride channels. *N Engl J Med* 350:1281-1283, 2004.

9 Behavior and Pain

Oral Glucose Before Venepuncture Relieves Neonates of Pain, but Stress Is Still Evidenced by Increase in Oxygen Consumption, Energy Expenditure, and Heart Rate
Bauer K, Ketteler J, Hellwig M, et al (Klinikum der Johann Wolfgang Goethe-Universität, Frankfurt, Germany; Freie Universität Berlin)
Pediatr Res 55:695-700, 2004   9–1

Background.—Although oral glucose appears to mitigate pain in neonates undergoing venepuncture, it is not know whether it mitigates stress. This prospective, randomized, double-blind trial analyzed whether 2 concentrations of glucose solution attenuated increases in oxygen consumption (Vo_2), energy expenditure (EE) and heart rate (HR) in neonates undergoing venepuncture.

Study Design.—The study group consisted of 58 neonates who were undergoing venepuncture as part of their care. Infants were randomly assigned to 2 mL 30% glucose, 0.4 mL 30% glucose, or 2mL water orally. When a venepuncture was scheduled, oral solution was administered in 1 minute, then venepuncture was performed within 2 minutes. Vo_2, carbon dioxide output volume, ECG, HR, and EE were measured for 30 minutes. Both crying time and the Premature Infant Pain Profile score (a validated pain measure for infants) were assessed and compared among the 3 study groups.

Findings.—Prior oral administration of 2 mL of glucose reduced both pain score and crying in neonates after venepuncture compared to those of both the placebo and the 0.4 mL glucose solution groups. However, administration of 2 mL of glucose solution did not affect Vo_2 increase, EE, nor HR.

Conclusion.—Although prior oral administration of 2 mL of 30% glucose solution appears to have been effective pain therapy for neonates undergoing a venepuncture, it did not ameliorate the stress of the procedure. Therefore, venepuncture and other stressful handling of neonates should be kept to a minimum. Other interventions may be useful for reducing stress in neonates who must undergo stressful procedures.

► Bauer et al looked at physiologic responses as an index of pain. They found that 2 mL of 30% glucose applied orally did lower the subjective pain score and the amount of crying after venepuncture compared to placebo controls, though a smaller dose (0.4 mL) did not. However, even the larger dose of glucose did not prevent a significant increase from baseline for HR, EE, or Vo_2. The study groups were small (20, 20, and 18 subjects in each group), and measurements of EE and Vo$_2$ are difficult, with some intrinsic variability. Perhaps the lower results in the treated infants would have reached significance with larger groups.

The authors theorized that the increase in the metabolic measurements were due to the physiologic response to both pain and handling, and perhaps the oral sweetener only decreased the first component. This seems plausible and perhaps could be addressed by additional studies with a control group exposed to "sham" venepuncture involving holding and restraint alone. I would think that the restraint and handling involved in just doing the metabolic studies would be enough to elicit the same metabolic stress. Could an additional control group be found just by performing the metabolic studies without any venepuncture?

R. S. Cohen, MD

Can Daily Repeated Doses of Orally Administered Glucose Induce Tolerance When Given for Neonatal Pain Relief?

Eriksson M, Finnström O (Örebro Univ Hosp, Sweden; Univ Hosp, Linköping, Sweden)
Acta Paediatr 93:246-249, 2004   9–2

Background.—Although the pain-relieving effect of sweet solutions for neonates is well documented, the mechanism is not well understood. Whether repeated doses of sweet solution would induce opioid-like tolerance to its pain-relieving effects in newborns was investigated in a prospective, randomized, blinded study.

Study Design.—The study group consisted of 43 full-term, healthy neonates whose parents administered either 1 mL of oral 30% glucose or water 3 times daily from birth until the metabolic screening test 3 to 5 days after birth. At the time of the metabolic screening test, the infants returned to the hospital and were all given the glucose solution. They then had their heel pricked for the test 2 minutes later. Crying time, the Premature Infant Pain Profile score, and changes in heart rate were used to evaluate pain by a researcher blinded as to group membership.

Findings.—There was no difference in the response to the sweet solution between the neonates randomized to prior water or to sweet solution treatment.

Conclusion.—This study found that repeated administration of a sweet solution to healthy neonates did not induce tolerance to its antinociceptive effects.

▶ The oral application of sweet solutions (eg, concentrated sucrose or glucose) to ameliorate pain has become an increasingly accepted therapy in neonatal ICUs. The exact mechanism isn't clear, though it appears to involve opioid receptors in addition to the soothing effect of sucking on the pacifier. Furthermore, we know little about the "pharmacology" of this treatment, eg, dosing, timing, side effects, etc. These 2 articles (Abstracts 9–1 and 9–2) add interesting and important data to this area while leaving many questions yet unanswered.

Eriksson and Finnström could not demonstrate the development of tolerance after thrice daily dosing for more than 72 hours. They reported no difference in pain score between infants exposed either to thrice daily glucose or placebo when both groups experienced heel sticks after treatment with oral glucose. Perhaps more frequent exposure would have resulted in tolerance. Certainly, in the neonatal ICU, noxious stimuli can and do happen more than 3 times a day with our sicker infants. Also, there was no control group that had their heels lanced without oral glucose treatment. Though unlikely, it is possible that their glucose treatment was ineffective and the pain score would not have differed significantly from completely untreated infants.

R. S. Cohen, MD

Randomised Controlled Trial of Swaddling Versus Massage in the Management of Excessive Crying in Infants With Cerebral Injuries
Ohgi S, Akiyama T, Arisawa K, et al (Nagasaki Univ, Japan)
Arch Dis Child 89:212-216, 2004   9–3

Background.—Infants with neonatal cerebral insults are susceptible to excessive crying as a result of difficulties with self-regulation.

Aims.—To compare the effectiveness of swaddling versus massage therapy in the management of excessive crying of infants with cerebral insults

Methods.—Randomised three-week parallel comparison of the efficacy of two intervention methods. Infants with symptoms of troublesome crying and their parents were randomly assigned to a swaddling intervention group (n = 13) or a massage intervention group (n = 12).

Results.—The amount of total daily crying decreased significantly in the swaddling group, but did not decrease significantly in the massage group. Infant behavioural profiles and maternal anxiety levels improved significantly in the swaddling group post-intervention. Parents in the swaddling group were more satisfied with the effectiveness of the intervention in reducing crying than parents in the massage group.

Conclusion.—Results indicate that swaddling may be more effective than massage intervention in reducing crying in infants with cerebral injuries.

▶ Infants with neonatal cerebral insults are susceptible to excessive crying, which prompted this randomized trial to compare the effectiveness of swaddling and massage to calm them. The amount of total daily crying decreased significantly in the swaddling group, and the parents were more satisfied. Swaddling is a reasonable and harmless intervention for infants with cerebral injuries who cry excessively. As I scanned this article it stimulated me to look at the bigger picture of developmental care.

Developmental care is a broad category of interventions designed to minimize the stress of the neonatal ICU environment. These interventions may include one or more elements, such as control of external stimuli (vestibular, auditory, visual, tactile), clustering of nursery care activities, and positioning or swaddling of the preterm infant. Symington and Pinelli[1] reviewed the available data (32 eligible randomized controlled trials involving 4 major groups of developmental care interventions, 19 subgroups, and multiple clinical outcomes) for promoting development and preventing morbidity in preterm infants. Some benefits of developmental interventions included improved short-term growth and feeding outcomes, decreased respiratory support, decreased length and cost of hospital stay, and improved neurodevelopmental outcomes to 24 months' corrected age. They concluded, "The results of the review indicate that developmental care interventions demonstrate some benefit to preterm infants with respect to: improved short-term growth and feeding outcomes, decreased respiratory support, decreased length and cost of hospital stay, and improved neurodevelopmental outcomes to 24 months corrected age. These findings were based on two or three small trials for each outcome, and did not involve meta-analyses of more than two trials for any one outcome. Although a number of other benefits were demonstrated, those results were from single studies with small sample sizes. The lack of blinding of the assessors was a significant methodological flaw in half of the studies. The cost of the interventions and personnel was not considered in any of the studies.

Although there is evidence of some benefit of developmental care interventions overall, and no major harmful effects reported, there were a large number of outcomes for which no or conflicting effects were demonstrated. The single trials that did show a significant effect of an intervention on a major clinical outcome were based on small sample sizes, and the findings were often not supported in other small trials. Before a clear direction for practice can be supported, evidence demonstrating more consistent effects of developmental care interventions on important short- and long-term clinical outcomes is needed. The economic impact of the implementation and maintenance of developmental care practices should be considered by individual institutions."

A. A. Fanaroff, MD

References

1. Symington A, Pinelli J: Developmental care for promoting development and preventing morbidity in preterm infants. *Cochrane Database Syst Rev* 4:CD001814, 2003.

Specific Newborn Individualized Developmental Care and Assessment Program Movements Are Associated With Acute Pain in Preterm Infants in the Neonatal Intensive Care Unit

Holsti L, Grunau RE, Oberlander TF, et al (British Columbia Research Inst for Children's and Women's Health, Vancouver, BC, Canada; Univ of British Columbia, Vancouver, Canada)

Pediatrics 114:65-72, 2004   9–4

Objective.—The Newborn Individualized Developmental Care and Assessment Program (NIDCAP) is widely used in neonatal intensive care units and comprises 85 discrete infant behaviors, some of which may communicate infant distress. The objective of this study was to identify developmentally relevant movements indicative of pain in preterm infants.

Methods.—Forty-four preterm infants were assessed at 32 weeks' gestational age (GA) during 3 phases (baseline, lance/squeeze, and recovery) of routine blood collection in the neonatal intensive care unit. The NIDCAP and Neonatal Facial Coding System (NFCS) were coded from separate continuous bedside video recordings; mean heart rate (mHR) was derived from digitally sampled continuous electrographic recordings. Analysis of variance (phase × gender) with Bonferroni corrections was used to compare differences in NIDCAP, NFCS, and mHR. Pearson correlations were used to examine relationships between the NIDCAP and infant background characteristics.

Results.—NFCS and mHR increased significantly to lance/squeeze. Eight NIDCAP behaviors also increased significantly to lance/squeeze. Another 5 NIDCAP behaviors decreased significantly to lance/squeeze. Infants who had lower GA at birth, had been sicker, had experienced more painful procedures, or had greater morphine exposure showed increased hand movements indicative of increased distress.

Conclusions.—Of the 85 NIDCAP behaviors, a subset of 8 NIDCAP movements were associated with pain. Particularly for infants who are born at early GAs, addition of these movements to commonly used measures may improve the accuracy of pain assessment.

► Although the NIDCAP has been used widely in neonatal ICUs throughout North America and Europe since the 1980s, this study is the first to examine whether the NIDCAP catalog behaviors can be used to identify acute pain in preterm infants under well-controlled conditions with a relatively large sample. The infants in this study showed facial, behavioral state, and heart rate responses similar to responses documented in other studies of responses of preterm infants to acute pain. Limitations of the study include lack of blinding to body movements, but facial coding was conducted blinded to events. The authors were thrilled to find a subset of 8 NIDCAP movements that seem to be associated with acute pain in preterm infants, including some that have not been described as behavioral pain cues before this study. They also noted 5 behaviors that decreased, including jitteriness and startles, which are behaviors associated with normal fetal sleep state rather than pain.

Fisting, flexing, and extending the extremities and finger splay increased during the lance phase. Finger splay was more common before 30 weeks' gestation, not only during lance/squeeze, but also during the baseline phase; they may therefore be a developmentally specific distress cue and may indicate more stress for these infants. Fisting is another sensitive distress cue in infants less than 30 weeks' gestation. In addition to fisting and finger splaying, which have been previously associated with painful experiences in the neonatal ICU, the movement of hand on face (which involves a defensivelike action, with the infant placing a hand on its face) may represent an additional pain cue in the preterm population. Frowning (brow lowering) also increased during the lance, as did foot clasping and mouthing.

A concern of the authors was that the foot lance was applied with the infants in the prone position and whether position affected the response. However, the same investigators examined this question[1] and reported that although the prone position promotes deep sleep in preterm neonates at 32 weeks' postconceptional age when they are undisturbed, placement in prone position is not a sufficient environmental comfort intervention for painful invasive procedures such as heel lance for blood sampling in the neonatal ICU. No significant differences were found in premature infants' responses to pain if they were prone or supine.

A. A. Fanaroff, MD

Reference

1. Grunau RE, Linhares MB, Holsti L, et al: Does prone or supine position influence pain responses in preterm infants at 32 weeks gestational age? *Clin J Pain* 20:76-82, 2004.

Parental Concern and Distress About Infant Pain
Franck LS, Cox S, Allen A, et al (Inst of Child Health, London; King's College, London; Great Ormond Street Hosp for Children NHS Trust, London)
Arch Dis Child Fetal Neonatal Ed 89:F71-F75, 2004   9–5

Objective.—To describe parent views on infant pain care and to explore relations between parents' experience of their infant's pain care and parental stress.

Design.—Descriptive, cross sectional survey.

Setting.—Nine neonatal units (196 parents) in the United Kingdom and two neonatal units in the United States (61 parents).

Participants.—Parents of preterm and full term infants admitted to hospital.

Interventions.—Parents completed a three part questionnaire after the second day of the infant's admission and after they had made at least one previous visit to see their infant in the neonatal unit.

Main Outcome Measures.—Parent concerns about infant pain; parental stress; parent state and trait anxiety.

Results.—Parents reported that their infants had experienced moderate to severe pain that was greater than they had expected ($p < 0.001$). Few parents (4%) received written information, although 58% reported that they received verbal information about infant pain or pain management. Only 18% of parents reported that they were shown signs of infant pain, but 55% were shown how to comfort their infant. Parents had numerous worries about pain and pain treatments. Parental stress was independently predicted by parents' estimation of their infant's worst pain, worries about pain and its treatment, and dissatisfaction with pain information received, after controlling for state anxiety and satisfaction with overall care ($F = 29.56$, df 6, $p < 0.001$, $R^2 = 0.44$). The findings were similar across sites, despite differences in infant characteristics.

Conclusions.—Parents have unmet information needs about infant pain and wish greater involvement in their infant's pain care. Parent concerns about infant pain may contribute to parental stress.

▶ Infants in neonatal ICUs all experience a lot of pain, and our management of pain in the neonatal ICU leaves much to be desired. In addition, it is not surprising that parents who witness many of the painful episodes in a neonate's stay express substantial anxiety about the effects of pain on their infant.

For parents, the neonatal ICU is a very stressful experience, and we might be able to mitigate this stress to some extent if we took the trouble to inform parents that although we need to perform some painful procedures on their infant, we will do everything we can to prevent and ameliorate pain when such procedures are unavoidable. In addition, we should encourage greater involvement of parents and enlist their support in helping alleviate pain in their infants. It is only relatively recently that we have emerged from the dark ages with respect to our understanding of pain in infants and children and our interventions to relieve it. The relief of pain in the sick neonate is still a controversial subject and, in many areas, the optimal approaches are yet to be defined.[1,2]

M. J. Maisels, MB, BCh

References

1. American Academy of Pediatrics, Committee on Fetus and Newborn: Prevention and management of pain and stress in the neonate. *Pediatrics* 105:454, 2000.
2. Anand KJ: Consensus statement for the prevention and management of pain in the newborn. *Arch Pediatr Adolesc Med* 155:173-180, 2001.

The Effect of Skin-to-Skin Contact (Kangaroo Care) Shortly After Birth on the Neurobehavioral Responses of the Term Newborn: A Randomized, Controlled Trial

Ferber SG, Makhoul IR (Univ of Haifa, Israel; Meyer Children's Hosp, Haifa, Israel)

Pediatrics 113:858-865, 2004   9–6

Background.—The initial postnatal period is highly stressful for neonates. The effects of skin-to-skin contact (kangaroo care [KC]) on the postdelivery behavioral responses of the healthy, term newborn were investigated in a randomized, blinded study.

Study Design.—The study group consisted of 50 consecutive healthy, term singleton newborns whose mothers had spontaneous vaginal deliveries. Newborns and mothers were randomly assigned to either standard care (control) or KC care. KC consisted of an hour of skin-to-skin contact in the delivery room before the newborn was taken to the nursery. Four hours after delivery, all infants were evaluated for 1 hour in the nursery by observers blinded as to treatment group.

Findings.—During the observation period, KC infants were observed to sleep longer, be in a quieter state, and to have more flexor and less extensor movements and postures compared with control newborns.

Conclusions.—KC seems to reduce stress in the immediate postoperative period for healthy term neonates. The medical staff should consider providing this type of care after delivery.

▶ Ferber and Makhoul have done a prospective, randomized, controlled trial on the effects of KC on term infants. The effect of skin-to-skin contact (or KC) on preterm infants is well studied. Daily KC in the neonatal ICU helps to improve bonding between the mother and preterm infant during the long stay of these infants in the nursery. One expects the same procedure may also be beneficial during the short stay of the term infant in the hospital. However, the findings of this study make one wonder whether the effect results from depriving controls from the natural mother-infant bonding in the immediate hours after delivery rather than from KC. After being weighed, infants who received KC remained with their mothers for 1 hour, whereas control infants were deprived and joined their mothers after the study was completed (5 hours postpartum). Among 10 variables studied, the authors found a rather modest effect on sleep, cry, and movement, which given the large standard deviations and the small sample size raises questions about the value of the statistical significance of the data. Many neonatal neurologic examinations, including the one used in this study, include sleep and alertness. However, recording sleep and alertness in newborn infants needs special expertise. The lack of familiarity of the observers with infant sleep studies, the lack of polysomnographic recordings, and the short period of observation (for quantitative sleep studies) make the sleep findings in this study less convincing. Furthermore, since the frequency of crying and the quality of movements are influenced by newborn sleep states, these results may be a consequence of sleep rather than independent findings. Although group randomization is the best way to investigate the effect of any intervention, the expectation is that differences will not be found between the control and experimental groups before the intervention. Therefore, it is worth mentioning that in this study, the sample size studied differed (22 control infants vs 25 infants receiving KC), and more girls were in the control group. Nevertheless, the conclusion of the study may well be to encourage changing the practice of care in hospitals by increasing interactions between mothers and infants for both preterm and term infants from the moment of birth onward.

M. Mirmiran, MD, PhD

Effects of Morphine Analgesia in Ventilated Preterm Neonates: Primary Outcomes From the NEOPAIN Randomised Trial
Anand KJS, for the NEOPAIN Trial Investigators Group (Univ of Arkansas, Little Rock; et al)
Lancet 363:1673-1682, 2004   9–7

Background.—Opioid analgesia is commonly used during neonatal intensive care. We undertook the Neurologic Outcomes and Pre-emptive Analgesia in Neonates (NEOPAIN) trial to investigate whether pre-emptive morphine analgesia decreases the rate of a composite primary outcome of neonatal death, severe intraventricular haemorrhage (IVH), and periventricular leucomalacia (PVL) in preterm neonates.

Methods.—Ventilated preterm neonates (n=898) from 16 centres were randomly assigned masked placebo (n=449) or morphine (n=449) infusions. After a loading dose (100 µg/kg), morphine infusions (23-26 weeks of gestation 10 µg kg^{-1}h^{-1}; 27-29 weeks 20 µg kg^{-1}h^{-1}; 30-32 weeks 30 µg kg^{-1} h^{-1}) were continued as long as clinically justified (maximum 14 days). Open-label morphine could be given on clinical judgment (placebo group 242/443 [54.6%], morphine group 202/446 [45.3%]). Analyses were by intention to treat.

Findings.—Baseline variables were similar in the randomised groups. The placebo and morphine groups had similar rates of the composite outcome (105/408 [26%] vs 115/419 [27%]), neonatal death (47/449 [11%] vs 58/449 [13%]), severe IVH (46/429 [11%] vs 55/411 [13%]), and PVL (34/367 [9%] vs 27/367 [7%]). For neonates who were not given open-label morphine, rates of the composite outcome (53/225 [24%] vs 27/179 [15%], p=0.0338) and severe IVH (19/219 [9%] vs 6/189 [3%], *p*=0.0209) were higher in the morphine group than the placebo group. Placebo-group neonates receiving open-label morphine had worse rates of the composite outcome than those not receiving open-label morphine (78/228 [34%] vs 27/179 [15%], *p*<0.0001). Morphine-group neonates receiving open-label morphine were more likely to develop severe IVH (36/190 [19%] vs 19/219 [9%], *p*=0.0024).

Interpretation.—Pre-emptive morphine infusions did not reduce the frequency of severe IVH, PVL, or death in ventilated preterm neonates, but intermittent boluses of open-label morphine were associated with an increased rate of the composite outcome. The morphine doses used in this study decrease clinical signs of pain but can cause significant adverse effects in ventilated preterm neonates.

▶ There has been much progress in the understanding of pain and its consequences for the newborn infant; however, there is still a great deal of missing information, misunderstanding, and even misinterpretation of the available data. Furthermore, pain in the newborn infant is under recognized and under treated. Neonatal caretakers must remain aware that sedation does not provide pain relief and may mask the newborn infant's ability to express pain. The ability to recognize and monitor pain has improved substantially, but there is a disconnect between recognizing that a procedure may be painful and attempts to alleviate pain. This is exemplified by the data from Simons et al.[1] They documented that on average, each of 156 neonates was subjected to a mean ± SD of 1414 procedures per day, most commonly suctioning. The highest exposure to painful procedures occurred during the first day of admission. Preemptive analgesic therapy was provided to fewer than 35% of neonates per study day, whereas 40% of the neonates did not receive any analgesic therapy in the neonatal ICU. They correctly concluded, "Despite the accumulating evidence that neonatal procedural pain is harmful, analgesic treatment for painful procedures is limited. Systematic approaches are required to reduce the occurrence of pain and to improve the analgesic treatment of repetitive pain in neonates." These are indeed ongoing, but the data have been discouraging.

The NOPAIN Study abstracted above, for example, is a wonderful multicenter, multinational collaborative effort designed to investigate whether preemptive morphine analgesia decreases the rate of a composite primary outcome of neonatal death, severe IVH, and PVL in preterm neonates. The answer is that it did not; indeed, the primary outcome was worse when open-labeled morphine was used.

Morphine did decrease clinical signs of pain, but at what price? In a similar trial Simons et al,[2] in The Netherlands in a randomized double-blind controlled trial, evaluated the effects of continuous IV morphine infusion on pain responses, incidence of IVH, and poor neurologic outcome (severe IVH, PVL, or death) on 150 newborn infants who required assisted ventilation. IV morphine (100 μg/kg and 10 μg/kg per hour) or placebo infusion was given for 7 days (or less because of clinical necessity in several cases). According to the various pain scales (Premature Infant Pain Scale; Neonatal Infant Pain Scale and Visual Analog Scale), the analgesic effect did not differ between the morphine and placebo groups. Routine morphine infusion decreased the incidence of IVH (23% vs 40%, $P = .04$), but did not influence poor neurologic outcome (10% vs 16%, $P = .66$). Hence, with evidence of neither a measurable analgesic effect nor better neurologic outcome, the routine use of morphine for preterm infants requiring ventilatory support cannot be recommended.

So, the database has expanded. We are wiser, but no closer to knowing how best to preempt painful procedures or to manage pain for ventilated preterm infants. We should all recognize the potential sources of pain, prevent unnecessary procedures, use specific and sensitive methods for the assessment of pain, and develop specific protocols to manage pain. A combination of environmental, behavioral, and pharmacologic approaches may provide the best pain relief.

A. A. Fanaroff, MD

References

1. Simons SH, van Dijk M, Anand KS, et al: Do we still hurt newborn babies? A prospective study of procedural pain and analgesia in neonates. *Arch Pediatr Adolesc Med* 157:1058-1064, 2003.
2. Simons SH, van Dijk M, van Lingen RA, et al: Routine morphine infusion in preterm newborns who received ventilatory support: A randomized controlled trial. *JAMA* 290:2419-2427, 2003.

Postoperative Pain Assessment in the Neonatal Intensive Care Unit
McNair C, Ballantyne M, Dionne K, et al (Univ of Toronto)
Arch Dis Child Fetal Neonatal Ed 89:F537-F541, 2004   9–8

Introduction.—The subjective nature of pain makes its measurement difficult in infants. No composite measures of infant pain have been evaluated for validity in the clinical context of real-time postoperative pain management. The combined validity of 2 measures of pain (premature infant pain profile [PIPP] and crying, need for oxygen, increased vital signs, expression, and sleepiness [CRIES]) were assessed in real-life postoperative pain evaluation in infants.

Methods.—Using a prospective, repeated-measures correlational design, the authors randomly assigned 2 staff nurses to use either the PIPP or CRIES measure. An expert rater evaluated each infant postoperatively and once daily using the visual analogue scale (VAS) at a level III neonatal ICU.

Results.—Pain was evaluated in 51 neonates (28-42 weeks' gestational age) postoperatively. No significant differences were noted in the rates of change between the pain assessment measures across time, using repeated-measures analysis of variance ($F_{50,2} = 0.62$; $P = .540$). Convergent validity analysis, using intraclass correlation, demonstrated a positive correlation, which was most evident in the initial 24 hours immediately, and 4, 8, 20, and 24 hours postoperatively. Correlations were more divergent at 40 and 72 hours postoperatively. No significant interactions were identified between gestational age and measure ($F_{304,4} = 0.75$; $P = .563$) and surgical group and measure ($F_{304,2} = 0.39$; $P = .680$).

Conclusion.—Both PIPP and CRIES are valid measures that correlate positively with pain during the initial 72 hours postoperatively in both term and preterm infants. Both measures together would provide health care professionals with an objective measure of neonatal pain.

▶ The assessment of postoperative pain in the term and preterm newborn is complex, and our knowledge is incomplete. Numerous tools have been reported but none have become the standard as they have not been evaluated in all patient populations after all types of surgery. Nor have most of these tools been adequately evaluated in the clinical arena. This article provides support for the clinical validation of 2 pain assessment tools, PIPP and CRIES, in term and premature infants of more than 28 weeks' gestation. However, what is desperately needed, are similar data for the postoperative evaluation of premature infants who are less than 28 weeks' gestation. These infants are our most vulnerable patients for whom suboptimal pain management probably has the most significant consequences.

D. Batton, MD

Postoperative Pain in the Neonate: Age-related Differences in Morphine Requirements and Metabolism
Bouwmeester NJ, Hop WCJ, van Dijk M, et al (Sophia Children's Hosp, Rotterdam, The Netherlands; Erasmus Med Ctr, Rotterdam, The Netherlands; et al)
Intensive Care Med 29:2009-2015, 2003   9–9

Introduction.—Health care professionals are becoming increasingly aware of the need for pain management in neonates and infants. Morphine doses that provide adequate postoperative analgesia in newborn infants have not been determined. The age-associated differences in morphine requirements and metabolism after thoracic or abdominal surgery were investigated in full-term neonates.

Methods.—The study included 68 neonates, 0 to 4 weeks old (gestational age 35-42 weeks) who were admitted to the surgical ICU after thoracic or abdominal surgery. Fifty-two neonates were younger than 7 days; 16 were 7 days or older. Postoperatively, patients were selected randomly to either continuous morphine (10 µg/kg per hour) or intermittent morphine (30 µg/kg every 3 hours). Additional morphine was administered, on the basis of pain scores. Pain was measured via the Comfort behavior scale and visual analog scale. Morphine and morphine-6-glucuronide (M6G) plasma concentrations were ascertained before surgery and at 0, 6, 12, and 24 hours postoperatively.

Results.—Younger neonates had significantly different median morphine values than those of older neonates: morphine requirements (10 vs 10.8 µg/kg per hour), morphine plasma concentration (23.0 vs 15.3 ng/mL), and M6G/morphine ratio (0.6 vs 1.5). Pain scores did not vary significantly between age groups or morphine treatment groups. Neonates who were mechanically ventilated longer than 24 hours had significantly higher morphine plasma concentration, compared with that of spontaneously breathing neonates 12 and 24 hours postoperatively (29.1 vs 13.1 ng/mL and 26.9 vs 12.0 ng/mL, respectively). Morphine plasma concentrations were not associated with analgesia or respiratory depression. Five neonates (intermittent morphine) experienced respiratory insufficiency ($P = NS$).

Conclusion.—Neonates, 7 days old or younger, need significantly less morphine postoperatively, compared with the need of older neonates. No significant differences were noted in the effectiveness and safety of continuous versus intermittent morphine regimens. Mechanical ventilation reduced morphine metabolism and clearance.

▶ Morphine and other opioids are used routinely for postoperative pain management in newborns although we have an incomplete understanding of their pharmacokinetics in this population. This article provides important data on morphine doses for term or near-term infants who are greater than or less than 1 week old at the time of their surgery. These data suggest that a lower dose of morphine can be used for younger newborns, and this information will be helpful to clinicians as we strive to provide effective postoperative pain relief without undesirable side effects. We desperately need similar data for our most vulnerable patients—those with a gestational age less than 28 weeks—in whom the consequences of over- or underdosing with morphine postoperatively may be the most significant.

D. Batton, MD

10 Gastrointestinal Health and Nutrition

Parenteral Glutamine Supplementation Does Not Reduce the Risk of Mortality or Late-onset Sepsis in Extremely Low Birth Weight Infants
Poindexter BB, for the National Institute of Child Health and Human Development Neonatal Research Network (Indiana Univ, Indianapolis; et al)
Pediatrics 113:1209-1215, 2004   10–1

Background.—Glutamine is one of the most abundant amino acids in both plasma and human milk, yet it is not included in standard intravenous amino acid solutions. Previous studies have suggested that parenteral nutrition (PN) supplemented with glutamine may reduce sepsis and mortality in critically ill adults. Whether glutamine supplementation would provide a similar benefit to extremely low birth weight (ELBW) infants is not known.

Methods.—We performed a multicenter, randomized, double-masked, clinical trial to assess the safety and efficacy of early PN supplemented with glutamine in decreasing the risk of death or late-onset sepsis in ELBW infants. Infants 401 to 1000 g were randomized within 72 hours of birth to receive either TrophAmine (control) or an isonitrogenous study amino acid solution with 20% glutamine whenever they received PN up to 120 days of age, death, or discharge from the hospital. The primary outcome was death or late-onset sepsis.

Results.—Of the 721 infants who were assigned to glutamine supplementation, 370 (51%) died or developed late-onset sepsis, as compared with 343 of the 712 infants (48%) assigned to control (relative risk: 1.07; 95% confidence interval: 0.97-1.17). Glutamine had no effect on tolerance of enteral feeds, necrotizing enterocolitis, or growth. No significant adverse events were observed with glutamine supplementation.

Conclusions.—Parenteral glutamine supplementation as studied did not decrease mortality or the incidence of late-onset sepsis in ELBW infants. Consequently, although no harm was demonstrated, routine use of parenteral glutamine supplementation cannot be recommended in this population.

A Randomized, Controlled Trial of Parenteral Glutamine in Ill, Very Low Birth-Weight Neonates

Thompson SW, McClure BG, Tubman TRJ (Craigavon Area Hosp, County Armagh, Northern Ireland; Royal Maternity Hosp, Belfast, Northern Ireland)
J Pediatr Gastroenterol Nutr 37:550-553, 2003   10–2

Objective.—The role of "novel substrates" in neonatal nutrition has generated much interest in recent years. Glutamine has been recognized as a "conditionally essential" amino acid in critically ill adults, particularly for gut and immune function; however, its potential role in the neonate remains unclear. The authors examined the safety and benefits of parenteral glutamine in ill, preterm neonates.

Design.—Randomized controlled trial.

Methods.—Thirty-five ill preterm neonates of <1000 g birth-weight were randomized to receive either glutamine-supplemented parenteral nutrition (PN) (n = 17) or standard PN (n = 18).

Results.—There were no significant differences in birth-weight, gestational age, male-to-female ratio, or Clinical Risk Index for Babies (CRIB) score between the two groups. During PN there were no significant differences between the groups in white cell count, differential white cell count, blood urea nitrogen, plasma ammonia, lactate, pyruvate, plasma glutamine, or glutamate. The median time to achieving full enteral nutrition (FEN) was shorter in the study group (13 days vs. 21 days, $P < 0.05$). The number of episodes of culture-positive sepsis or age at discharge did not differ between groups.

Conclusions.—Parenteral glutamine appears to be well tolerated and safe in the ill, preterm neonate. It may reduce the time to achieving FEN.

▶ Sepsis is a major cause of morbidity and mortality in low–birth weight infants. Hence the prospect of enhancing the immune system either enterally or parenterally is very attractive. The gastrointestinal tract is the largest surface area of the body and the primary entry site for microorganisms and foreign antigens. The use of enteral feedings enriched with immune-enhancing ingredients, or "prebiotics," such as glutamine, arginine, omega-3 fatty acids, nucleotides, probiotics, and lactoferrin, have attracted much interest. Furthermore, the re-emergence of probiotics such as *Lactobacillus* raises intriguing possibilities of reducing gastrointestinal disorders as well as sepsis in this vulnerable population. Glutamine has been recognized as a "conditionally essential" amino acid in critically ill adults, particularly for gut and immune function; however, its potential role in the neonate remains unclear.

Ball and Hardy[1] in 2002 reviewed the literature and examined the issues surrounding the use of glutamine in pediatrics and neonatology. Evidence showed that glutamine levels are affected in a number of life stages and conditions. Useful, indicative studies are emerging, but many fail to demonstrate significant differences. They identified the need for a great deal of further research in this area, including larger multicenter trials. Well, the trials have been done (the studies by Poindexter et al and Thompson et al), more basic research has been concluded, and we remain bereft of evidence of the benefit of glutamine supplementation either enterally or parenterally for low–birth weight infants.

Glutamine is one of the most abundant amino acids in both plasma and human milk, yet it is not included in standard intravenous amino acid solutions for neonates. Poindexter et al, in a large prospective trial, hypothesized that PN supplemented with glutamine may reduce sepsis and mortality rate in ELBW infants, akin to its action in critically ill adults. Alas, parenteral glutamine supplementation, as studied, did not decrease mortality rate or the incidence of late-onset sepsis in ELBW infants. They correctly concluded that although no harm was demonstrated, routine use of parenteral glutamine supplementation cannot be recommended in this population. In examining the safety of glutamine supplementation, Thompson et al found no evidence of harm, but neither did they find benefit other than a shorter time to full enteral nutrition. So although breast milk is loaded with glutamine, Parimi et al[2] in Cleveland noted that glutamine administered enterally to growing preterm infants was entirely metabolized in the gut and had no discernable effect on whole-body protein and nitrogen kinetics. Glutamine, therefore, remains an enigma with regard to preterm infants.

A. A. Fanaroff, MD

References

1. Ball PA, Hardy G: Glutamine in pediatrics—Where next? *Nutrition* 18:451-454, 2002.
2. Parimi PS, Devapatla S, Gruca LL, et al: Effect of enteral glutamine or glycine on whole-body nitrogen kinetics in very-low-birth-weight infants. *Am J Clin Nutr* 79:402-409, 2004.

Survey of Vitamin A Supplementation for Extremely-Low-Birth-Weight Infants: Is Clinical Practice Consistent With the Evidence?
Ambalavanan N, Kennedy K, Tyson J, et al (Univ of Alabama, Birmingham; The Univ of Texas, Houston)
J Pediatr 145:304-307, 2004   10–3

Objective.—To survey the attitudes and practices among level III neonatal intensive care units in the United States regarding vitamin A supplementation for extremely-low-birth-weight (ELBW; birth weight ≤1000 g) infants.

Study design.—A pretested questionnaire regarding vitamin A supplementation was distributed to all (n = 102) neonatal-perinatal training program directors (TPD) and 105 randomly selected directors of level III neonatal intensive care units (nontraining program directors, NTPD).

Results.—Ninety-nine percent of TPD and 94% of NTPD responded. In a minority of programs (20% TPD, 13% NTPD), >90% of eligible extremely-low-birth-weight neonates are supplemented with vitamin A, whereas in most programs (69% TPD, 82% NTPD), routine supplementation is not practiced. Most centers (91% TPD, 81% NTPD) supplementing vitamin A use a dose of 5000 IU IM 3 times per week for 4 weeks. The most common reason that TPD give for not supplementing vitamin A is the perceived small benefit, whereas the most common reason for NTPD is that they consider the intervention unproven.

Conclusions.—These findings indicate inconsistency in practicing evidence-based medicine in neonatal practice, where therapies are often administered on the basis of weaker evidence of safety and benefit than supports vitamin A supplementation. Educational interventions may be required to endorse the benefits and safety of vitamin A supplementation.

▶ "Evidenced-based neonatology": if we all practice it, why does it turn out so differently in different neonatal ICUs (NICUs)? Why does it depend on whether a NICU has a training program? Let me first admit my bias: after participating in the large, National Institutes of Health Neonatal Network vitamin A supplementation trial,[1] our NICU routinely gives it to ELBW infants to try to reduce bronchopulmonary dysplasia. The current article's survey reveals that three fourths of the nation's NICUs view the same evidence and come to a different clinical conclusion. As not all of these centers can have lower than average bronchopulmonary dysplasia rates, it is intriguing that they would not opt to give this inexpensive medication, even if administered subcutaneously. It can't be a money issue; compared with surfactant and inhaled nitric oxide, vitamin A costs peanuts. It would indeed be unfortunate if adoption of vitamin A supplementation suffered from a lack of a corporate sponsor and the attendant marketing. The reported survey results indicate that most nonusers claim that the benefits of vitamin A are either too small or unproven. As the authors suggest, perhaps some neonatologists are expecting that our treatments should be more of a magic bullet; in which case we should not be using even more unproven therapies such as bronchodilators or diuretics to treat bronchopulmonary dysplasia. Given the biologic basis of its action, I can understand an approach that restricts vitamin A supplementation of ELBW infants to be based on vitamin A levels; however, such an approach should be considered experimental until proven by clinical trial. Until such a study demonstrates a better way to supplement vitamin A, or a different study demonstrates a heretofore risk of such supplementation, this article continues to speak to the wide variability and distinction between evidence and practice.

W. D. Rhine, MD

Reference

1. Tyson JE, Wright LL, Oh W, et al: Vitamin A supplementation for extremely-low-birth-weight infants. National Institute of Child Health and Human Development Neonatal Research Network. *N Engl J Med* 340:1962-1968, 1999.

Paradoxical Impact of Body Positioning on Gastroesophageal Reflux and Gastric Emptying in the Premature Neonate
Omari T, Rommel N, Staunton E, et al (Univ of Adelaide, Australia; Women's and Children's Hosp, North Adelaide, Australia; Royal Adelaide Hosp, Adelaide, Australia)
J Pediatr 145:194-200, 2004
10–4

Objectives.—To combine manometry and impedance to characterize the mechanisms of gastroesophageal reflux (GER) and to explore their relation to the rate of gastric emptying (GE) and body position.

Study Design.—Ten healthy preterm infants (35 to 37 weeks' postmenstrual age) were studied with the use of a micromanometric/impedance assembly. Episodes of GER were identified by impedance, and the mechanism (s) of GER triggering and GER clearance were characterized. GE was determined with a C13Na-octanoate breath test.

Results.—Gastroesophageal reflux episodes (n = 89) were recorded, consisting of 74% liquid, 14% gas, and 12% mixed. Transient lower esophageal sphincter relaxation (TLESR) was the predominant mechanism of reflux, triggering 83% of GER. Of 92 TLESRs recorded, 27% were not associated with reflux. Infants studied in the right lateral position had significantly (*P* < .01) more GER, a higher proportion of liquid GER (*P* < .05), and faster GE (*P* < .005) when compared with infants studied in the left lateral position.

Conclusions.—In healthy preterm infants, GER is predominantly liquid in nature. Right-side positioning is associated with increased triggering of TLESR and GER despite accelerating GE.

▶ This is an elegant study that uses newer technology to confirm the pathophysiology of GER in premature neonates and the effect of positioning on its severity. Following the American Academy of Pediatrics' recommendations against the prone position (to prevent sudden infant death syndrome), when faced with GERD, most pediatricians have advised parents to use the left lateral position to help their children. The study data would have been more convincing if the same patients had been studied in both the right and left lateral positions.

The ability to miniaturize medical equipment to fit a premature newborn is impressive. Nevertheless, we need to remember that we still do not have appropriate normative data for impedance monitoring, although it is helpful in correlating the presenting symptoms with the episodes of reflux.

S. Gebara, MD

Systematic Review of Transpyloric Versus Gastric Tube Feeding for Preterm Infants

McGuire W, McEwan P (Ninewells Hosp, Dundee, Scotland)
Arch Dis Child Fetal Neonatal Ed 89:F245-F248, 2004   10–5

Background.—Preterm infants may have difficulty with oral feeding because of poor coordination of sucking and swallowing. Enteral nutrition may be delivered through a catheter by way of the gastric or transpyloric route. A meta-analysis was done to determine whether feeding by the transpyloric rather than the gastric route improves feeding tolerance and growth and development, without increasing adverse consequences, in preterm infants who require tube feeding.

Study Design.—The standard collaborative search strategy of the Cochrane Neonatal Collaborative Review group was used. The Cochrane Controlled Trials Register (2003), Medline (1966 to April 2003) and Embase (1980 to April 2003) were searched. A fixed effect model was used for meta-analysis.

Findings.—Eight trials with a total of 340 preterm infants were included. There was no difference between gastric and pyloric tube feeding for growth or development. Transpyloric feeding was associated with a greater incidence of gastrointestinal disturbances and an increased mortality rate. There was no difference between these 2 feeding methods for other adverse events.

Conclusions.—There is no benefit to transpyloric enteral feeding of preterm infants, but there may be increased risks associated with use of this route. Transpyloric feeding cannot be recommended for this vulnerable patient group.

▶ One of the most difficult challenges facing the neonatologist is providing enteral nutrition for the very low birth weight infant. In most situations, discoordinated gastrointestinal motility is the limiting factor in this process. While all the muscular layers of the intestine and appropriate innervation are in place by the 24th week of gestation, these infants have significant gastroesophageal reflux, delayed gastric emptying time, and either quiescence or paucity of the normal migrating motor complexes necessary for the propulsion of intraluminal contents. To obviate some of these problems, transpyloric feeds have been used, and in some centers this has become a routine method of feeding the immature infant.

These authors have performed a thorough and comprehensive search by using the Cochrane Neonatal Collaborative Review process, and have stated that the transpyloric route has not shown any benefit over the nasogastric route of feeding. Although most of the data that were reviewed are from studies carried out in the 1970s, with two in the 1980s and one in 1992, the benefits of transpyloric feeds did not decrease the incidence of aspiration pneumonia, improve rapidity of weight gain, or result in earlier discharge from the hospital. Although these studies did not demonstrate an increased incidence of intestinal perforation, this problem has been encountered by many who have used either silastic or polyurethane transpyloric feeding catheters.

In lieu of the transpyloric feeding tube, what could one use to mitigate the poor intestinal motility? Cisapride, which was used with great enthusiasm, has been removed from the market because of its potential for producing prolongation of the QTc interval and serious arrhythmias. Metoclopramide has been used with some success in infants, but the medication has had some serious side effects such as extrapyramidal reactions.

Recently, erythromycin, a motilin agonist, given enterally in 10-mg/kg dose every 6 hours, has improved gastric emptying and shortened whole-gut transmit time in premature infants.[1] Judchula and Berseth,[2] using lower doses of 1 to 3 mg/kg, did not demonstrate induction of mature migrating motor complexes or of increasing the amplitude and frequency of antral contractions in infants of less than 31 weeks' gestation. They demonstrated that more mature preterm and term infants had significant responses to this agent.

Few prokinetic agents are available for the very immature infant, but eythromycin in a dosage of 3 to 10 mg/kg every 6 hours has some promise in facilitating enteral motility. There are still potential problems, such as an increase in the incidence of pyloric stenosis, risks of bacterial overgrowth, and cardiac arrhythmias.[3] Thus, while erythromycin has potential in facilitating gastrointestinal motility, it should be reserved for infants with significant motility problems and not be used routinely in all infants until further studies have been carried out and documented that it is beneficial without causing significant side effects.[4]

P. Sunshine, MD

References

1. Costales C, Gounaris A, Varhalama E, et al: Erythromycin as a prokinetic agent in preterm infants. *J Pediatr Gastroenterol Nutr* 34:23-25, 2002.
2. Jadcherla SR, Berseth CL: Effect of erythromycin on gastroduodenal contractile activity in developing neonates. *J Pediatr Gastroenterol Nutr* 34:16-22, 2002.
3. Kaul A: Erythromycin as a prokinetic agent. *J Pediatr Gastroenterol Nutr* 34:13-15, 2002.
4. Ng PC, SO KW, Fung KSC, et al: Randomised controlled study of oral erythromycin for treatment of gastrointestinal dysmotility in preterm infants. *Arch Dis Child Fetal Neonatal Ed* 84:F177-F182, 2001.

Randomized Double-Blind Study of the Nutritional Efficacy and Bifidogenicity of a New Infant Formula Containing Partially Hydrolyzed Protein, a High β-Palmitic Acid Level, and Nondigestible Oligosaccharides
Schmelzle H, Wirth S, Skopnik H, et al (Univ of Greifswald, Germany; Children's Hosp, Wuppertal, Germany; Municipal Hosp, Worms, Germany; et al)
J Pediatr Gastroenterol Nutr 36:343-351, 2003   10–6

Objectives.—The aim of this study was to evaluate the nutritional efficacy and bifidogenic characteristics of a new infant formula containing partially hydrolyzed whey protein, modified vegetable oil with a high β-palmitic acid content, prebiotic oligosaccharides, and starch.

Methods.—In a double-blind study, healthy formula-fed term infants aged younger than 2 weeks were randomized to receive either the new infant formula (NF) or a standard formula (SF) until the age of 12 weeks. Anthropometric measurements were taken at enrollment, 6 weeks, and 12 weeks. In a subsample of infants, blood samples were taken at 6 weeks and stool samples were taken at enrollment and 6 weeks. Blood samples were analyzed for biochemical measures of protein status and amino acids, and stools were analyzed for total bacteria and bifidobacteria. Mothers completed a feeding diary and questionnaire at 6 and 10 weeks.

Results.—One hundred fifty-four infants were enrolled in the study; 102 completed the trial. The growth of infants in both formula groups was in line with published growth curves. During the first 6 weeks, NF girls gained more weight and head circumference than the SF girls. These velocity differences were not maintained throughout the 12-week study period. The NF stools had a higher proportion of bifidobacteria at 6 weeks compared with the SF stools, and they were softer. There were no clinically significant differences in the blood biochemical and amino acid values between groups. Both formulas were well tolerated by the infants.

Conclusions.—When compared with a standard infant formula, the new formula supported satisfactory growth, led to higher counts of bifidobacteria in the feces, produced blood bio-chemical values typical of formula-fed infants, and was well tolerated.

▶ Judging from the bombardment of information on nutrition in the various media, you would have guessed that jazzing up the formula with hydrolyzed whey protein, modified vegetable oil with high β-palmitic acid content, prebiotic oligosaccharides, and starch would result in enhanced growth. And of course you have been proven wrong by Schmelzle and associates. The prebiotics served their function well, and the infants receiving NF did have softer stools containing microflora with more bifidobacteria. Both formulae were well tolerated and the growth and biochemical parameters were not different. One can speculate, as the authors did, that having a higher proportion of bifidobacteria may protect against gastrointestinal infections and allergy, but that would require another set of studies. Yes, you guessed it, that is what the authors suggest; but of course, human breast milk is best.

A. A. Fanaroff, MD

Effect of Bottles, Cups, and Dummies On Breast Feeding in Preterm Infants: Randomised Controlled Trial
Collins CT, Ryan P, Crowther CA, et al (Women's and Children's Hosp, North Adelaide, South Australia; Univ of Adelaide, South Australia; Mercy Hosp for Women, Melbourne, Victoria, Australia)
BMJ 329:193-196, 2004   10–7

Objective.—To determine the effect of artificial teats (bottle and dummy) and cups on breast feeding in preterm infants.

Design.—Randomised controlled trial.

Setting.—Two large tertiary hospitals, 54 peripheral hospitals.

Participants.—319 preterm infants (born at 23-33 weeks' gestation) randomly assigned to one of four groups: cup/no dummy (n = 89), cup/dummy (n = 72), bottle/no dummy (n = 73), bottle/dummy (n = 85). Women with singleton or twin infants < 34 weeks' gestation who wanted to breastfeed were eligible to participate.

Interventions.—Cup or bottle feeding occurred when the mother was unable to be present to breast feed. Infants randomised to the dummy groups received a dummy on entry into the trial.

Main Outcome Measures.—Full breast feeding (compared with partial and none) and any breast feeding (compared with none) on discharge home.

Secondary outcomes: prevalence of breast feeding at three and six months after discharge and length of hospital stay.

Results.—303 infants (and 278 mothers) were included in the intention to treat analysis. There were no significant differences for any of the study outcomes according to use of a dummy. Infants randomised to cup feeds were more likely to be fully breast fed on discharge home (odds ratio 1.73, 95% confidence interval 1.04 to 2.88, $P = 0.03$), but had a longer length of stay (hazard ratio 0.71, 0.55 to 0.92, $P = 0.01$).

Conclusions.—Dummies do not affect breast feeding in preterm infants. Cup feeding significantly increases the likelihood that the baby will be fully breast fed at discharge home, but has no effect on any breast feeding and increases the length of hospital stay.

▶ Despite the limitations of poor compliance, this is a valuable study. Little objective data are available on how to manage feedings in preterm infants whose mothers seek to breastfeed, but the mother is not there or the infant is too immature to nurse effectively at the breast.

Rocha et al[1] compared cup to bottle feeding beginning at 37 weeks' postconceptional age in low birth weight (LBW) infants and found no difference in the rate of any breastfeeding, but a higher rate of breastfeeding at 3 months postdischarge. Other data on cup feeding suggest that, although safe, intake is so small as to bring its usefulness into question.[2,3] Certainly the reluctance of both staff and parents in this study to use exclusive cup feeding makes it a less feasible intervention. These factors, when combined with the increase in length of hospital stay associated with cup feeding, support the conclusion that cup feeding is not a strategy that will significantly impact rates of breastfeeding among preterm infants.

Other interventions to circumvent bottle feeding that have been tried include the use of nasogastric feeds. Kliethermes et al[4] found that tube feeding, as compared with bottle feeding, improved breastfeeding rates at discharge in LBW infants, but this study has neither been repeated nor conducted in a population of smaller (very LBW) infants whose mothers will be pumping for much longer before discharge.

Certainly this is a difficult clinical problem. It is possible that individual infants will be "talented" or flexible enough to tolerate bottle feeding and still learn to nurse effectively, whereas others cannot—any method of prospectively identifying such infants would be helpful. At least we know that there is no reason to avoid pacifiers, and possibly a trial of nasogastric feeds combined with pacifier suckling, and at least daily attempted nursing at the breast would be supported by both the data and mothers, and neonatal professionals.

L. Furman, MD

References

1. Rocha NM, Martinez FE, Jorge SM: Cup or bottle for preterm infants: Effects on oxygen saturation, weight gain and breastfeeding. *J Human Lact* 18:132-138, 2002.
2. Marinelli KA, Burke GS, Dodd VL: A comparison of the safety of cupfeedings and bottlefeedings in premature infants whose mothers intend to breastfeed. *J Perinatol* 21:350-355, 2001.
3. Dowling DA, Meier PP, Di Fiore JM, et al: Cup-feeding for preterm infants: Mechanics and safety. *J Human Lact* 18:13-20, 2002.
4. Kliethermes PA, Cross ML, Lanese MG, et al: Transitioning preterm infants with nasogastric tube supplementation: increased likelihood of breastfeeding. *J Obstet Gynecol Neonatal Nurs* 28:264-273, 1999.

▶ The terminology on either side of the Atlantic creates interesting situations. Collins et al show that "dummies," ie, pacifiers, have no significant effect on establishing breast feeding in preterm infants. Cups, on the other hand, improve the likelihood of establishing breast feeding, but delay discharge. Is this cost effective, and whose costs are we examining? Prolonging hospital stay is not desirable for many reasons. The philosophy in both the United States and the United Kingdom is that feeding human milk to preterm infants is highly desirable. It presents a challenge to both the mothers and staff, but if there are benefits, then it is surely worth the effort.

There are few who would argue about either the short- or long-term benefits of breast feeding for term infants. Indeed, it is gospel that feeding human milk reduces all sorts of infections and even sudden infant death syndrome. Is there similar evidence for preterm infants? Despite intensive research in infant nutrition uncertainty persists over many aspects of practice. Whereas Lucas et al[1] has suggested that the intelligence is higher in preterm infants fed human milk with fortifiers, it is somewhat distressing to read the systematic review by de Silva et al[2] on the question: "Does human milk (HM) reduce infection rates in preterm infants?" They included a total of 9 reports, including 6 cohorts and 3 randomized controlled trials. They concluded that "Methodological problems included poor study design, inadequate sample size, failure to adjust for confounding variables, and inadequate definitions of HM feeding and outcome measures. In conclusion, the advantage of HM in preventing infection in preterm (VLBW) infants is not proven by the existing studies. Recommendations are made regarding the methodology required for further study of this important topic." The risks of human milk feeding may include transmission of cytomegalovirus, but I remain of the opinion that in the long run the benefits outweigh the risks and we should continue to encourage women who deliver prematurely to provide human milk for their offspring. The evidence is accumulating that the way a preterm infant is fed, in just the early weeks postpartum, may have a major impact on later growth and development and program the cardiovascular system. For example, breast milk consumption was associated with lower later blood pressure in children born prematurely.[3]

A. A. Fanaroff, MD

References

1. Lucas A, Morley R, Cole TJ: Randomised trial of early diet in preterm babies and later intelligence quotient. *BMJ* 317:1481-1487, 1998.
2. de Silva A, Jones PW, Spencer SA: Does human milk reduce infection rates in preterm infants? A systematic review. *Arch Dis Child Fetal Neonatal Ed* 89:F509-F513, 2004.
3. Singhal A, Cole TJ, Lucas A: Early nutrition in preterm infants and later blood pressure: Two cohorts after randomised trials. *Lancet* 357:413-419, 2001.

The Effect of Prenatal Consultation With a Neonatologist on Human Milk Feeding in Preterm Infants

Friedman S, Flidel-Rimon O, Lavie E, et al (Rehovot and Hebrew Univ, Jerusalem)
Acta Paediatr 93:775-778, 2004

10–8

Objective.—To study the effect of prenatal consultation (PC) with a neonatologist on the incidence and duration of human milk feeding (HMF) in preterm infants.

Design/Methods.—A retrospective matched case-control study was preformed at a perinatal centre. Study infants were preterm infants (23-35 wk) whose mothers had received PC emphasizing the importance of HMF. Control infants were matched by birthweight, gestational age and multiplicity.

Results.—Each group included 29 mothers and 46 preterm infants. Mean gestational age was 30.1 ± 3 wk in both groups. Mean birthweight was 1 329 ± 489 (PC) and 1 334 ± 441 g (control). PC infants received HMF for significantly longer, both in the hospital and after discharge (hospital: PC 37 ± 34 d vs control 15 ± 19 d, $p = 0.001$; discharge PC 60 ± 57 d vs control 21 ± 32 d; $p = .0001$). No significant difference in neonatal morbidity was detected between the groups.

Conclusions.—PC is associated with significantly longer HMF in preterm infants, both in hospital and after discharge.

▶ For mothers threatening to deliver a preterm infant, there are several important advantages to having a PC with a neonatologist. First, the neonatologist can prepare the parents on what to expect in the delivery room as well as the neonatal ICU. Second, by engaging in discussion with the parents, the neonatologist can both assist the parents in making informed decisions and inform the health care team of those decisions, whether they are for full resuscitation or comfort care.[1] Finally, the neonatologist can become a source of "continuity and comfort" as the parents transition from the obstetrical ward to the neonatal ICU.

Previous studies have validated the usefulness of a PC with a neonatologist.[2] The authors of this study, however, are the first to report 2 additional findings: first, an absolute increase in the number of mothers who choose to breastfeed; and second, those who choose to breastfeed do so for a longer period of time. These are important benefits. The American Academy of Pediatrics recently updated guidelines on breastfeeding emphasize the myriad advantages of breastfeeding, listing "health, nutritional, immunologic, developmental, psychologic, social, economic, and environmental benefits."[3] These advantages apply to preterm infants as well, but mothers of preterm infants face additional challenges not encountered by mothers of healthy term infants and therefore require close support.

There are several limitations to the study, which the authors readily acknowledge. First, the study was retrospective in design and thus could not control for the information delivered. Second, the study involved a single institution in which all consultation was provided by 2 attendings who were interested and skilled in counseling on breastfeeding. This speaks well to the quality of consultation at that institution but may have limited applicability to other places with a variety of professionals performing consultations. Finally, because the study group was defined by the initiation of a PC, there was a selection bias in favor of preterm labor as the cause of delivery in the study group. Despite these limitations, however, this article should be commended for highlighting the PC as a key opportunity to promote HMF for preterm infants.

J. M. Fanaroff, MD, JD

References

1. Committee on Bioethics, American Academy of Pediatrics: Ethics of the care of critically ill infants and children. *Pediatrics* 98:149-152, 1996.
2. Halamek LP. Prenatal consultation at the limits of viability. *NeoReviews* 4(6):e153, 2003.
3. Section on Breastfeeding, American Academy of Pediatrics: Breastfeeding and the use of human milk. *Pediatrics* 115:496-506, 2005.

Factors Influencing Initiation of Breast-Feeding Among Urban Women
Noble L, Hand I, Haynes D, et al (Jacobi Med Ctr, Bronx, NY; Bronx Lebanon Hosp, NY)
Am J Perinatol 20:477-483, 2003   10–9

The objective of our study was to identify factors associated with the initiation of breast-feeding in a poor urban area. One hundred postpartum, nonadolescent, non-drug using mothers, 50 breast-feeding and 50 formula feeding, were consecutively interviewed. Breast-feeding women were more likely to be born outside of the United States (42 versus 14%, $p = 0.002$), have more years of education (12.1 ± 1.9 versus 10.9 ± 1.7, $p = 0.002$), be employed either prior to or during pregnancy (38 versus 16%, $p = 0.000$), be married (46 versus 26%, $p = 0.037$), be a nonsmoker (86 versus 64%, $p = 0.011$), have more prenatal visits (8.4 ± 7.3 versus 5.0 ± 5.9, $p = 0.010$), or have a breast-feeding mother (48 versus 26%, p = 0.023). There were no differences in age or ethnicity. The father of the breast-feeding baby was more likely to be better educated (12.0 ± 2.8 versus 10.5 ± 3.6 years, p = 0.022) and to work full-time (68 versus 40%, p = 0.005). Eighty-four percent of formula feeders knew that breast milk was better for their babies but decided not to breast-feed due to concerns of pain, smoking, and work. Sixty-three percent of women made the choice to breast-feed prior to the pregnancy, 26% during the pregnancy, and 11% after delivery. Significantly more multiparas decided prior to the pregnancy compared with primiparas. We recommend that breast-feeding education should be started prior to the first pregnancy and tailored to the concerns of the women.

▶ The objective of this study was to identify factors associated with the initiation of breastfeeding in a poor, urban area of New York City. Comparing 50 mothers who chose to formula feed exclusively to 50 mothers who chose to breastfeed (partially or exclusively), factors associated with formula feeding, which are consistent with other reports, were poverty, lower education, unemployment, single marriage status, smoking, and nonimmigrant status. Factors not consistently reported in other studies include no ethnic differences between African American and Hispanics, no positive influence of prenatal classes on breastfeeding initiation, and fathers of formula-fed infants being less supportive of the feeding decision than those of breastfed infants.

What information does this study contribute to the important question of how and when to influence the feeding decisions of mothers who are statistically most likely to formula feed? The study report that "84% of formula feeders knew that breast milk was better for their babies, but decided not to breastfeed due to concerns of pain, smoking, and work." As the majority of mothers made feeding choices before pregnancy, these investigators recommend that breastfeeding education be started before the first pregnancy and tailored to the concerns of the women. Yet if prenatal education had no impact, it is difficult to imagine that preconception breastfeeding education, in a low-education population, would be more persuasive.

In this study, 21% of primiparous women made feeding decisions after delivery, while still in the hospital. It has been demonstrated that in an inner-city hospital that provides care to poor, minority, and immigrant families, full implementation of the Ten Steps to Successful Breastfeeding, initially conceived by the World Health Organization and United Nations Children's Emergency Fund, can strongly influence initiation rates.[1] At Boston Medical Center, initiation rates increased among U.S.-born black mothers from 34% (1998) to 64% (1998) to 74% (1999). The American Academy of Pediatrics recently revised policy statement on breastfeeding strongly supports these steps.[2] It is clear from this and many other studies that women, including those less educated, are quite aware of the superiority of human milk. From the Boston example, what is needed are hospitals, which provide new mothers with accurate information and skilled support, at a time when behavioral changes are most likely to be adopted.

J. Morton, MD

References

1. Philipp BL, Merewood A, Miller L, et al: Baby-friendly hospital initiative improves breastfeeding initiation rates in a US hospital setting. *Pediatrics* 108:677-681, 2001.
2. American Academy of Pediatrics, Section on Breastfeeding. Policy statement: Breastfeeding and the use of human milk. *Pediatrics* 115:496-506, 2005.

Suppressive Effects of Breast Milk on Oxidative DNA Damage in Very Low Birthweight Infants

Shoji H, Shimizu T, Shinohara K, et al (Juntendo Univ, Tokyo)

Arch Dis Child Fetal Neonatal Ed 89:F136-F138, 2004   10–10

Background.—Premature infants are exposed to many potential sources of oxygen free radical production, including high concentrations of inspired oxygen, frequent alterations in blood flow to major organs, and inflammation with accumulation of neutrophils and macrophages. Premature infants are also known to have a poorly developed antioxidant system, which may place them at risk of radical damage. An imbalance between oxidant generating systems and antioxidants in very low birthweight (VLBW) infants has been implicated in the pathogenesis of the major complications of prematurity. Many kinds of antioxidant are present in human milk, which is thought to prevent diseases mediated by oxygen free radicals in VLBW infants. 8-Hydroxydeoxyguanosine (8-OHdG) has been accepted as a sensitive marker for oxidative DNA damage. The purpose of the present study was to examine the antioxidant effects of breast milk in VLBW infants.

Methods.—The infants in this study had a birth weight of less than 1500 g and no major congenital abnormalities and were born in or transported to the neonatal ICU of one hospital in Tokyo. The breast-fed group included 15 infants (8 boys and 7 girls) with a mean gestational age of 29.2 (2.3) weeks

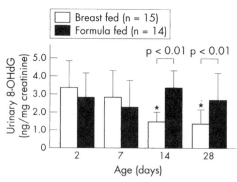

FIGURE 1.—Change in urinary 8-hydroxydeoxyguanine (8-OHdG) excretion at 2, 7, 14, and 28 days of age in breast fed and formula fed very low birthweight infants. Values are mean (SD). *p<0.01 compared with 2 and 7 days. (Courtesy of Shoji H, Shimizu T, Shinohara K, et al: Suppressive effects of breast milk on oxidative DNA damage in very low birthweight infants. *Arch Dis Child Fetal Neonatal Ed* 89:F136-F138, 2004, with permission from the BMJ Publishing Group.)

and a mean birth weight of 1231 (298) g who received more than 90% of their intake as breast milk. The formula-fed group was composed of 14 infants (8 boys, 6 girls) with a mean gestational age of 28.7 (2.0) weeks and a mean birth weight of 1182 (281) g who received 90% of their intake in the form of commercial formula for premature infants. Urinary 8-OHdG concentrations were measured in both groups at 2, 7, 14, and 28 days of age.

Results.—The excretion of urinary 8-OHdG at 14 and 28 days of age was significantly lower than at age 2 and days of age in the breast-fed group and significantly lower than in the formula-fed group (Fig 1).

Conclusions.—This study shows the first direct evidence of the antioxidant action of human milk by measurement of urinary 8-OHdG in VLBW infants, showing that oxidative DNA damage is significantly more suppressed in breast-fed VLBW infants than in formula-fed VLBW infants at 14 and 28 days of age.

▶ It is getting positively tiresome to reiterate repeatedly the benefits of human milk for human infants of all birth weights, shapes, and sizes. But there is no harm in doing so again. For the first time, we now have direct evidence of the antioxidant action of human milk in VLBW infants and we know that VLBW infants are susceptible to oxidative free radical damage. Urinary 8-OHdG is a noninvasive marker for in vivo oxidative DNA damage, and these investigators previously showed lower excretion of urinary 8-OHdG in breast-fed term neonates (2004 YEAR BOOK OF NEONATAL AND PERINATAL MEDICINE, page 238). They now demonstrate similar findings in a group of VLBW infants. The VLBW infants who received breast milk had significantly lower levels of urinary 8-OHdG excretion at 14 and 28 days of age. Nature still knows best.

M. J. Maisels, MB, BCh

Effect of Storage on Breast Milk Antioxidant Activity

Hanna N, Ahmed K, Anwar M, et al (Univ of Medicine and Dentistry of New Jersey, New Brunswick; St Peter's Univ, New Brunswick)
Arch Dis Child Fetal Neonatal Ed 89:F518-F520, 2004   10–11

Background.—Human milk, which contains compounds beneficial to infants, is often expressed and stored before use. Changes in its antioxidant activity with storage have not been studied.

Objectives.—To measure antioxidant activity of fresh, refrigerated (4°C), and frozen human milk (-20°C), stored for two to seven days; to compare the antioxidant activity of milk from mothers delivering prematurely and at term; to compare the antioxidant activity of infant formulas and human milk.

Methods.—Sixteen breast milk samples (term and preterm) were collected from mothers within 24 hours of delivery and divided into aliquots. Fresh samples were immediately tested for antioxidant activity, and the rest of the aliquots were stored at -20°C or 4°C to be analysed at 48 hours and seven days respectively. The assay used measures the ability of milk samples to in-

TABLE 1.—Comparison of the Antioxidant Capacity of Human Milk and Formula

	Fresh	4°C (48 Hours)	4°C (7 Days)	−20°C (48 Hours)	−20°C (7 Days)
Human milk (n = 16)	1.66 (0.06)	1.58 (0.06)	1.48 (0.05)	1.45 (0.05)	1.34 (0.04)
Formula (n = 5)	1.07 (0.02)*	1.08 (0.04)*	1.05 (0.02)*	1.05 (0.02)*	1.07 (0.04)*

Data are presented as Trolox equivalent antioxidant capacity.
*$p < 0.05$ compared with human milk.
(Courtesy of Hanna N, Ahmed K, Anwar M, et al: Effect of storage on breast milk antioxidant activity. *Arch Dis Child Fetal Neonatal Ed* 89:F518-F520, 2004, with permission from the BMJ Publishing Group.)

hibit the oxidation of 2,2'-azino-di-3-(ethylbenzthiazolinesulphonate) to its radical cation compared with Trolox.

Results.—Antioxidant activity at both refrigeration and freezing temperatures was significantly decreased (Table 1). Freezing resulted in a greater decrease than refrigeration, and storage for seven days resulted in lower antioxidant activity than storage for 48 hours. There was no difference in milk from mothers who delivered prematurely or at term. Significantly lower antioxidant activity was noted in formula milk than in fresh human milk.

Conclusions.—To preserve the antioxidant activity of human milk, storage time should be limited to 48 hours. Refrigeration is better than freezing and thawing.

▶ The comprehensive statement recently issued by the American Academy of Pediatrics on breastfeeding and the use of human milk recommends that human milk be given to premature and other high-risk infants either by direct breastfeeding or by using the mother's own expressed milk.[1] Because preterm infants have reduced antioxidant capacity, it would be nice if the antioxidant activity of human milk could be preserved until it is given to the infant.

This study shows that both refrigeration and freezing significantly decrease the antioxidant activity of human milk, and this decrease in activity increased with longer storage time. In addition, refrigeration affected the antioxidant capacity less significantly than did freezing. The conclusion is clear: if we want to preserve antioxidant activity we should endeavor to refrigerate rather than freeze expressed breast milk and give it to the babies within 48 hours after its collection. Because of the anti-infective, anti–necrotizing enterocolitis properties and other benefits of human milk for low birth weight infants, we should make every effort to get the maximum benefit from this unique source of human nutrition.

M. J. Maisels, MB, BCh

Reference

1. American Academy of Pediatrics, Section on Breastfeeding: Breastfeeding and the use of human milk. *Pediatrics* 115:496-506, 2005.

Increased Osmolality of Breast Milk With Therapeutic Additives

Srinivasan L, Bokiniec R, King C, et al (Imperial College London; Hammersmith Hosp, London; Queen Charlottes and Chelsea Hosp, London)
Arch Dis Child Fetal Neonatal Ed 89:F514-F517, 2004   10–12

Aim.—To evaluate the changes in the osmolality of expressed breast milk (EBM) after the addition of seven additives and four proprietary fortifiers commonly used during neonatal intensive care.

Methods.—The osmolality of 5 ml EBM was measured with increasing doses of 6% NaCl, caffeine, sodium ironedetate, folic acid, and multivitamin drops. Sodium acid phosphate and chloral hydrate were added to 8 ml EBM, and the fortifiers were added to standard volumes of EBM. Dose-effect curves were plotted, and the volume of milk that must be added to the above additives to maintain osmolality below 400 mOsm/kg was calculated.

Results.—The osmolality of the pure additives ranged from 242 to 951 mOsm/kg. There was a significant increase in the osmolality of EBM with increasing doses of all additives except caffeine. The osmolality of EBM with many additives in clinically used dosages potentially exceeded 400 mOsm/kg. The greatest increase occurred with sodium ironedetate syrup, where the osmolality of EBM increased to 951.57 (25.36) mOsm/kg. Proprietary fortifiers increased the osmolality of EBM to a maximum of 395 mOsm/kg.

Conclusion.—Routine additives can significantly increase the osmolality of EBM to levels that exceed current guidelines for premature infant feeding. A simple guide for clinical use is presented, which indicates the amount of milk required as diluent if hyperosmolality is to be avoided.

▶ We sometimes add medications to the expressed breast milk that our mothers provide for their infants in the neonatal ICU. These authors show that by so doing we might significantly increase the osmolality of the expressed breast milk beyond safe limits. They provide us with a useful and practical guide to the amount of breast milk that is required as a solvent for various additives to maintain osmolality below 400 mOsm/kg.

M. J. Maisels, MB, BCh

Why Are Babies Weaned Early? Data From a Prospective Population Based Cohort Study

Wright CM, Parkinson KN, Drewett RF (Univ of Glasgow, Scotland; Univ of Newcastle upon Tyne, England; Univ of Durham, England)
Arch Dis Child 89:813-816, 2004   10–13

Background.—The recommended age of introduction of solids food to the diet of infants (weaning) has recently been increased in the UK to 6 months, but most babies are still weaned before the age of 4 months.

Aims.—To examine what predicts the age of weaning and how this relates to weight gain and morbidity using data from a population based cohort.

Methods.—Parents of 923 term infants born in a defined geographical area and recruited shortly after birth were studied prospectively using postal questionnaires, weaning diaries, and routinely collected weights, of whom 707 (77%) returned data on weaning.

Results.—The median age of first weaning solids was 3.5 months, with 21% commencing before 3 months and only 6% after 4 months of age. Infants progressed quickly to regular solids with few reported difficulties, even when weaned early. Most parents did not perceive professional advice or written materials to be a major influence. The strongest independent predictors of earlier age at weaning were rapid weight gain to age 6 weeks, lower socioeconomic status, the parents' perception that their baby was hungry, and feeding mode. Weight gain after 6 weeks was unrelated to age of weaning. Babies weaned before 3 months, compared to after 4 months, had an increased risk of diarrhoea.

Conclusions.—Social factors had some influence on when weaning solids were introduced, but the great majority of all infants were established on solids before the previously recommended age of 4 months, without difficulty. Earlier weaning was associated with an increased rate of minor morbidity.

▶ A growing body of research reporting the association of improved outcomes of breastfed children and the exclusivity and duration of breast milk feedings provides strong support for the recommendations of the American Academy of Pediatrics and World Health Organization for 6 months of exclusive breastfeeding before the introduction of solids.[1]

To examine why the majority of children in the United Kingdom are introduced to solids earlier than even 4 months, this prospective study examined the social and biologic correlates of early introduction of solid food. Out of a sample size of 707 subjects, 21% were introduced to solids before 3 months, and only 6% were given solids after 4 months. Significant predictors of early introduction were lower socioeconomic status, bottle feeding, rapid weight gain from birth to 6 weeks, and the perception that the "baby seemed hungry." Predictors of "delayed" introduction of solids (after 4 months) included any breastfeeding and disagreement with the statement "baby seemed hungry." Parents were more influenced by the perceived needs of their child than external advice. The study reported an increased rate of minor short-term morbidity, notably diarrhea, in those weaned earlier.

The findings in this study have been reported elsewhere, except for one: the children introduced to solids earlier (those who were predominately rapidly growing, formula-fed infants), were more likely perceived by their parents as "hungry." In contrast, the parents of breastfed children did not perceive their children as requiring more than breast milk for satiety. Having the option of providing an unlimited supply of formula coupled with documentation of rapid weight gain, the question arises as to why parents of bottle-fed children believed that formula alone was insufficient. The explanation could be either a physiologic one or an infant-parent psychosocial dynamic. Some studies suggest a protective effect between breastfeeding and obesity, although genetic factors and environmental influences play a strong role.[2,3] Studies demonstrate that after the first few months, breastfed babies have a slower rate of growth, different metabolic rates, and trimmer proportions. Whether breast-feeding influences metabolic programming or early learned self-regulation of food intake remains unclear. Poorly understood neuroendocrine interactions exist between systems that control satiety and those that control relative body fat mass.[4] In rat models, nutritional alterations early in life, such as overfeeding of calorie-dense foods, may contribute to metabolic programming and obesity-related diseases such as diabetes and cardiovascular disease.[5] Further investigation into why formula-fed infants grow faster, and yet are perceived as "hungry," may uncover a relationship between early diet and physiologic influences on satiety.

J. Morton, MD

References

1. Policy statement: Breastfeeding and the use of human milk, section on breast-feeding. *Pediatrics* 115:496-506, 2005.
2. Dewey KG: Is breastfeeding protective against child obesity? *J Hum Lact* 19:9-18, 2003.
3. Toschke AM, Vignerova J, Lhotska L, et al: Overweight and obesity in 6-14 year old Czech children in 1991: Protective effect of breast-feeding. *J Pediatr* 141:764-769, 2002.
4. Singhal A, Farooqi IS, O'Rahilly S, et al: Early nutrition and leptin concentrations in later life. *Am J Clin Nutr* 75:993-999, 2002.
5. Srinivasan M, Laychock SG, Hill DJ, et al: Neonatal nutrition: Metabolic programming of pancreatic islets and obesity. *Exp Biol Med* 228:15-23, 2003.

TGF-β in Human Milk Is Associated With Wheeze in Infancy
Oddy WH, Halonen M, Martinez FD, et al (Curtin Univ of Technology, Perth, Australia; Univ of Western Australia, Perth; Univ of Arizona, Tucson)
J Allergy Clin Immunol 112:723-728, 2003   10–14

Background.—Cytokines secreted in human milk might play important roles in newborn health and in the development of infant immune responses. We investigated the relationship of the concentration and dose of cytokines in human milk to infant wheeze at 1 year of age.

Objective.—Our objective was to test whether the cytokines in milk could account for some of the apparent protective effect of breast-feeding against wheeze in the first year of life.

Methods.—Data on breast-feeding and infant wheeze were collected prospectively from birth to 1 year from 243 mothers participating in the Infant Immune Study in Tucson, Arizona. Breast milk samples obtained at a mean age of 11 days postpartum were assayed by means of ELISA for concentrations of TGF-β1, IL-10, TNF-α, and the soluble form of CD14. The dose of each cytokine was assessed for a relationship with wheeze in bivariate and logistic regression analyses.

Results.—Increasing duration of breast-feeding was significantly associated with a decreased prevalence of wheeze ($P = .039$). There was wide variability in levels of each cytokine in milk as well as variability between women in the amount of each cytokine produced. There was a significant inverse association between the dose of TGF-β1 received through milk with the percentage of wheeze ($P = .017$), and the relationship was linear ($P = .006$). None of the other cytokines showed a linear relationship with wheeze. In multivariate analyses the risk of wheeze was significantly decreased (odds ratio, 0.22; 95% CI 0.05-0.89; $P = .034$) with increasing TGF-β1 dose (long breast-feeding and medium-high TGF-β1 level compared with short breast-feeding and low TGF-β1 level).

Conclusion.—This analysis shows that the dose of TGF-β1 received from milk has a significant relationship with infant wheeze, which might account for at least some of the protective effect of breast-feeding against wheeze.

▶ Breastfeeding remains superior to infant formula despite the best efforts of industry to simulate human milk by recently adding compounds such as 3-omega fatty acids, oligosaccharides, nucleotides, and even lactoferrin. In addition to the ideal nutrient composition, human milk provides hormones, growth factors, and cytokines that modulate or prevent disease. Furthermore, human milk enhances the neonate's immature immunologic system and strengthens host defense mechanisms against infective and other foreign agents, even after breastfeeding has ceased. Factors in human milk that contribute to host defense include immunoglobulins, kappa-casein, lysozyme, lactoferrin, haptocorrin, alpha-lactalbumin, and lactoperoxidase. Also, prebiotic activity by human milk proteins promotes the growth of beneficial bacteria such as *Lactobacilli* and *Bifidobacteria*, which, by decreasing pH, inhibit the growth of pathogens. Additionally, cytokines and lactoferrin have immunomodulatory activity.

Questions remain whether and how exposure to human milk protects against wheeze and asthma. The task for Oddy et al was to test whether the cytokines in milk could account for some of the apparent protective effect of breastfeeding against wheeze in the first year of life. They found that the longer the duration of breastfeeding, the less likely the infants were to wheeze in the first year of life.

After a number of analyses the only cytokine implicated was TGF-β1, with the risk of wheeze reduced proportionally to the dose of TGF-β1. On the other hand, Bottcher et al,[1] who examined the relationships among breastfeeding, immunoglobulin A (IgA) production, and the development of atopic disease in children, noted that differences in the composition of cytokines, chemokines, and secretory IgA in breast milk did not, to any major degree, affect the development of a positive skin prick testing, atopic symptoms, or salivary IgA antibody production during the first 2 years of life.

A. A. Fanaroff, MD

Reference

1. Bottcher MF, Jenmalm MC, Bjorksten B: Cytokine, chemokine and secretory IgA levels in human milk in relation to atopic disease and IgA production in infants. *Pediatr Allergy Immunol* 14:35-41, 2003.

Early Enteral Feeding and Nosocomial Sepsis in Very Low Birthweight Infants

Flidel-Rimon O, Friedman S, Lev E, et al (Kaplan Med Ctr, Rehovot, Israel; Hebrew Univ, Jerusalem; Schneider Children's Hosp, Petach-Tiqva, Israel)

Arch Dis Child Fetal Neonatal Ed 89:F289-F292, 2004   10–15

Background.—Early introduction of enteral feeding is associated with improved growth in preterm infants, but it has been implicated in the pathogenesis of necrotizing enterocolitis (NEC). At the neonatology unit of the Kaplan Medical Center in Rehovot, Israel, enteral feeding has been initiated at earlier ages and progressed in larger daily increments. The impact of this change on the rate of nosocomial sepsis (NS) and NEC in very low birth weight infants was evaluated retrospectively.

Study Design.—A retrospective chart review was performed of 385 very low birth weight infants born during 1995-2001. Enteral feeding was initiated as soon as the infant was considered stable. Contraindications to feeding including NEC, feeding intolerance, and suspected sepsis. Enteral feeding was initiated with either breast milk or preterm formula. Parenteral feeding was initiated with glucose, protein, and lipid. The amount and timing of enteral and parenteral feedings were compared between infants with and without NEC or NS. An infection control task force was established during the study period to reduce sepsis.

Findings.—Of the 385 preterm infants, 42% developed NS and 9% developed NEC. Enteral feeding was initiated at a significantly earlier age in infants who did not develop NS. The timing of feedings had no effect on the development of NEC. Multiple logistic regression analysis indicated that the timing of enteral feeding, respiratory distress syndrome, and birth weight were significant prognostic factors for NS.

Conclusions.—Earlier enteral feeding of preterm infants was associated with a reduced risk of NS. A large randomized trial should be performed to confirm this finding.

▶ Although this was a retrospective analysis, it supports the data accumulated from previously reported studies that have demonstrated the benefits of initiating early enteral feeds and "priming the gut" in very low birth weight infants. These gut-stimulating feeds have been shown to enhance gastrointestinal development and function while the infants are still receiving parenteral nutrition as well. The major concern of introducing these early feeds was that they increased infants' chances of developing NEC, but the studies showed no such increased risk. While Rayyis et al[1] showed no increased risk of NEC in slow versus rapid increases in volumes given to the infant, Berseth and co-workers[2] found that rapid increases in feeding volumes of 20 mL/kg per day increased the incidence of NEC in their babies. They recommended limiting the feeding volumes as the intestine adapts to extrauterine life.

Nevertheless, any technique that can hasten intestinal adaptation and decrease the necessity and duration of IV nutrition would be most welcome, especially if by doing so, the incidence and risks of nosocomial infection could be reduced. Recent data from the Neonatal Research Network of the National Institute of Child Health and Human Development documented that infections among the extremely low birth weight infant are associated with poor growth and neurodevelopmental outcomes.[3]

We still have to walk a very tight rope between early introduction of enteral feeds and trying to increase volumes without causing any more mischief than necessary.

P. Sunshine, MD

References

1. Rayyis SF, Ambalavanan N, Wright L, et al: Randomized trial of "slow" versus "fast" feed advancements on the incidence of necrotizing entercolitis in very low birth weight infants. *J Pediatr* 134:293-297, 1999.
2. Berseth Cl, Bisquera JA, Paje VU: Prolonged small feeding volumes early in life decreases the incidence of necrotizing entercolitis in very low birth weight infants. *Pediatrics* 111:529-534, 2003.
3. Stoll BJ, Hansen NI, Adams-Chapman I, et al: Neurodevelopmental and growth impairment among extremely low-birth-weight infants with neonatal infection. *JAMA* 292:2357-2365, 2004.

Variations in Incidence of Necrotizing Enterocolitis in Canadian Neonatal Intensive Care Units

Sankaran K, for the Canadian Neonatal Network (Univ of Saskatchewan, Canada; et al)

J Pediatr Gastroenterol Nutr 39:366-372, 2004   10–16

Objectives.—Necrotizing enterocolitis (NEC) is the most common acquired intestinal disease of neonates. Previous reports on incidence have generally examined small cohorts of extremely low-birth-weight infants and have not examined risk-adjusted variations among neonatal intensive care units (NICUs). The authors examined risk-adjusted variations in the incidence of NEC in a large group of Canadian NICUs and explored possible therapy-related risks.

Methods.—The authors obtained data on 18,234 infants admitted to 17 tertiary level Canadian NICUs from January 1996 to October 1997. They used multivariate logistic regression analysis to examine the inter-NICU variation in incidence of NEC, with adjustment for population risk factors and admission illness severity, and explored therapy-related variables.

Results.—The incidence of NEC was 6.6% (n = 238) among 3,628 infants with birth weight ≤1,500 g (VLBW), and 0.7% (n = 98) among 14,606 infants with birth weight >1,500 g (HBW). Multivariate logistic regression analysis showed that for VLBW infants, NEC was associated with lower gestational age and treatment for hypotension and patent ductus arteriosus. Among HBW infants, NEC was associated with lower gestational age, presence of congenital anomalies (cardiovascular, digestive, musculoskeletal, multiple systems) and need for assisted ventilation. There was no significant variation in the risk-adjusted incidence of NEC among NICUs, with the exception of one NICU reporting no cases of NEC.

Conclusions.—Risk factors for NEC were different in VLBW and HBW infants. There was no significant variation in the risk-adjusted incidence of NEC among Canadian NICUs, with one possible exception.

▶ It has been exciting to watch the proliferation of neonatal networks and the flurry of publications that this has generated. The NICHHD Neonatal Network and the large and ever-expanding Vermont Oxford Network have collaborated so that their data collection and definitions are consistent. This permits internetwork comparison, which is a reasonable goal for some of the other national networks.

This report from the Canadian Network on NEC documents an incidence of 6.6%, which is identical to the NICHHD Neonatal Network (6%-7%) for the period 1997 to 2002. Whereas mortality rate and other major morbidities have declined, the incidence of NEC has remained constant. Regrettably, NEC retains its preeminence as the most common surgical emergency in the NICU. In the NICHHD Network the incidence of NEC for all infants less than 1500 g ranges from 0% to 11% among the various units. I was therefore intrigued to learn that the Canadian Network, on a risk-adjusted basis, found that there was no center variation. Indeed, center variation has been a constant feature in all multicenter trials.

NEC is considered to be caused by the coincidence of intestinal ischemia-reperfusion injury and systemic inflammation from the colonization of pathogenic bacteria. Interleukin (IL)-8, a proinflammatory cytokine, has been implicated in the pathogenesis of NEC. IL-1β activates the IL-8 gene by regulating the transcriptional nuclear factor κB (NF-κB) signaling pathways in intestinal cells. Platelet activating factor is another potent initiator of the inflammatory cascade that results in NEC. Human milk has a protective role but does not entirely prevent NEC. Minekawa et al[1] reported that human breast milk dramatically suppressed the IL-1β–induced activation of the IL-8 gene promoter by inhibiting the activation pathway of NF-κB and also induced the production of IκBα. This suggests one of the pathways by which human breast milk could be protective against NEC.

A. A. Fanaroff, MD

Reference

1. Minekawa R, Takeda T, Sakata M, et al: Human breast milk suppresses the transcriptional regulation of IL-1β-induced NF-κB signaling in human intestinal cells. *Am J Physiol Cell Physiol* 287:C1404-C1411, 2004.

Surgical Management of Bowel Perforations and Outcome in Very Low-Birth-Weight Infants (≤1,2000 g)

Sharma R, Tepas JJ III, Mollitt DL, et al (Univ of Florida, Jacksonville)
J Pediatr Surg 39:190-194, 2004   10–17

Purpose.—The efficacy of peritoneal drainage (PD) as an alternative to laparotomy (LAP) in the management of bowel perforation (PRF) in very low-birth-weight infants (VLBW ≤1,200 g) remains uncertain. The authors hypothesized that survival of VLBW infants with PRF depends on the severity of illness rather than on the initial surgical approach.

Methods.—Demographic, clinical, and outcome data on all VLBW infants were abstracted prospectively over a 12½-year period. Infants with PRF were stratified by PD or by LAP. Illness acuity was compared using the sum of a 7-point scoring system based on the clinical signs determined to be of prognostic significance. The factors associated with adverse outcome and the epidemiology of PRF were also examined.

Results.—Of 937 infants, 78 with PRF required surgical intervention, consisting of PD in 32 (41%) and LAP in 46 (59%). Mean birth weight, illness acuity score, and the number of infants with NEC were significantly lower in PD ($P = .0005$). A higher proportion of PD infants received indomethacin ($P = .01$). There were no other differences between the 2 groups. Regardless of the choice of procedure, birth weight did not affect mortality rate; however, a shorter interval between PRF identification and surgical intervention was associated with improved survival rate ($P = .001$). Postoperative liver dysfunction, short gut syndrome, and enteric stricture were more common among LAP. Mortality rate, however, did not differ. When severe thrombocytopenia ($P < .03$) or neutropenia was present ($P < .03$), outcome of LAP was better than PD. Rescue LAP for 8 of rapidly deteriorating PD infants saved 5. Regardless of surgical approach, coagulopathy ($P < .003$), severe thrombocytopenia ($P < .005$), neutropenia ($P < .0001$), and multiple organ failure ($P < .0001$) were all predictive of fatality.

Conclusions.—Choice of surgical approach should be based on the underlying illness and not on birth weight. In the presence of clinical indication of necrotic gut, or profound abdominal infection, LAP is a better choice. PD, however, is far less morbid and should be considered for isolated PRF. Rescue LAP must be considered without delay when PD fails.

▶ Although necrotizing enterocolitis remains the most common cause of gastrointestinal perforation, in preterm infants perforation may also rarely be seen with duodenal atresia, Hirschsprung disease, inspissated meconium, Meckel's diverticulum, traumatic passage of gastric tubes, transpyloric feeding tubes, and milk curd syndrome.

Corticosteroids and indomethacin must also be considered. Whereas classic radiographs had always been the preferred diagnostic method, sonography is an effective tool in the diagnosis of pneumoperitoneum, with sensitivity and specificity equal to those of radiography. The scissors maneuver may be a useful adjunct for improving the diagnostic yield of sonography. This consists of applying and then releasing slight pressure onto the abdominal wall with the caudal part of a parasagittally oriented linear-array probe. It is helpful to detect intraperitoneal free air superficial to the liver.[1]

Sharma et al, in the opening sentence of their abstract, state that the "efficacy of peritoneal drainage as an alternative to laparotomy in the management of bowel perforation in very low-birth-weight infants (VLBW ≤1,200 g) remains uncertain." By reviewing a series over more than a decade at their own institution, they attempt to shed some light on this problem. And to an extent, they do, but the issue is far from resolved. Common sense mandates that the choice of surgical approach be determined by the underlying cause.

Necrotizing enterocolitis, to everyone's frustration, remains the most common and most severe gastrointestinal disorder in neonates; if there is evidence of peritonitis or necrotic bowel, laparotomy is indicated. Peritoneal drainage may be considered for isolated perforations that assumed epidemic proportions with the use of early corticosteroids, particularly when combined with indomethacin. Gollin et al[2] reported a consecutive series of 29 extremely low-birth-weight infants in which PD was intended as definitive treatment for intestinal perforation. Survival was comparable with that found in a series in which immediate laparotomy and resection were used. Few secondary abdominal procedures were required. The interval between PD and full enteral nutrition, however, was long (69 days), and the incidence of nonabdominal infectious complications and cholestasis was substantial. The issue will not easily be resolved; however, follow-up data from some of the prospective trials comparing PD and laparotomy should be available soon and may provide the definitive answers.

A. A. Fanaroff, MD

References

1. Karahan OI, Kurt A, Yikilmaz A, et al: New method for the detection of intraperitoneal free air by sonography: Scissors maneuver. *J Clin Ultrasound* 32:381-385, 2004.
2. Gollin G, Abarbanell A, Baerg JE: Peritoneal drainage as definitive management of intestinal perforation in extremely low-birth-weight infants. *J Pediatr Surg* 38:1814-1817, 2003.

11 Hematology and Bilirubin

Blood Transfusion Increases Functional Capillary Density in the Skin of Anemic Preterm Infants
Genzel-Boroviczény O, Christ F, Glas V (Ludwig-Maximilian Univ, Munich)
Pediatr Res 56:751-755, 2004   11–1

Direct visualization of the microcirculation at the level of the skin capillaries may provide information on the quality of tissue perfusion. Orthogonal polarization spectral imaging (OPS) enables noninvasively direct observation of those blood vessels. OPS was applied to the upper arm of 13 preterm anemic infants [median (95% confidence interval) gestational age: 26 wk (25–26 wk); birth weight: 730 g (652–789 g)] before and 2 and 24 h after transfusion (Tx). OPS images of skin perfusion were continuously recorded on video. Off-line quantitative data of microvascular perfusion were obtained by measuring functional capillary density, vessel diameter, red blood cell velocity, and flow. We found a significant increase in functional capillary density 2 h after transfusion with an additional significant rise after 24 h [before: 142 (134–155); 2 h after Tx: 185 (166–196); 24 h after Tx: 206 (185–219) cm/cm^2; $p < 0.001$), thus indicating improved microvascular perfusion. Vessel diameter, red blood cell velocity, and flow did not change significantly. There were no significant changes in clinical variables, such as blood pressure, heart rate, or body temperature Whereas conventional monitoring methods did not show any changes after transfusion, quantitative analyses of OPS images indicated improved perfusion; hence, it seems a useful monitor for assessing the response to therapies aimed to improve tissue perfusion.

▶ Decisions regarding whether to transfuse preterm infants in the neonatal ICU are often difficult. Efforts to conserve blood by limiting the number of tests and volume of blood drawn from extremely low birth weight infants have decreased the numbers of red blood cell transfusions in recent years; nevertheless, transfusions are still a common occurrence. For each infant, the advantages of transfusion must be balanced against the consequences and potential risks. Traditionally we have directed our attention to the effects of the blood transfusion on the red cell parameters, hematocrit and hemoglobin levels, as well as clinical parameters including temperature, respiratory rate, heart rate, blood pressure, and acid-base balance. Genzel-Boroviczény et al present a new and unusual end point to observe after a blood transfusion. Whereas the clinical parameters did not change, use of orthogonal polarization spectral imaging documented markedly improved perfusion. The figures tell the whole story. I am in agreement with the authors that this is a neat way to monitor improved perfusion, but it is a stretch to think that this will become "a useful monitor for assessing the response to therapies aimed to improve tissue perfusion."

A. A. Fanaroff, MD

Human Platelet Antigen-Specific Alloantibodies Implicated in 1162 Cases of Neonatal Alloimmune Thrombocytopenia
Davoren A, Curtis BR, Aster RH, et al (Blood Ctr of Southeastern Wisconsin, Milwaukee)
Transfusion 44:1220-1225, 2004   11–2

Background.—Neonatal alloimmune thrombocytopenia (NATP) caused by fetomaternal mismatch for human platelet (PLT) alloantigens (HPAs) complicates approximately 1 in 1000 to 1 in 2000 pregnancies and can lead to a serious bleeding diathesis, intracranial hemorrhage, and sometimes death of the fetus or neonate. As a national reference center for NATP investigations, our experience with this entity over a 12-year period was reviewed.

Study design and Methods.—The laboratory records of all cases of suspected NATP referred for evaluation from January 1, 1990, to December 31, 2002, were analyzed. The spectrum of PLT alloantibody specificities identified was compared with an earlier reported series of serologically verified NATP cases.

Results.—HPA-specific alloantibodies were identified in 1162 (31%) of 3743 sera of mothers of infants with clinically suspected NATP. Maternal HPA-1a (Pl^{A1}) alloimmunization accounted for the majority (79%) of confirmed NATP cases, with HPA-5b (Br^a), HPA-3a (Bak^a), and HPA-1b (PL^{A2}) alloantibodies accounting for 9, 2, and 4 percent of cases, respectively. In addition, an increase in the number of cases in which multiple HPA-specific alloantibodies were present in maternal sera was observed during the study period.

Conclusion.—Although, as with the earlier series, maternal HPA-1a alloimmunization was the dominant cause of NATP, the identification of an increasing number of cases due to alternative HPA polymorphisms suggests that investigation for HPA-1 incompatibility alone is no longer sufficient to fully evaluate clinically suspect NATP cases.

▶ Thrombocytopenia is a malady well known to neonatologists everywhere. Only 1% to 2% of term neonates have a platelet count below 150,000, which defines thrombocytopenia in neonates as well as adults. However, nearly 25%

of all neonates admitted to neonatal ICUs have thrombocytopenia develop (up to 50% of the sickest infants). The condition can be fatal in onset as noted in congenital infections (TORCH, HIV), in chromosomal aneuploidies (trisomy 13, 18, 21, triploidy), in inherited platelet defects, (Wiskott Aldrich syndrome), maternal autoimmune disease (ITP, SLE), and in alloimmune disease, the subject of this article.

Early onset thrombocytopenia, defined as presenting in the first 72 hours of life, is frequently noted in all the aforementioned conditions as well as placental insufficiency states (pregnancy-induced hypertension [PIH], intrauterine growth retardation [IUGR], maternal diabetes), perinatal asphyxia, and perinatal infection (group B *Streptoccus*, *Escherichia coli*, *Haemophilus influenza*).

Alloimmune thrombocytopenia (AIT) is the platelet equivalent to Rh disease in the newborn infant. Unlike Rh disease, however, first-born infants can be affected; there is no Rhogam equivalent yet available to prevent the mother's mounting an antibody response against the fetus' platelet antigens. The diagnosis of AIT initially enters the differential when a complete blood count (CBC) performed in an otherwise healthy newborn infant reveals severe thrombocytopenia.

Intracranial hemorrhage (ICH) is the most feared complication in AIP, and occurs in 7% to 15% of affected infants (see text). Twenty-five percent to 50% of these bleeds occur in utero. In the "old days" we seldom transfused the lucky majority of these infants who were well clinically and had no ICH by US, even when the platelet counts were below 20,000. Our thinking was that if the infant had emerged unscathed from the birthing battle without a brain bleed, she/he was unlikely to face a more serious risk during the sedentary first weeks of infancy. The infant's platelet count will, of course, gradually recover as the maternally acquired antibodies dissipate. Even today, a clear correlation between degree of thrombocytopenia and the resulting bleeding risk has not been demonstrated.[1] However, few hematologists or neonatologists boast the intestinal fortitude to do nothing when the platelet count plunges below 20,000 in an otherwise healthy newborn infant. Random platelet transfusion will do no good in this scenario as most donors will have the same offending HPAs as the infant, and be rapidly destroyed. Only maternal platelets, or platelets from a known compatible HPA donor will restore an affected infant's platelet count. Likewise, immune IVIG can increment the infant's platelet count over time by blocking splenic clearance of antibody-laden platelets from the infant's circulation.

Identification of the antiplatelet antibody profile is key to nailing the correct diagnosis in the thrombocytopenic infant in whom AIT is suspected. As shown in this study, a diagnosis can be made in up to a third of cases. Subsequent pregnancies are likely to be affected, and AIT, if confirmed, necessitates increased fetal surveillance. The efficacy of antenatal screening for AIT has been raised in the literature.[2] The jury is still out on this question, however.

A. A. Fanaroff, MD

References

1. Sola MC: Evaluation and treatment of severe and prolonged thrombocytopenia in neonates [Review]. *Clin Perinatol* 31:1-14, 2004.
2. Murphy MF, Williamson LM, Urbaniak SJ: Antenatal screening for fetomaternal alloimmune thrombocytopenia: Should we be doing it? [Review]. *Vox Sanguinis* 83 Suppl 1:409-416, 2002.

Effects of Intralipid Infusion on Blood Viscosity and Other Haemorheological Parameters in Neonates and Children
Kessler U, Poeschl J, Raz D, et al (Univ of Heidelberg, Germany)
Acta Paediatr 93:1058-1062, 2004   11–3

Background.—Intralipid, a soybean triglyceride emulsion, is used for parenteral nutrition in adults and infants. Pulmonary complications have been reported after intralipid infusion in preterm infants. The hemorheological effects of intralipid were studied in preterm and full-term neonates, both in vivo and in vitro.

Study Design.—The study group consisted of 10 preterm infants, 10 full-term infants, and 10 children. Blood viscosity, hematocrit, plasma viscosity, red blood cell (RBC) aggregation, and RBC deformability were analyzed before and after intralipid infusion. Hemorheological parameters were also studied in vitro with blood from preterm neonates, full-term neonates, and healthy adults before and after the addition of intralipid.

Findings.—During intralipid infusion, plasma triglycerides increased in all neonates and children. Whole blood viscosity decreased by about 10% in all 3 groups. RBC aggregation decreased by about 20% after intralipid infusion in all 3 groups. Plasma proteins, plasma viscosity, and RBC deformation were unaffected by intralipid infusions. When blood was incubated with intralipid in vitro, there was a significant, dose-dependent reduction in RBC aggregation

Conclusions.—Infusion of intralipid (0.6 g/kg over 4 hours) does not impair blood flow, but reduces RBC aggregation. Previously described side effects of intralipid infusion cannot be related to impaired blood flow.

▶ Despite the common use of intralipid infusion in the course of parenteral nutrition for preterm infants, old beliefs still linger and contribute to hesitation around the use of intralipids. One example is a concern that free fatty acids become elevated with the infusion of intralipids, putting infants at risk for the allosteric effects of free fatty acids binding to albumin with the consequent displacement of bilirubin from albumin, thus increasing the risk of kernicterus. However, at the doses and infusion rates recommended, free fatty acid levels do not reach a level at which such effects are of any practical consequence, and "free" bilirubin levels might actually decrease in the circumstance of intralipid infusion as bilirubin binds to the intralipid. Another concern has been the potential effect on blood viscosity that might contribute to resistance to blood flow and problems with pulmonary function.

For this reason, the authors investigated the effects of IV fat on blood viscosity and its determinants (hematocrit, plasma viscosity, RBC aggregation and deformability) in preterm and full-term neonates as well as children before and after intralipid infusion. They confirmed previous findings that show that whole blood viscosity at a given hematocrit, plasma viscosity, and RBC aggregation are lower in preterm infants compared with full-term infants and lower in full-term infants than in children and adults. The bottom line is that they found no impairment of flow properties of blood. In fact, RBC aggregation appears to decrease with intralipid infusion, suggesting improved blood flow properties at low shear forces, for example, in the veins. Thus, any suspected adverse pulmonary effects are not the result of impaired flow properties of blood caused by intralipid infusion. Intralipid infusion remains a mainstay of parenteral alimentation in preterm infants. Fortunately, we continue to be reassured by systematic studies of the effect of this nutrient source on other aspects of transitional biology and physiology.

D. K. Stevenson, MD

Short-term Use of Umbilical Artery Catheters May Not Be Associated With Increased Risk for Thrombosis
Coleman MM, Spear ML, Finkelstein M, et al (Thomas Jefferson Univ, Philadelphia; Christiana Care Health Services, Newark, Del)
Pediatrics 113:770-774, 2004   11–4

Background.—The use of umbilical arterial catheters (UACs) can be complicated by the development of neonatal thrombosis. Two serum markers, specifically, fibrinogen 1.2 (F1.2) and thrombin–antithrombin (TAT), have potential diagnostic value and can be assayed and correlated with abdominal US views of the UAC thrombosis. F1.2 and TAT levels were determined longitudinally and compared with platelet count values and US evidence of thrombi in infants younger than 1 week who had UACs.

Methods.—All 33 infants had a UAC placed in the first 24 hours of life, and all received equal heparin doses. F1.2 and TAT levels, platelet counts, and abdominal aorta US scans were assessed every other day from age 24 hours or less. Longitudinal production of F1.2 and TAT was related to thrombus formation in or around the UACs over time.

Results.—No significant difference in F1.2 and TAT levels were noted over the 5-day study period. Platelet counts fell, but the decline was not statistically significant. Birth weight and gestational age showed no significant correlation with F1.2 and TAT levels on multiple linear regression. In 61 US studies, only 1 thrombus and 1 case of decreased aortic flow were detected, and both were in the same patient. The patient's F1.2 level was 5.5 nM/L, which was higher than the mean for the study population. The TAT level was consistent with the study population's mean value. The first platelet count was 141,000. Although no evidence of intraventricular hemorrhaging was found premortem, the patient died before 48 hours of age.

Conclusions.—During the first 5 days of use, indwelling UACs may not present an increased risk of thrombus formation.

▶ It is difficult to balance the risks and benefits of a procedure as "standard" as UAC placement when we don't know whether the associated thrombosis rate is 1 or 60%. Fortunately, it appears that the permanent injury rate from UAC-related thromboses is much closer to the lower figure. However, this article points out some of the dilemmas of defining the problem. Traditionally, the diagnosis of a thrombus is made by US; however, unless a patient is in a clinical trial or has complications that are thought to be related to a thrombus, most babies with UACs aren't routinely screened for this complication. Given the further uncertainty about what to do if one finds the problem, who could blame the clinician for not looking? The present article reveals an intriguing and presumably sensitive means of looking for UAC-associated thrombi, that is, the biochemical tests for serum markers of thrombogenesis: F1.2 and TAT. Following their neonatal ICU practice guidelines, the investigators found no elevation of these markers in the studied population after UACs were in place for several days. However, given the relative absence of UAC-related clots in this study population as determined by US, there is no good way of knowing whether these chemical tests correlate with such thrombi. Whether it was the effect of infusing only 0.2 normal saline with heparin, the brand of catheter, the duration of UAC use, or something else cannot be determined, and it is impossible to fully explain the authors' "negative" result (which was fortunately "positive" for their patients). Perhaps, with the expanded use of chemical assays of thrombosis, we will better understand the incidence and natural course of catheter-related clots.

W. D. Rhine, MD

Evaluation of Plasma Ionized Magnesium Levels in Neonatal Hyperbilirubinemia

Sarici SU, Serdar MA, Erdem G, et al (Hacettepe Univ, Turkey; Gulhane Med Academy, Ankara, Turkey)
Pediatr Res 55:243-247, 2004   11–5

Introduction.—Deposition of unbound bilirubin or its acid form in the neuron membrane produces permanent neuronal injury with a distinctive regional topography throughout the CNS. Increased and prolonged activation of the N-methyl-D-aspartate (NMDA) receptor results in brain cell injury despite its physiologic roles in brain plasticity; neuronal growth; synaptogenogenesis; and development of learning, memory, and vision. Magnesium (Mg) ion, like MK-801, is one of the most significant antagonistic regulators of the NMDA receptor/ion channel complex.

It protects the CNS against hypoxia and exerts its neuroprotective effects by blocking excitotoxic and NMDA receptor-mediated neuronal injury mechanisms. Plasma levels of ionized magnesium (IMg), measured by ion-selective electrode, were assessed in neonatal hyperbilirubinemia by comparing the newborn with (205 µM or more) and without (less than 205 µM) significant hyperbilirubinemia (groups of severe and moderate hyperbilirubinemia, respectively).

Methods.—Serum bilirubin, plasma IMg, and ionized calcium (ICa) levels were ascertained in 165 healthy term infants with nonhemolytic indirect hyperbilirubinemia during the first 10 days of life.

Results.—Mean serum bilirubin, plasma IMg, and ICa levels were 200.1 µM, 0.54 mM, and 1.15 mM, respectively, in 165 newborn infants with a mean postnatal age of 156.1 hours. A significant positive association was seen between the mean serum bilirubin and plasma IMg levels (r = 0.535; $P < .001$). Serum bilirubin levels (304.4 µM vs 94.1 µM) and plasma IMg levels (0.6 mM vs 0.49 mM) were significantly higher and plasma ICa levels (1.13 mM vs 1.18 mM) were significantly lower in 83 infants with severe hyperbilirubinemia, compared to 82 infants with moderate hyperbilirubinemia.

Seventeen of the 83 infants with severe hyperbilirubinemia had IMg levels greater than the normal range (0.69 mM or greater), compared to none of the 82 infants with moderate hyperbilirubinemia. Fifteen of the 17 infants with high IMg levels had bilirubin levels above 290 µM.

Conclusion.—An increase in plasma IMg may be due to extracellular movement of Mg. Considering the neuroprotective functions and beneficial effects of Mg ion in improving neurologic outcome, it is possible that there is a neuroprotective role or a compensatory mechanism of increased IMg levels to decrease bilirubin toxicity.

▶ Although the toxicity of bilirubin in the CNS is undisputed, various mechanisms of injury have been proposed. One of the more intriguing proposed mechanisms for bilirubin toxicity is analogous to that proposed for hypoxic-ischemic injury, that is, increased and prolonged activation of the NMDA receptor. Bilirubin in a newborn piglet model can also increase activation of the NMDA receptor by modifying its binding characteristics, increasing the receptor's affinity for NMDA receptor antagonists, and thus causing neuronal injury. Moreover, antagonists like MK-801 are able to block neuronal injury caused by hypoxia-ischemia as well as by bilirubin.

Such observations give credibility to the teleologic argument presented in this article. The argument goes something like this: The Mg ion is one of the most important antagonistic regulators of the NMDA receptor ion channel complex; thus, Mg is a logical subject of investigation as a neuroprotective agent; elevated IMg levels are associated with severe hyperbilirubinemia, defined as serum bilirubin levels of 205 µM or greater.

The etiologic stretch comes with the argument that the elevation in IMg is an adaptive response which might protect neurons. In fairness to the authors, the other possibility that they acknowledge is that significant erythrocyte destruction—which may be a prominent factor in pathologic causes of jaundice—could be responsible for the observed alterations in Mg metabolism and increased levels of IMg in circulation, leading to the association of elevated IMg levels with severe hyperbilirubinemia. Nonetheless, this is an intriguing observation and introduces another level of complexity into the investigations of bilirubin-induced neurotoxicity.

D. K. Stevenson, MD

Glucose-6-Phosphate Dehydrogenase Activity in Male Premature and Term Neonates

Mesner O, Hammerman C, Goldschmidt D, et al (Bnai Zion Med Ctr, Haifa, Israel; Technion Science Inst, Haifa, Israel; Shaare Zedek Med Ctr, Jerusalem; et al)

Arch Dis Child Fetal Neonatal Ed 89:F555-F557, 2004   11–6

Background.—Neonates have higher glucose-6-phosphate dehydrogenase (G6PD) activity than adults. Some studies have suggested even higher activity in preterm infants. Whether G6PD activity is higher in premature than in term neonates was determined, as well as whether higher activity would interfere with the diagnosis of G6PD deficiency.

Study Design.—The study group consisted of 118 male neonates, of whom 94 were premature (23-36 weeks' gestation). G6PD activity was determined in the first 48 hours after delivery. The study was limited to boys, as G6PD deficiency is an X-linked condition.

Findings.—Of the 94 premature infants, 4 had G6PD activity below 2 U per gram of hemoglobin and were clearly deficient. G6PD activity in the remaining preterm infants was significantly higher than in the term infants. Subgroup analysis revealed that G6PD activity was primarily elevated in those born between 29 and 32 weeks' gestation (Fig 1).

Conclusions.—G6PD activity is elevated in premature infants born between 29 and 32 weeks' gestation. The higher G6PD activity does not appear to affect the diagnosis of G6PD deficiency.

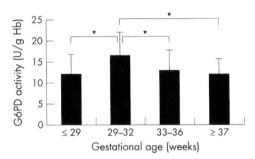

FIGURE 1.—Glucose-6-phosphate dehydrogenase (*G6PD*) activity (mean [SD]) for the 3 subgroups of premature infants and the term and near term neonates. *Asterisk*, P < .001. (Courtesy of Mesner O, Hammerman C, Goldschmidt D, et al: Glucose-6-phosphate dehydrogenase activity in male premature and term neonates. *Arch Dis Child Fetal Neonatal Ed* 89:F555-F557, 2004, with permission from the BMJ Publishing Group.)

► One of the most intriguing findings of this study is an apparent developmental pattern of G6PD activity that increases from less than 29 weeks to 29 to 32 weeks of gestational age and then decreases again towards term. The authors admit that they do not understand this pattern, which of course will need to be confirmed. Nonetheless, the underlying hypothesis that G6PD activity might be higher in preterm infants than in term and near-term neonates, at least for those between 29 and 32 weeks of gestational age, was proven correct. From a practical perspective, the ability to diagnose G6PD deficiency is not compromised by this apparent pattern of G6PD activity in the premature infant. Also, the simple explanation that an increased number of immature red blood cells is associated with increased G6PD activity is not supported by these observations. The fact that there might be a maturational or developmental effect contributing to the control of red blood cell G6PD activity leaves open for now the question of its significance for the developing fetus.

D. K. Stevenson, MD

Cost-Effectiveness of Strategies That Are Intended to Prevent Kernicterus in Newborn Infants
Suresh GK, Clark RE (Med Univ of South Carolina, Charleston; Univ of Massachusetts, Worcester)
Pediatrics 114:917-924, 2004   11–7

Objective.—There is concern about an increasing incidence of kernicterus in healthy term neonates in the United States. Although the incidence of kernicterus is unknown, several potential strategies that are intended to prevent kernicterus have been proposed by experts. It is necessary to assess the costs, benefits, and risks of such strategies before widespread policy changes are made. The objective of this study was to determine the direct costs to prevent a case of kernicterus with the following 3 strategies: (1) universal follow-up in the office or at home within 1 to 2 days of early newborn discharge, (2) routine predischarge serum bilirubin with selective follow-up and laboratory testing, and (3) routine predischarge transcutaneous bilirubin with selective follow-up and laboratory testing.

Methods.—We performed an incremental cost-effectiveness analysis of the 3 strategies compared with current practice. We used a decision analytic model and a spreadsheet to estimate the direct costs and outcomes, including the savings resulting from prevented kernicterus, for an annual cohort of 2 800 000 healthy term newborns who are eligible for early discharge. We used a modified societal perspective and 2002 US dollars. With each strategy, the test and treatment thresholds for hyperbilirubinemia are lowered compared with current practice.

Results.—With the base-case assumptions (current incidence of kernicterus 1:100 000 and a relative risk reduction [RRR] of 0.7 with each strategy), the cost to prevent 1 case of kernicterus was 10 321 463 dollars, 5 743 905 dollars, and 9 191 352 dollars respectively for strategies 1, 2, and 3 listed above. The total annual incremental costs for the cohort were, respectively, 202 300 671 dollars, 112 580 535 dollars, and 180 150 494 dollars. Sensitivity analyses showed that the cost per case is highly dependent on the population incidence of kernicterus and the RRR with each strategy, both of which are currently unknown. In our model, annual cost savings of 46 179 465 dollars for the cohort would result with strategy 2, if the incidence of kernicterus is high (1:10,000 births or higher) and the RRR is high (≥ 0.7). If the incidence is lower or the RRR is lower, then the cost per case prevented ranged from 4 145 676 dollars to as high as 77 650 240 dollars.

Conclusions.—Widespread implementation of these strategies is likely to increase health care costs significantly with uncertain benefits. It is premature to implement routine predischarge serum or transcutaneous bilirubin screening on a large scale. However, universal follow-up may have benefits beyond kernicterus prevention, which we did not include in our model. Research is required to determine the epidemiology, risk factors, and causes of kernicterus; to evaluate the effectiveness of strategies intended to prevent kernicterus; and to determine the cost per quality-adjusted life year with any proposed preventive strategy.

▶ This is an important addition to our ongoing quest to understand the problem of kernicterus, to develop strategies for its prevention, and to know how much each of these strategies might cost. Furthermore, although the recent American Academy of Pediatrics Guideline is quite prescriptive in its requirements for risk assessment and follow up,[1] we currently have no data on either the efficacy or effectiveness of these recommendations for preventing kernicterus. The potential estimated relative risk reduction of 0.7 (as a result of the interventions) could, as noted by the authors, be optimistic and, depending on the degree of risk reduction actually achieved and the overall incidence of kernicterus, there is as much as a 20-fold difference in the range of the cost to prevent 1 case.

Because we have a system for documenting the incidence of sudden infant death syndrome (SIDS), it was possible to demonstrate that the introduction of a simple intervention (having infants sleep on their backs) approximately halved the incidence of SIDS. Of course, the baseline incidence was about 1 in 1000, perhaps 100 times more frequent than kernicterus. Demonstrating that the introduction of (and compliance with) guidelines has had an impact on the incidence of kernicterus is going to be difficult, and this is all the more reason why the Centers for Disease Control and Prevention should develop a strategy for identifying and recording cases when they do occur.

M. J. Maisels, MB, BCh

Reference

1. Maisels MJ, Baltz RD, Bhutani V, et al: Management of hyperbilirubinemia in the newborn infant 35 or more weeks of gestation. *Pediatrics* 114:297-316, 2004.

▶ Readers should note that the trace element in the heme oxygenase inhibitor, stannsoporfin, is very tightly bound to the porphyrin ring structure and that there is no known physiological mechanism by which the free metal can be released in vivo. This contrasts with certain synthetic heme analogues, in which the metal may be labile. The natural compound iron protoporphyrin, ie, the heme moiety of hemoglobin, is a substrate for heme oxygenase, which releases the iron atom by enzymic action. If the released iron is not seques-tered promptly by iron-binding proteins, the free metal can produce tissue oxi-dative injury. This cannot happen with stannsoporfin.

Stannsoporfin has not shown any evidence of the toxicities displayed by the agricultural and industrial organotins in which the metal is complexed through metal-carbon bonding. Stannsoporfin has no metal-carbon bonds; its complex-ing with the porphyrin ring structure occurs solely through the nitrogen moi-eties, as is the case for the iron atom of heme. The best analogy to make for stannsoporfin is to consider it similar to vitamin B-12, in which cobalt, essential for the biological function of the vitamin (but which in the free metal form can be toxic) is similarly bound to a porphyrin ring through metal-nitrogen bonds.

In any case, tin, even in the free form, is highly biocompatible as it is an ele-ment found widely in animal and human tissues and in foods. The metal has also had significant medial uses, and there is some evidence that it is an es-sential trace element for growth. The amount of the element in a single dose of stannsoporfin administered to a 4 kg infant is less than 3 mg. The normal di-etary intake of the metal in humans averages 17 mg/day. The agreed-upon limit for the trace element in foods in the United States has been set at 300 mg/kg.

A. Kappas, MD

Ursodeoxycholic Acid (UDCA) Therapy in Very-Low-Birth-Weight Infants With Parenteral Nutrition–Associated Cholestasis

Chen C-Y, Tsao P-N, Chen H-L, et al (Natl Taiwan Univ, Taipei)
J Pediatr 145:317-321, 2004

11–8

Background.—Cholestasis is an important side effect of prolonged paren-teral nutrition in infants. Ursodeoxycholic acid (UDCA) is a bile acid used to

TABLE 2.—The Serum Biochemistries of Cholestatic Infants Treated With or Without UDCA

	Treated Group (n = 12)	Control Group (n = 18)	P Value
Initial total bilirubin (mg/dL)	5.8 ± 0.5	6.2 ± 0.6	.899
Initial direct bilirubin (mg/dL)	3.5 ± 0.3	4.0 ± 0.5	.397
Peak total bilirubin (mg/dL)*	8.8 ± 1.6	13.9 ± 1.6	.007
Peak direct bilirubin (mg/dL)*	5.3 ± 0.6	8.7 ± 1.1	.023
Peak AST (mg/dL)	204.4 ± 26.7	209.8 ± 25.6	.849
Peak ALT (mg/dL)	94.8 ± 13.4	101.6 ± 20.5	.626
Peak GGT (mg/dL)	214.2 ± 29.7	218.2 ± 33.0	1.000
Peak ALP (mg/dL)	1205.8 ± 137.8	1411.5 ± 103.1	.189

Value presented as mean ± SEM.
*$P < .05$.
Abbreviations: AST, Aspartate aminotransferase; *ALT,* alanine aminotransferase; *GGT,* γ-glutamyl transpeptidase; *ALP,* alka-line phosphatase.

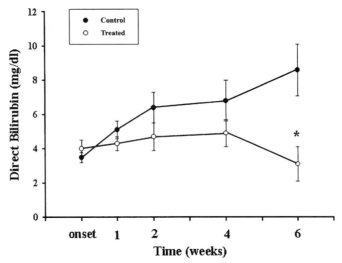

FIGURE 1.—Comparison of serum direct bilirubin level between the treatment and the control groups measured at onset and at 1, 2, 4, and 6 weeks after cholestasis developed. The level in the control group was significantly higher than that of the treatment group at 6 weeks (*asterisk*). (Reprinted by permission of the publisher from Chen C-Y, Tsao P-N, Chen H-L, et al: Ursodeoxycholic acid [UDCA] therapy in very-low-birth-weight infants with parenteral nutrition–associated cholestasis. *J Pediatr* 145:317-321. Copyright 2004 by Elsevier.)

treat cholestasis in adults. The effect of UDCA on very low birth weight (VLBW) infants with parenteral nutrition-associated cholestasis (PNAC) was examined retrospectively.

Study Design.—The study group consisted of 30 VLBW infants who developed PNAC from January 1999 to December 2002 at a single institution. Cholestasis was defined as an elevated direct bilirubin level of more than 2 mg/dL. The treatment group received UDCA within 14 days of onset, whereas the control group did not receive medical treatment.

Findings.—VLBW infants who developed PNAC and received UDCA therapy had a shorter duration of cholestasis and significantly lower peak serum levels of direct bilirubin than did infants in the control group (Table 2, Fig 1).

Conclusions.—Treatment with UDCA ameliorated the effects of PNAC in VLBW infants. A placebo-controlled trial of UDCA should be performed to confirm its effects in this vulnerable population.

▶ Although the authors conclude that UDCA therapy in VLBW infants with PNAC can decrease the duration and extent of jaundice and shorten the clinical course of PNAC, the study leaves more questions unanswered than it answers. Moreover, the treatment group showed no differences in other liver function tests, besides total and direct bilirubin levels, compared with the control group. Of what clinical consequence is the change in bilirubin profile, if cytoprotection is not commensurate with this effect? It is unlikely that elevations of the magnitude observed in direct bilirubin represent a threat to the

CNS of the infant. Cholestasis has been associated with increased hemolytic rates, which could contribute to anemia of prematurity in this context, but it is unlikely that the direct bilirubin itself is responsible for this effect. Thus, the demonstration of improved cholestasis in the UDCA-treated infants in this retrospective study (originally designed as a prospective study) leads the authors to conclude appropriately that a randomized controlled trial of UDCA is still needed. Moreover, biochemical end points are probably not the best ones to consider in this high-risk group of infants. In infants without an absolute contraindication to feeding, small (trophic) amounts of enteral feeds may provide a similar stimulus to that of UDCA for bile flow. The fact that a medicine works does not necessarily mean that it is good. I think the jury is still out on this one.

D. K. Stevenson, MD

Cost-Effectiveness of Postnatal Home Nursing Visits for Prevention of Hospital Care for Jaundice and Dehydration

Paul IM, Phillips TA, Widome MD, et al (Pennsylvania State Univ, Hershey)
Pediatrics 114:1015-1022, 2004   11–9

Objectives.—(1) To describe the relationship between postnatal home nursing visitation and readmissions and emergency department (ED) visits for neonatal jaundice and dehydration in the first 10 days of life. (2) To evaluate the cost-effectiveness of providing home nursing visits after newborn discharge with specific attention to prevention of jaundice and dehydration that require hospital-based services.

Methods.—A retrospective analysis of a financial database allowed for review of the discharge disposition and subsequent care for all neonates who were born at a single center from January 2000 through December 2002. Financial data reflect reimbursement values and costs of care from the payers' perspective at the single center. We performed a deterministic cost-effectiveness analysis using a decision tree that reflected the costs and probabilities of infants in each particular health state after nursery discharge.

Results.—A total of 73 (2.8%) of 2641 newborns who did not receive a home visit were readmitted to the hospital in the first 10 days of life with jaundice and/or dehydration compared with 2 (0.6%) of 326 who did re-

TABLE 2.—Readmissions and ED Visits in the First 10 Days of Life

	Home Visit, n (%)	No Home Visit, n (%)	P
Total patients	326 (11.0)	2641 (89.0)	—
Readmissions	2 (0.6)	73 (2.8)	.0141
ED visits	0 (0)	92 (3.5)	<.0001
Readmission or ED visit	2 (0.6)	144* (5.5)	<.0001

*Twenty-one infants were readmitted from the ED and were counted only once.

(Courtesy of Paul IM, Phillips TA, Widome MD, et al: Cost-effectiveness of postnatal home nursing visits for prevention of hospital care for jaundice and dehydration. *Pediatrics* 114:1015-1022, 2004. Reprinted by permission of *Pediatrics*.)

ceive a home visit (Table 2). Similarly, 92 (3.5%) of 2641 newborns who were discharged without subsequent home nursing care had an ED visit for these reasons in the first 10 days of life compared with 0 (0%) of 326 who did have such a visit. Of infants who received a home visit, 324 (99.4%) of 326 did not require subsequent hospital services in this time period compared with 2497 (94.5%) of 2641 of those who did not receive a visit. After nursery discharge, the average cost per child who received a home health visit was 109.80 dollars compared with 11870 dollars for each newborn who did not receive a visit. The incremental cost-effectiveness ratio of a routine home visit strategy compared with a no visit strategy was −81.82 dollars.

Conclusions.—A home nursing visit after newborn nursery discharge is highly cost-effective for reducing the need for subsequent hospital-based services.

▶ This study confirms that if we pay attention to the needs of mothers and infants in the first few days after hospital discharge, we can have a significant impact on the quality of their care. In addition, we can save money. What more logical approach could there be than to provide a home visit by a nurse? In this study a single home visit by a nurse within 48 hours of discharge significantly reduced the likelihood of the infant being readmitted for jaundice or dehydration and significantly reduced the likelihood of a visit to an emergency department in the first 10 days of life. When it comes to follow-up, nurses do it better than doctors. They spend more time with family, they are more apt to discuss psychosocial issues, they help mothers with their breastfeeding, and they are generally more sensitive to patients' concerns. In addition, the home visit spares the mother the necessity of being transported to the physician's office. Although, as demonstrated in this study, these visits are cost effective, the question is who is paying? If the hospital has to provide the home visit, then it is bearing the cost. As hospitals desperately try to cut costs to stay afloat, this type of service is one of the first to be cut. We also don't know exactly which interventions on the part of the visiting nurses resulted in a decreased need for admission. These interventions could range from advice regarding breastfeeding (which should reduce the risk of dehydration and jaundice) to the use of home phototherapy in a jaundiced newborn. Whatever was done, the difference in outcomes in the 2 groups was striking and suggests that the American Academy of Pediatrics guidelines[1] should place even more emphasis on the importance of home visits by nurses in ensuring a "safe first week of life."

M. J. Maisels, MB, BCh

Reference

1. Maisels MJ, Baltz RD, Bhutani V, et al: Management of hyperbilirubinemia in the newborn infant 35 or more weeks of gestation. *Pediatrics* 114:297-316, 2004.

12 Renal, Metabolism, and Endocrine Disorders

Central Congenital Hypothyroidism Due to Gestational Hyperthyroidism: Detection Where Prevention Failed
Kempers MJE, van Tijn DA, van Trotsenburg ASP, et al (Univ of Amsterdam)
J Clin Endocrinol Metab 88:5851-5857, 2003   12–1

Much worldwide attention is given to the adverse effects of maternal Graves' disease on the fetal and neonatal thyroid and its function. However, reports concerning the adverse effects of maternal Graves' disease on the pituitary function, illustrated by the development of central congenital hypothyroidism (CCH) in the offspring of these mothers, are scarce. We studied thyroid hormone determinants of 18 children with CCH born to mothers with Graves' disease. Nine mothers were diagnosed after pregnancy, the majority after their children were detected with CCH by neonatal screening. Four mothers were diagnosed during pregnancy and treated with antithyroid drugs since diagnosis. Another four mothers were diagnosed before pregnancy, but they used antithyroid drugs irregularly; free T_4 concentrations less than 1.7 ng/dl (<22 pmol/liter) were not encountered during pregnancy. All neonates had decreased plasma free T_4 concentrations (range 0.3-0.9 ng/dl, 3.9-11.5 pmol/liter); plasma TSH ranged between 0.1 and 6.6 mU/liter. TRH tests showed pituitary dysfunction. Seventeen children needed T_4 supplementation. Because all mothers were insufficiently treated during pregnancy, it is hypothesized that a hyperthyroid fetal environment impaired maturation of the fetal hypothalamic-pituitary-thyroid system. The frequent occurrence of this type of CCH (estimated incidence 1:35000) warrants early detection and treatment to minimize the risk of cerebral damage. A T_4-based screening program appears useful in detecting this type of CCH. However, the preferential and presumably best strategy to prevent CCH caused by maternal Graves' disease is preserving euthyroidism throughout pregnancy.

▶ Traditionally we have come to anticipate hyperthyroidism in the newborn when the mother's condition has neither been recognized nor treated. This series from Kempers et al was a revelation for me as I became more aware of CCH, a rare form of hypothyroidism, with an estimated frequency of no more than 1 in 50,000 newborns. In addition to the mechanism reported by Kempers et al, central hypothyroidism can be due to recessive inheritance of loss-of-function mutations of the TSH-beta gene and to developmental defects of the hypothalamus or pituitary.

Neonatal screening programs have successfully identified many metabolic and endocrine disorders in a timely fashion so that appropriate pharmacologic and dietary interventions have resulted in normal development in most cases.[1] Congenital hypothyroidism is the most prevalent neonatal endocrine disorder and affects 1 in 3000 to 4000 newborns. Newborn screening for CCH is one of the most successful such programs because early diagnosis and hormone replacement therapy have resulted in normal development in the vast majority of cases. However, despite early intervention, up to 10% of patients with hypothyroidism have delayed mental development and persistent neurologic symptoms. Factors identified with poorer outcomes include late diagnosis, poor compliance, and inadequate thyroid hormone replacement.

The cause of CCH in the majority of newborns is unknown. More recently, in a few cases the molecular basis of CCH has been clarified. It has become evident that, in some patients with persistent mental retardation and neurologic symptoms, defects in transcription factors expressed in the thyroid gland as well as in the CNS during embryonic development cause both defective thyroid and CNS development.[2] The clarification of further molecular defects that affect the thyroid gland and brain development will help us understand the poor outcome of patients with CCH despite early interventions and force us to develop new diagnostic and therapeutic strategies that will ensure adequate counseling and care for these patients.

A. A. Fanaroff, MD

References

1. Zamboni G, Zaffanello M, Rigon F, et al: Diagnostic effectiveness of simultaneous thyroxine and thyroid-stimulating hormone screening measurements. Thirteen years' experience in the Northeast Italian Screening Programme. *J Med Screen* 11:8-10, 2004.
2. Gruters A, Jenner A, Krude H: Long-term consequences of congenital hypothyroidism in the era of screening programmes. *Best Pract Res Clin Endocrinol Metab* 16:369-382, 2002.

Iodothyronine Levels in the Human Developing Brain: Major Regulatory Roles of Iodothyronine Deiodinases in Different Areas

Kester MHA, Martinez de Mena R, Obregon MJ, et al (Erasmus Univ, Rotterdam, The Netherlands; Consejo Superior de Investigaciones Cientificas-UAM, Madrid; Yorkhill Natl Health Service Trust, Glasgow, Scotland)
J Clin Endocrinol Metab 89:3117-3128, 2004   12–2

Thyroid hormones are required for human brain development, but data on local regulation are limited. We describe the ontogenic changes in T_4, T_3, and rT_3 and in the activities of the types I, II, and III iodothyronine deiodinases (D1, D2, and D3) in different brain regions in normal fetuses (13-20 wk postmenstrual age) and premature infants (24-42 wk postmenstrual age). D1 activity was undetectable.

The developmental changes in the concentrations of the iodothyronines and D2 and D3 activities showed spatial and temporal specificity but with divergence in the cerebral cortex and cerebellum. T_3 increased in the cortex between 13 and 20 wk to levels higher than adults, unexpected given the low circulating T_3. Considerable D2 activity was found in the cortex, which correlated positively with T_4 ($r = 0.65$). Cortex D3 activity was very low, as was D3 activity in germinal eminence and choroid plexus. In contrast, cerebellar T_3 was very low and increased only after midgestation. Cerebellum D3 activities were the highest (64 fmol/min·mg) of the regions studied, decreasing after midgestation. Other regions with high D3 activities (midbrain, basal ganglia, brain stem, spinal cord, hippocampus) also had low T_3 until D3 started decreasing after midgestation. D3 was correlated with T_3 ($r = -0.682$) and rT_3/T_3 ($r = 0.812$) and rT_3/T_4 ($r = 0.889$).

Our data support the hypothesis that T_3 is required by the human cerebral cortex before midgestation, when mother is the only source of T_3. D2 and D3 play important roles in the local bioavailability of T_3. T_3 is produced from T_4 by D2, and D3 protects brain regions from excessive T_3 until differentiation is required.

▶ Our understanding of the role of thyroid hormone in fetal brain development has evolved greatly over the past 15 years. We now know that thyroid hormone is required for normal in utero brain development and that the fetus is protected from a lack of its own thyroid hormone by placental transfer of maternal thyroxine (T_4).[1-4] Maternal transfer of T_4 is critical during early pregnancy when the fetus cannot yet synthesize its own hormone, and throughout pregnancy in infants with congenital hypothyroidism. The systemic levels of T_4 in infants with congenital hypothyroidism are, however, substantially lower than those in normal infants. How is it that these low levels of maternally derived T_4 can protect fetal brain development?

Kester et al report data from human fetuses that clarify some of the protective mechanisms. The data demonstrate that the enzymes that metabolize thyroid hormone are temporally and spatially regulated, and that the regulation results in preferential synthesis of the active thyroid hormone [triiodothyronine (T_3)] in areas of the brain that require T_3 for normal development. Specifically, during important development windows, the fetal cerebral cortex is largely protected from hypothyroxinemia by increases in levels of type 2 iodothyronine deiodinase (which converts T_4 to T_3) and decreases in levels of type 3 deiodinase (which inactivates T_4 and T_3).

This study underscores the importance of thyroid hormone for fetal brain development and elucidates one mechanism that ensures that human fetal brain tissues are exposed to the needed levels of active thyroid hormone.

M. B. Koontz, MD

M. R. Palmert, MD, PhD

References

1. Vulsma T, Gons MH, de Vijlder JJ: Maternal-fetal transfer of thyroxine in congenital hypothyroidism due to a total organification defect or thyroid agenesis. *N Engl J Med* 321:13-16, 1989.
2. Calvo R, Obregon MJ, Ruiz de Ona C, et al: Congenital hypothyroidism, as studied in rats. Crucial role of maternal thyroxine but not of 3,5,3'-triiodothyronine in the protection of fetal brain. *J Clin Invest* 86:889-899, 1990.
3. Haddow JE, Palomaki GE, Allan WC, et al: Maternal thyroid deficiency during pregnancy and subsequent neuropsychological development of the child. *N Engl J Med* 341:549-555, 1999.
4. Bianco AC, Salvatore D, Gereben B, et al: Biochemistry, cellular and molecular biology, and physiological roles of the iodothyronine selenodeiodinases. *Endocrine Reviews* 23:38-89, 2002.

Hyperinsulinaemic Hypoglycaemia in Preterm Neonates

Hussain K, Aynsley-Green A (NHS Trust, London; Univ College London)
Arch Dis Child Fetal Neonatal Ed 89:F65-F67, 2004   12–3

Introduction.—Hyperinsulinism in infancy (HI) is an important cause of severe and recurrent hypoglycaemia among newborns. It typically appears in infants born at term; only 1 case in a premature infant has been reported as an incidental finding. Reported are 7 infants born at 31-36 wk gestation who experienced severe persistent hyperinsulinism.

TABLE 1.—Clinical Details of the Seven Preterm Babies with Hyperinsulinism

	1	2	3	4	5	6	7
Sex	M	F	F	M	M	M	F
Gestational age (weeks)	31	34	36	33	36	36	36
Birth weight (g)	1740	1800	2150	3300	3780	4250	4040
Apgar scores (1 and 5 min)	8, 9	7, 9	7, 9	7, 9	8, 9	9, 9	8, 9
Age of presentation (h)	3	1	2	72	1	<1	1
Mode of delivery	CS	CS	CS	CS	NVD	NVD	NVD
Maximum glucose required (mg/kg/min)	22	19	19	14	21	19	21
Treatment	SP	D/C	D/C	SP	SP	SP	D/C

CS, Caesarean section; NVD, normal vaginal delivery; SP, subtotal pancreatectomy; D, diazoxide; C, chlorothiazide.

(Courtesy of Hussain K, Anysley-Green A: Hyperinsulinemia hypoglycemia in preterm neonates. *Arch Dis Child Fetal Neonatal Ed* 89:F65-F67, 2004, with permission from the BMJ Publishing Group.)

TABLE 2.—Results of the Diagnostic Fast and Intermediary Metabolites in Seven Preterm Babies with Hyperinsulinemia

	1	2	3	4	5	6	7
Glucose (mmol/l)	1.1	2.5	2.2	1.8	1.7	1.8	1.7
Insulin (mU/l)	15	16.4	13.1	12.6	8.0	13.8	28.5
NEFA (mmol/l)	0.13	0.16	0.14	0.05	0.12	0.17	0.05
3β-Hydroxybutyrate (mmol/l)	<0.05	<0.05	<0.05	<0.05	<0.05	<0.05	<0.05
Cortisol (nmol/l)	75	155	67	NM	111	NM	350
Growth hormone (mU/l)	60	23.6	36.6	NM	11.1	12.4	68.8
Ammonia (μmol/l) (normal 50)	45	45	40	50	48	42	50
Lactate (mmol/l)	1.3	1.2	1.5	1.9	2.0	1.5	1.9
Branched chain amino acids	Suppressed branch chain amino acids in all cases						
Urine organic acids	Normal for all						
Acylcarnitines	Normal for all						

NM, not measured; NEFA, non-esterified fatty acids.
(Courtesy of Hussain K, Anysley-Green A: Hyperinsulinemia hypoglycemia in preterm neonates. *Arch Dis Child Fetal Neonatal Ed* 89:F65-F67, 2004, with permission from the BMJ Publishing Group.)

Findings.—All 7 infants developed hypoglycaemia between 1 h to 72 h of age. Birth weights were 1740 to 4040 g (Table 1). Two infants were macrosomic, and 5 were appropriate size for gestational age. All infants experienced markedly increased glucose infusion requirement, ranging between 14 to 22 mg/kg/min. The highest glucose requirement occurred in an infant with a weight that was appropriate for gestational age. All infants exhibited exquisite sensitivity to being deprived of energy administered in the form of IV glucose administration. The laboratory blood glucose dropped to <2.6 mmol/L within 30 min of the reduction in glucose infusion rate; all infants had biochemical profiles that reflected hyperinsulinemic, hypoketotic, hypofattyacidemic hypoglycaemia with increased need for glucose. Plasma concentrations were normal. All 5 infants in whom plasma cortisol levels were measured had inappropriately low levels at the time of hypoglycaemia (Table 2). Diazoxide (5-20 mg/kg/d) and chlorothiazide (7-10 mg/kg/d) were administered to all infants. Of these, 3 responded adequately to a starting dose of diazoxide 10 mg/kg/d with chlorothiazide 7 mg/kg/d to allow IV glucose support to be discontinued; treatment effect was obvious within 48 h. It was possible to discontinue medical treatment in these 3 infants after 3 to 6 mo. The other 4 infants failed to become glucose drip independent, even in the presence of increased dose of diazoxide to 20 mg/kg/d and introduction of continuous IV or subcutaneous infusion of glucagon (1.0 μg/kg/h) and octreotide (10 μg/kg/d). All 4 of these infants underwent 95% pancreatectomy to control hypoglycaemia. Nifedipine (0.75 mg/kg/d) was necessary in 1 infant to prevent recurrence of hypoglycaemia. Histological examination of the pancreas revealed changes consistent with the diffuse form of HI. Electrophysiology examination using patch clamp techniques on the resected pancreas revealed complete loss of function of the K_{ATP} channel in the β cell membrane, which is the most common cause of HI.

Conclusion.—Hyperinsulinemia hypoglycaemia should be suspected in the diagnosis of any preterm infant who presents with severe hypoglycaemia. Of particular note for diagnosis is the importance of the glucose infusion requirement. Near total pancreatectomy may be necessary to control hypoglycaemia.

▶ We have all had the frustrating experience of caring for an infant with persistent hyperinsulinism leading to recurrent and severe hypoglycemia. These infants are almost always full term and some of them are large for gestation (LGA). The LGA infants resemble infants of diabetic mothers suggesting that hyperinsulinism was present for sometime before birth.

A similar clinical picture in the preterm infant is extremely rare, but because these investigators work at a national and international referral center for such infants, they were able to assemble a group of 7 infants born at 31-36 weeks gestation who experienced severe hyperinsulinism. They emphasize some important clinical points. Although all of the reported infants had the typical biochemical profile of hyperinsulinism (elevated free fatty acid levels, increased glucose requirements) as well as raised insulin concentrations, in this situation the diagnosis of hyperinsulinism does not require very high insulin levels. A normal insulin concentration (for normoglycemia) is inappropriate in the presence of hypoglycemia. Thus, "the demonstration of any measurable insulin in a hypoglycaemic sample is strong evidence for a failure of basal insulin control."

We need to pay attention to the glucose infusion requirements in preterm infants who are hypoglycemic. Those who need an excessive glucose infusion rate are likely to be hyperinsulinemic and require further investigation. Some will respond to treatment with diazoxide but others will require subtotal pancreatectomy.

M. J. Maisels, MB, BCh

Both Relative Insulin Resistance and Defective Islet β-cell Processing of Proinsulin Are Responsible for Transient Hyperglycemia in Extremely Preterm Infants
Mitanchez-Mokhtari D, Lahlou N, Kieffer F, et al (Hôpital Necker-Enfants Malades, Paris; Hôpital Saint Vincent de Paul, Paris; Institut de Puériculture, Paris)
Pediatrics 113:537-541, 2004   12–4

Objective.—Many extremely preterm infants develop hyperglycemia in the first week of life during continuous glucose infusion. The objective of this study was to determine whether defective insulin secretion or resistance to insulin was the primary factor involved in transient hyperglycemia of extremely preterm infants.

Methods.—A prospective comparative study was conducted in appropriate-for-gestational-age preterm infants <30 weeks of gestational age with the aim specifically to evaluate the serum levels of proinsulin, insulin, and C-peptide secreted during transient hyperglycemia by specific immunoassays. Three groups of infants were investigated hyperglycemic (*n* = 15) and normoglycemic preterm neonates (*n* = 12) and normal, term neonates ($n = 21$). In addition, the changes in β-cell peptide levels were analyzed during and after intravenous insulin infusion in the hyperglycemic group. Data were analyzed using analysis of variance and analysis of variance for repeated measures.

Results.—At inclusion, insulin and C-peptide levels did not differ in hyperglycemic subjects and in preterm controls. Proinsulin concentration was significantly higher in the hyperglycemic group (36.5 ± 3.9 vs 23.2 ± 0.9 pmol/L). Compared with term neonates, proinsulin and C-peptide levels were higher in normoglycemic preterm infants (23.2 ± 0.9 vs 18.9 ± 2.71 pmol/L and 1.67 ± 0.3 vs 0.62 ± 0.12 nmol/L, respectively). During and after insulin infusion in hyperglycemic neonates, plasma glucose concentration fell and proinsulin and C-peptide levels were lowered (18.4 ± 7.6 and 20.7 ± 4.5 pmol/L, respectively).

Conclusion.—These data suggest that 1) preterm neonates are sensitive to changes in plasma glucose concentration, but proinsulin processing to insulin is partially defective in hyperglycemic preterm neonates; 2) hyperglycemic neonates are relatively resistant to insulin because higher insulin levels are needed to achieve euglycemia in this group compared with normoglycemic neonates. These results also show that insulin infusion is beneficial in extremely preterm infants with transient hyperglycemia.

▶ We often see hyperglycemia in our extremely low birth weight population. These infants develop hyperglycemia even though their glucose infusion rate is appropriate for their basal requirements (4-7 mg/kg per minute). These investigators wanted to know whether this hyperglycemia was the result of defective insulin secretion or resistance to insulin. To do this they investigated a group of hyperglycemic and normoglycemic preterm neonates as well as a group of normal term neonates. They evaluated the serum levels of proinsulin, insulin, and C-peptide secreted during transient hyperglycemia in infants younger than 30 weeks' gestation. Compared with term neonates, proinsulin and C-peptide levels were higher in normoglycemic preterm infants. Their data suggest that there is a defect in the processing of proinsulin in β-cells as well as a partial resistance to insulin in hyperglycemic infants younger than 30 weeks' gestation. If these are the defects responsible for the altered glucose homeostasis found in these infants, then we need to give them more insulin. Although many neonatologists are hesitant about using continuous insulin infusion to treat transient hyperglycemia in this population, these data suggest that this is, indeed, the appropriate intervention.

M. J. Maisels, MB, BCh

Mild Gestational Hyperglycemia, the Metabolic Syndrome and Adverse Neonatal Outcomes

Bo S, Menato G, Gallo M-L, et al (Univ of Turin, Italy)
Acta Obstet Gynecol Scand 83:335-340, 2004   12–5

Background.—The aim of this study was to evaluate the prevalence of the metabolic syndrome and its effect on neonatal outcomes in pregnancies with different degrees of hyperglycemia.

Methods.—One hundred and fifty women with gestational diabetes, 100 with one abnormal value on the oral glucose tolerance test, 100 with a normal oral glucose challenge test and 350 with an abnormal challenge test and normal tolerance test were enrolled.

Results.—The prevalence of the metabolic syndrome was: 0%, 4.9%, 20% and 18% in the normal challenge test, abnormal challenge and normal tolerance test, one abnormal value and gestational diabetes patients, respectively. Offspring birth weights, prevalence of large-for-gestational age babies and icterus were significantly higher in women with an abnormal challenge test (both with a normal tolerance test or one abnormal value or gestational diabetes). Metabolic syndrome was the best predictor of the presence of large-for-gestational age babies in patients with an abnormal challenge and normal tolerance test (OR = 3.15), one abnormal value (OR = 3.53) and gestational diabetes (OR = 4.15).

Conclusions.—Metabolic syndrome in mid-pregnancy was an independent predictor of macrosomia in women with any degree of gestational hyperglycemia; the oral glucose challenge test identifies pregnancies with metabolic abnormalities and adverse neonatal outcomes also in the presence of a normal oral glucose tolerance test.

▶ The association between maternal hyperglycemia, worsening metabolic control in diabetes, and fetal macrosomia has been known ever since Pedersen[1] proposed the maternal hyperglycemia and fetal hyperinsulinemia hypothesis. Freinkel[2] later extended this concept by proposing the significance of transfer of other metabolic substrates, such as fats and amino acids, to the fetus and their contribution to fetal macrosomia. The concentration of these substrates increases in maternal circulation as a consequence of decompensation in metabolism in diabetic pregnancy.[3] Additionally, Knopp et al[4] have demonstrated correlation between maternal hyperlipidemia and fetal macrosomia. Later studies demonstrated normal pregnancy to be a state of insulin resistance. The magnitude of resistance to insulin action described as decreased peripheral (primarily skeletal muscle) uptake of glucose in response to a sustained steady-state level of insulin.[5] Whether insulin resistance is an adaptation for accretion of nitrogen by the mother or to divert nutrients to the fetus or both remains to be ascertained.[6] Other studies showed that the magnitude of insulin resistance was much higher in women with gestational diabetes.[7] A significant correlation (albeit weak, $r^2 = 0.28$), was shown between maternal insulin resistance and infant birth weight.[8] Other studies have demonstrated an association between lack of development of insulin resistance or higher insulin sensitivity and intrauterine growth retardation.[9]

Whether the relationships among maternal hyperglycemia, dyslipidemia, insulin resistance, and fetal macrosomia represent worsening metabolic regulation of the mother or a distinct new entity remains controversial. The study of Bo et al has grouped them together as "metabolic syndrome" of pregnancy.

Metabolic syndrome, or syndrome X, was proposed by Reaven[10] to describe a cluster of entities (hypertension, triglyceridemia, overactivity of sympathetic nervous system, and increased renal sodium reabsorption) with a common denominator of insulin resistance in nonpregnant adults. The metabolic syndrome is additionally associated with an increased risk of arteriosclerotic cardiovascular disease. The metabolic syndrome has now been specifically defined by the World Health Organization and the National Cholesterol Education Program Adult Treatment Panel III to include impaired fasting plasma glucose, impaired glucose tolerance test, and insulin resistance plus abdominal obesity, increased triglycerides, low high-density lipoprotein cholesterol levels, high blood pressure (>140/90 mm Hg), and microalbuminuria. Bo et al used some of these criteria to define the "metabolic syndrome" of pregnancy, essentially bringing together the severity of decompensation in glucose metabolism.

It is important to note that the frequency of metabolic syndrome in their population was the same in their class 3 women, with only 1 abnormal glucose value on oral glucose tolerance test (20/100 [20%]) and in their class 4 women who were positive for gestational diabetes mellitus (18/150 [12%]). The incidence of large for gestational age infants was the same across all women, from minimal evidence of glucose intolerance (positive oral glucose screen but negative glucose tolerance test; class 2) to those with established gestational diabetes mellitus. The incidence of LGA was 19% in class 2, 18.9% in class 3, and 20.7% in class 4. Nonetheless, statistical analysis of the data showed "metabolic syndrome to be an independent predictor of macrosomia." The mean blood pressure in all classes was in the normal range.

Thus, the question remains, should the cluster of events associated with decompensating glucose tolerance, with dyslipidemia and fasting hyperinsulinemia during late pregnancy, be termed metabolic syndrome, or simply worsening glucose intolerance of pregnancy, or gestational diabetes mellitus? Specifically, in the absence of hypertension, the above cluster will only prognosticate fetal macrosomia and long-term risk of type II diabetes in the mother, an association previously described. An association between the described metabolic syndrome in pregnancy and atherosclerotic cardiovascular disease in the mother remains to be established.

S. C. Kalhan, MD

References

1. Pedersen J. Hyperglycemia-hyperinsulinism theory and birth weight In Pedersen J (ed), *The pregnant diabetic and her newborn*, Baltimore, MD, Williams & Wilkins, 1977, pp 211-220.
2. Freinkel N: Banting Lecture 1980: Of pregnancy and progeny. *Diabetes* 29:1023-1035, 1980.

3. Metzger BE, Phelps RL, Freinkel N, et al: Effects of gestational diabetes on diurnal profiles of plasma glucose, lipids, and individual amino acids. *Diabetes Care* 3:402-409, 1980.
4. Knopp RH, Magee MS, Walden CE, et al: Prediction of infant birth weight by GDM screening tests. Importance of plasma triglyceride. *Diabetes Care* 15:1605-1613, 1992.
5. Ryan EA, O'Sullivan MJ, Skyler JA: Insulin action during pregnancy. Studies with the euglycemic clamp technique. *Diabetes* 34:380-389, 1985.
6. Kalhan SC, Devapatla S: Pregnancy, insulin resistance and nitrogen accretion. *Curr Opin Clin Nutr Metab Care* 2:359-363, 1999.
7. Catalano PM, Bernstein IM, Wolfe RR, et al: Subclinical abnormalities of glucose metabolism in subjects with previous gestational diabetes. *Am J Obstet Gynecol* 155:1255-1262, 1986.
8. Catalano PM, Drago NM, Amini SB: Maternal carbohydrate metabolism and its relationship to fetal growth and body composition. *Am J Obstet Gynecol* 172:1464-1470, 1995.
9. Sokol RJ, Kazzi GM, Kalhan SC, et al: Identifying the pregnancy at risk for intrauterine growth retardation: Possible usefulness of the intravenous glucose tolerance test. *Am J Obstet Gynecol* 143:220-223, 1982.
10. Reaven GM: Banting lecture 1988: Role of insulin resistance in human disease. *Diabetes* 37:1595-1607, 1988.

Circulating Adrenocorticotropic Hormone (ACTH) and Cortisol Concentrations in Normal, Appropriate-for-Gestational-Age Newborns Versus Those With Sepsis and Respiratory Distress: Cortisol Response to Low-Dose and Standard-Dose ACTH Tests

Soliman AT, Taman KH, Rizk MM, et al (Univ of Alexandria, Egypt; Ain Shams Univ, Cairo, Egypt)
Metabolism 53:209-214, 2004   12–6

Background.—Some neonates admitted to the neonatal ICU have circulatory and respiratory problems that are improved by administration of corticosteroids. However, it is unclear whether these symptoms could be caused

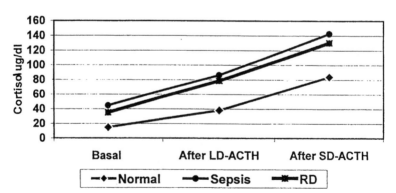

FIGURE 1.—Mean values of basal and stimulated cortisol responses to low-dose (LD) and standard-dose (SD) ACTH tests. *Abbreviations: ACTH*, Adrenocorticotropic hormone; *RD*, respiratory distress. (Courtesy of Soliman AT, Taman KH, Rizk MM, et al: Circulating adrenocorticotropic hormone (ACTH) and cortisol concentrations in normal, appropriate-for-gestational-age newborns versus those with sepsis and respiratory distress: Cortisol response to low-dose and standard-dose ACTH tests. *Metabolism* 53:209-214, 2004.)

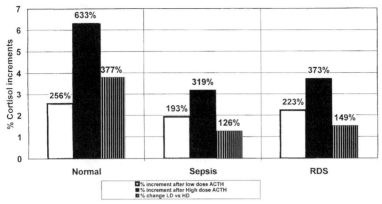

FIGURE 2.—Percent increments of cortisol concentrations after low-dose (LD) and standard-dose (SD) ACTH tests and percent difference of responses between LD and SD ACTH in normal newborns and those with sepsis and RD. *Abbreviations: ACTH,* Adrenocorticotropic hormone; *RD,* respiratory distress. (Courtesy of Soliman AT, Taman KH, Rizk MM, et al: Circulating adrenocorticotropic hormone (ACTH) and cortisol concentrations in normal, appropriate-for-gestational-age newborns versus those with sepsis and respiratory distress: Cortisol response to low-dose and standard-dose ACTH tests. *Metabolism* 53:209-214, 2004.)

or affected by adrenal insufficiency. Data on cortisol secretion by newborns during different types of stress are insufficient, and the cortisol responses of these infants to different doses of adrenocorticotropic hormone (ACTH) stimulation are not standardized. It has been suggested that the use of a supraphysiologic dose of exogenous ACTH (250 µg) may cause false-positive responses as a result of maximal stimulation of the adrenal cortex and that the test should be done with the use of lower doses of ACTH. It is possible that the low-dose ACTH test could diagnose early and mild cases of adrenal suppression in both infants and adults. Whether corticotroph cell hypofunctioning occurs in some stressed newborns, whether a difference is seen in the cortisol response to different stressful conditions, and whether the low-dose ACTH test can diagnose early, mild cases of adrenal insufficiency that might not be detected with the high-dose test were determined in newborns.

TABLE 1.—ACTH and Cortisol Secretion in Newborns With and Without Stress

	ACTH (ng/mL)	Basal Cortisol (µg/dL)	Cortisol After LD ACTH (µg/dL)	Cortisol After SD ACTH (µg/dL)
Normal (n = 30)	50.2 ± 6.9	14.8 ± 1.9	38.1 ± 5	84 ± 6.9
Sepsis (n = 30)	30.8 ± 4.4*	44.8 ± 12.2*†	86.3 ± 13.3*	142.8 ± 17.7*
RD (n = 30)	51.4 ± 8.5	35 ± 7.1*	78.6 ± 9.8*	130.6 ± 18.4*

*P < .05, sepsis and RD groups vs normal.
†P < .05, RD vs sepsis.
Abbreviations: LD, Low-dose; *SD,* standard dose; *ACTH,* adrenocorticotropic hormone; *RD,* respiratory distress.
(Courtesy of Soliman AT, Taman KH, Rizk MM, et al: Circulating adrenocorticotropic hormone (ACTH) and cortisol concentrations in normal, appropriate-for-gestational-age newborns versus those with sepsis and respiratory distress: Cortisol response to low-dose and standard-dose ACTH tests. *Metabolism* 53:209-214, 2004.)

TABLE 2.—Prognosis and Cortisol Secretion in Subgroups of Septic Newborns

	Mortality	Basal Cortisol	Cortisol After LD ACTH	Cortisol After SD ACTH
TLC > 5,000 (n = 20)	25.00	49.8 ± 14.2	94.4 ± 16.5	145.9 ± 19.5
TLC < 5,000 (n = 10)	50.00	38.2 ± 9.5*	72.4 ± 11.4*	141.7 ± 16.3
Without menengitis (n = 18)	11.11	51.7 ± 12.2	99.9 ± 15.7	141.5 ± 15.4
With menengitis (n = 12)	50.00	37.3 ± 11.9*	76.5 ± 12.2*	145.2 ± 18.7
Survived (n = 22)		46.3 ± 13.2	98.5 ± 13.5	147.8 ± 21.2
Died (n = 8)		42.8 ± 11.4	56.3 ± 10.2*	139.5 ± 15.7

*$P < .01$.

Abbreviations: LD, Low-dose; SD, standard-dose; ACTH, adrenocorticotropic hormone; TLC, total leukocyte count.
(Courtesy of Soliman AT, Taman KH, Rizk MM, et al: Circulating adrenocorticotropic hormone (ACTH) and cortisol concentrations in normal, appropriate-for-gestational-age newborns versus those with sepsis and respiratory distress: cortisol response to low-dose and standard-dose ACTH tests. *Metabolism* 53:209-214, 2004.)

Methods.—The peak responses of cortisol to low-dose and standard-dose ACTH stimulation tests were compared in 90 full-term newborns, including 30 with sepsis, 30 with respiratory distress, and 30 healthy infants. Basal cortisol and ACTH levels were measured in a fasting venous sample. Serum cortisol concentrations were measured 30 minutes after low-dose ACTH and 60 minutes after standard-dose ACTH administration by radioimmunoassay.

Results.—The mean basal circulating cortisol concentration and peak cortisol responses to low-dose and standard-dose ACTH tests were higher in stressed infants with sepsis and respiratory distress than in healthy infants (Fig 1). Basal but not ACTH-stimulated cortisol concentrations were significantly higher in newborns with sepsis than in those with respiratory distress (Fig 2). Circulating cortisol concentrations after the low-dose ACTH test were significantly higher in newborns with sepsis than in those with respiratory distress (Table 1).

Conclusions.—The low-dose ACTH test may be more discriminatory than the standard-dose test in infants under stress (Table 2). Additional studies are needed to determine whether supplementation with stress doses of hydrocortisone may improve the outcomes in these patients.

▶ The authors ambitiously set out to address 3 important questions in this study: (1) Does a state of relative adrenal insufficiency exist among "stressed" full-term newborns compared with normal full-term newborns? (2) Is there a difference in the degree of insufficiency depending on the type of "stress" experienced by the newborn (sepsis vs respiratory distress)? (3) Can low-dose ACTH stimulation testing detect subtle yet clinically significant adrenal insufficiency that would be missed by "standard dose" testing? The challenges to this type of investigation are many. Patient numbers will be relatively small, unless a multicenter effort is undertaken. It is also difficult to definitively separate one kind of stress (eg, respiratory distress) from another (eg, sepsis). As the authors point out, what adrenal insufficiency means for newborn infants in a variety of stressful conditions is difficult to define. Challenges are also inherent in the design of any crossover ACTH stimulation testing study with respect to the order of testing and the interval between tests.

The authors point out the significant difference in percentage change of serum cortisol levels in response to ACTH among the different diagnostic groups. Mean peak cortisol responses to ACTH were higher in the stressed groups overall than in the healthy group, and the absolute mean response appeared adequate overall (Fig 1). Of great interest, however, is the focused evaluation of the results from the sepsis group. After low-dose ACTH stimulation, a significantly lower peak cortisol level was noted among patients with sepsis who died than among those who survived. The difference between mean basal and mean peak cortisol levels after low-dose ACTH was less than 15 µg/dL among nonsurviving infants with sepsis compared with greater than 50 µg/dL among survivors. This was a demonstrably high-risk group (8/30 died), and clinical details beyond the assigned diagnostic category were not presented.

Clearly, it would be inappropriate to point to a poor cortisol response to low-dose ACTH as the single predictive variable for adverse outcomes in a complex multifactorial clinical scenario. Nonetheless, this is a hypothesis-generating investigation, the results are intriguing, and they require further prospective, observational study. The pendulum seems to have swung hard against any postnatal steroid use in recent years, but perhaps, the time has come for a careful and measured evaluation of the clinical conditions associated with relative adrenal insufficiency.

S. R. Hintz, MD

Can an Alternative Umbilical Arterial Catheter Solution and Flush Regimen Decrease Iatrogenic Hemolysis While Enhancing Nutrition? A Double-Blind, Randomized, Clinical Trial Comparing an Isotonic Amino Acid With a Hypotonic Salt Infusion

Jackson JK, Diondo DJ, Jones JM, et al (Univ of Missouri, Kansas City)
Pediatrics 114:377-383, 2004   12–7

Objective.—In the process of sampling blood through an umbilical arterial catheter (UAC), infant blood comes into stagnant contact with infusion solution in the "waste syringe" before being reinfused. We have previously demonstrated in vitro that this process is associated with less hemolysis of red blood cells (RBCs) with use of an isotonic solution compared with a hypotonic 0.25 normal saline (NS) solution. The objective of this study was to compare the in vivo effect on hemolysis of 2 UAC infusion/flush regimens (an isotonic regimen vs a hypotonic regimen) and to assess the early nutritional benefit of an amino acid solution as the isotonic UAC infusion solution.

Methods.—Infants who had a birth weight of ≤1.5 kg and were expected to have a UAC for ≥3 days were enrolled within 24 hours of life into this prospective, double-blind, randomized, clinical trial of 2 UAC infusion solution/flush regimens. Power analysis demonstrated that 40 infants were needed to determine differences in hemolysis quantified by plasma-free hemoglobin

(PFH) level. Nutrition from glucose was evaluated by measurement of daily dextrose calories. C-peptide was measured to evaluate endogenous insulin production. Adverse events and protein tolerance were tracked.

Results.—Twenty-two infants (mean gestational age: 27 weeks; 945 g birth weight) were enrolled in each group, for an average of 4.2 days (range: 2.5-8 days). There were no group differences in demographics. PFH levels were lower for infants who received isotonic amino acid (IAA) in comparison with 0.25 NS (33 ± 14 mg/dL vs 62 ± 27 mg/dL, respectively). C-peptide was higher in those who received IAA, as were nonprotein calories received on days 4 to 6 of the study (51 ± 11 kcal/kg/day vs 44 ± 12 kcal/kg/day, IAA vs 0.25 NS, respectively).

Conclusions.—Lower PFH levels in IAA versus 0.25 NS group were consistent with our hypothesis of decreased hemolysis with an isotonic infusion/flush regimen. IAA use may also allow greater early glucose nutrition, as indicated by the higher level of endogenous insulin production and improved glucose tolerance. IAA seems to be a superior UAC solution to 0.25 NS in that it is associated with less hemolysis and improved nutrition.

▶ Postnatal growth failure is extremely common in the very low birth weight (<1.5 kg) and extremely low birth weight infant (<1 kg). Although approximately 20% of extremely low birth weight infants are small for gestational age at birth, by 36 weeks' corrected age 89% have growth failure, and at 18 to 22 months 40% still have weights, lengths, and head circumferences less than the tenth percentile. Growth failure is associated with an increased risk of poor neurodevelopmental outcome.[1] To remedy this, aggressive nutritional support, beginning with amino acid supplementation on day 1 of life, has become commonplace. Jackson et al's well-designed, prospective, randomized, controlled trial addresses dual issues, namely which flush solution minimizes hemolysis, and is it feasible to provide caloric supplementation by the flush solution. There are unambiguous answers to the questions and, in both instances, the isotonic amino acid proved to be superior. There were direct measurements of hemolysis, and the combination of an elevated C-peptide and better glucose control were indicative of more endogenous insulin production. In this small series there was no evidence of harm. Although Poindexter et al[2,3] were unable to demonstrate that parenteral glutamine supplementation reduced the risk of mortality or late-onset sepsis, they were able to implement protocols of earlier and more aggressive amino acid supplementation. Growth was better during the initial hospitalization in the infants receiving the most amino acid supplementation early.

On the basis of the data gathered by Jackson et al, consideration should be given to modifying flush solutions. Isotonic solutions are preferred and the addition of amino acids should be strongly considered.

A. A. Fanaroff, MD

References

1. Dusick AM, Poindexter BB, Ehrenkranz RA, et al: Growth failure in the preterm infant: Can we catch up? *Semin Perinatol* 27:302-310, 2003.

2. Poindexter BB, et al for the National Institute of Child Health and Human Development Neonatal Research Network: Parenteral glutamine supplementation does not reduce the risk of mortality or late-onset sepsis in extremely low birth weight infants. *Pediatrics* 113:1209-1215, 2004.
3. Poindexter BB, et al for the National Institute of Child Health and Human Development Neonatal Research Network: Effect of parenteral glutamine supplementation on plasma amino acid concentrations in extremely low-birth-weight infants. *Am J Clin Nutr* 77:737-743, 2003.

Outcome of Isolated Antenatal Hydronephrosis

Cheng AM, Phan V, Geary DF, et al (Univ of Toronto)
Arch Pediatr Adolesc Med 158:38-40, 2004   12–8

Objective.—To define the clinical outcome in isolated antenatal hydronephrosis (ANH), defined as pelviectasis without vesicoureteral reflux or urinary tract obstruction.

Study Design and Patients.—We analyzed prospectively gathered data from patients with isolated ANH. Pelviectasis, graded using the anterior-posterior diameter reference criteria, was defined by the status of the more severely affected kidney. Urinary tract obstruction was ruled out by diethylenetriamine pentaacetic acid scan when clinically indicated Statistical differences were analyzed using the McNemar and χ^2 tests.

Results.—Isolated ANH was defined in 63 patients. The first postnatal ultrasonogram (mean ± SD age, 18.4 ± 17.8 days) revealed resolution of ANH in 16 (25%), mild pelviectasis in 34 (54%), and moderate or severe pelviectasis in 13 (21%). Ultrasonogram at the last follow-up visit (23.3 ± 14.8 months) in 57 patients demonstrated normal pelvic diameter or mild pelviectasis in 47 (82%) ($P =.002$). In the 13 patients with moderate or severe neonatal pelviectasis, severity decreased in 11 (85%) Deterioration of any grade of pelviectasis occurred in only 3 (5%) of 57 patients. Renal growth, measured by renal length, was normal in all 57 patients.

Conclusion.—Isolated ANH resolves or improves in most patients during the first 2 years of life.

▶ Because of the almost universal use of antenatal US, it is not rare to have the incidental finding of fetal hydronephrosis. The authors note that ANH has an incidence of 0.5% to 1%, but what happens to the kidneys in these infants and how much additional evaluation is necessary have not been well defined (unless they have uteropelvic junction obstruction or vesicoureteral reflux). In the absence of these abnormalities, we are left with the diagnosis of isolated ANH where the only abnormality is pelviectasis or pelvocaliectasis of varying degrees of severity.

The authors identified 63 infants who met this definition and monitored them for 23 ± 14.8 months. Their results clearly demonstrate that isolated ANH generally remains stable or resolves spontaneously in 4 of 5 infants. Even moderate or severe neonatal pelviectasis can be expected to improve in 85%. Only 3 (5%) of 57 infants showed any degree of deterioration in the grade of their pelviectasis. The investigators also demonstrated the previously described predominance of males among infants with hydronephrosis, although the outcome in the 2 sexes was equivalent.

These findings are reassuring. If we see an infant with isolated ANH who does not have uteropelvic junction obstruction or reflux we need only provide occasional US evaluation to be reassured that the condition is improving or remaining stable. Only the most severe cases require more frequent monitoring.

M. J. Maisels, MB, BCh

Long-Term Clinical Outcome of Infants With Mild and Moderate Fetal Pyelectasis: Validation of Neonatal Ultrasound as a Screening Tool to Detect Significant Nephrouropathies

Ismaili K, for the Brussels Free Univ Perinatal Nephrology Study Group (Hôpital Universitaire des Enfants—Reine Fabiola, Brussels, Belgium; et al)
J Pediatr 144:759-765, 2004   12–9

Objective.—To assess the long-term outcome of infants with mild and moderate fetal pyelectasis and to determine the predictive value of neonatal ultrasound imaging in identifying significant nephrouropathies (Fig 3).

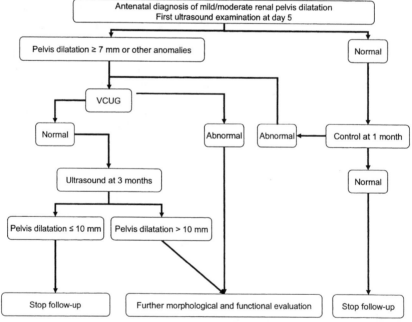

FIGURE 3.—Algorithm of a rational postnatal imaging strategy in infants with mild to moderate fetal renal pelvis dilatation. (Reprinted by permission of the publisher from Ismaili K, for the Brussels Free University Perinatal Nephrology Study Group: Long-term clinical outcome of infants with mild and moderate fetal pyelectasis: Validation of neonatal ultrasound as a screening tool to detect significant nephrouropathies. *J Pediatr* 144:759-765. Copyright 2004 by Elsevier.)

Study Design.—This prospective study included 213 infants with antenatal mild to moderate pyelectasis who were followed for up to 2 years. Postnatal renal ultrasound examinations were performed at day 5 and months 1, 3, 6, 12 and 24 after birth. Voiding cystourethrography was performed in all infants.

Results.—Normal or nonsignificant findings were diagnosed in 130 of 213 (61%) infants. Significant nephrouropathies were diagnosed in 83 of 213 (39%) infants. The sensitivity, specificity, positive predictive value, and negative predictive value of two successive neonatal renal ultrasound examinations performed at day 5 and 1 month to predict significant nephrouropathies were 96%, 76%, 72%, and 97%, respectively. In 102 of 213 (48%) infants with normal neonatal renal ultrasound scans, we later found only three of 102 (3%) cases with significant nephrouropathies.

Conclusions.—We found in a population of infants with mild to moderate fetal pyelectasis a 39% incidence of significant nephrouropathies. Ultrasound is an excellent screening tool with high sensitivity and negative predictive value that allows avoidance of unjustified medical follow-up in patients with two normal neonatal ultrasound scans.

▶ Renal abnormalities are common on the fetal US, but in many instances there is not an underlying pathologic entity. As water conservation is not a priority for the fetus and they are in a state of constant diuresis (15 mL/kg per hour), findings suggestive of hydronephrosis are common. How common is the subject of Ismaili et al's report on behalf of the Brussels Free University Perinatal Nephrology Study Group. In this prospective study 213 infants with antenatal mild to moderate pyelectasis were followed for up to 2 years with multiple postnatal US and voiding cystourethrograms. The optimists among us would emphasize that in 61% normal or nonsignificant findings were present postnatally, whereas the pessimists would stress that significant nephrouropathies were present in 39%. The consensus was that the use of 2 us examinations performed at 5 days and 1 month were both sensitive (96%) and had a high negative predictive value (97%). In only 3 of 102 infants with normal neonatal renal US scans was a significant nephrouropathy subsequently detected. They concluded that US is an excellent screening tool that allows avoidance of unjustified medical follow-up in patients with 2 normal neonatal US scans.

Acton et al[1] reported the results of a 5-year review of 778 neonatal renal scans seen in an obstetric hospital. Most infants were referred on the basis of antenatal US findings. In 92% of the cases pyelectasis was the reason for referral, this verifying the high prevalence noted by Ismaili et al. The good news was that majority of neonates (76%) had a normal postnatal scan; however, a number had vesicoureteric reflux found on micturating cystourethrogram. Persisting mild to moderate pyelectasis or hydronephrosis (15%) proved to be a normal variant in many infants but had a similar appearance to those with an early obstructive cause (1%). An additional 59 infants (8%) presented with a miscellaneous group of renal anomalies, many with a characteristic and distinctive antenatal US appearance that clinched the diagnosis.

We conclude that pyelectasis is a common finding on the fetal renal US scan. The majority of infants have a normal urinary tract, but significant pathology may be present, justifying close follow-up with postnatal US and liberal use of the voiding cystourethrogram.

A. A. Fanaroff, MD

Reference

1. Acton C, Pahuja M, Opie G, et al: A 5-year audit of 778 neonatal renal scans (part 2). Miscellaneous anomalies in 59 infants: A pictorial presentation. *Australas Radiol* 47:354-362, 2003.

13 Pharmacology

High Dose Caffeine Citrate for Extubation of Preterm Infants: A Randomised Controlled Trial
Steer P, Flenady V, Shearman A, et al (Univ of Queensland, Australia; Univ of Sydney, NSW, Australia; Royal Hobart Hosp, Tasmania, Australia; et al)
Arch Dis Child Fetal Neonatal Ed 89:F499-F503, 2004   13–1

Introduction.—Methylxanthines have been used to facilitate extubation among very low birth weight infants. The 2 existing methylxanthines, aminophylline and caffeine, have both been used in preterm infants. Caffeine has demonstrated the advantage of a longer half-life and less toxicity compared with theophylline. The standard lose of caffeine citrate is a loading dose of 20 mg/kg, with a maintenance dose of 5 mg/kg daily; at these dose levels, up to one third of preterm infants cannot be extubated. Two-dose regimens for caffeine citrate were used in the periextubation period for neonates born at fewer than 30 weeks' gestation in a multicenter, randomized, double-blind clinical investigation to determine if a higher dose was more effective than a standard dose regimen in facilitating successful extubation in a very preterm infant without an increase in adverse effects.

Methods.—Infants born at fewer than 30 weeks' gestation and ventilated for more than 48 hours were evaluated in 4 tertiary neonatal units. A total of 234 infants were randomly assigned to 1 of 2 dosing regimens for management of periextubation: 20 mg/kg per day versus 5 mg/kg per day of caffeine citrate. Treatment was initiated 24 hours before planned extubation or within 6 hours of unplanned extubation. The primary outcome measure was failure to extubate within 48 hours of caffeine loading or reintubation and ventilation or doxapram within 7 days of caffeine loading.

Results.—A significant decrease in failure to extubate was observed in the 20 mg/kg per day dosing group (15.0% vs 29.8%; relative risk, 0.51; 95% confidence interval, 0.31-0.85; number needed to treat, 7 [95% confidence interval, 4-24]). A significant difference in duration of mechanical ventilation was observed in infants of fewer than 36 weeks' gestation who received the 20-mg/kg per day dose (mean, 14.4 days vs 22.1 days; $P = .01$). The number of episodes of apnea within 7 days of initiation of treatment was significantly reduced in the high-dose caffeine group (median, 4 [range, 0-92] vs 7 [range, 0-56] episodes) (Table 2). No difference in adverse effects was seen in measures of mortality rate, major neonatal morbidity, death, or severe disability or general quotient at 12 months.

TABLE 2.—Analysis of Trial Data

	20 mg/kg (n = 113)	5 mg/kg (n = 121)	RR (95% CI)	P Value
Extubation failure	17 (15%)	36 (29.8%)	0.51 (0.31 to 0.85)	<0.01
Not extubated	6	7		
Reventilated	10	29		
Doxapram	1	0		
Duration of mechanical ventilation (days)	7.4 (3.3-16.5)	9.0 (0.5-77)		0.38
Duration of NCPAP (days)	10.1 (2.3-21.2)	9.8 (4.3-20.1)		0.56
Documented apnoea	4 (1-12)	7 (2-22)		<0.01
Documented apnoea (days)*	0.6 (0.1-2.1)	1.3 (0.3-4.3)		0.02

Values are median (interquartile range) unless otherwise indicated. Extubation failure defined as not extubated within 48 hours of caffeine, reintubation, or doxapram within 7 days of caffeine loading. Documented apnea is episodes of apnea recorded by nursing staff within 7 days of the start of caffeine treatment.
*Nonventilated days in successfully extubated infants (85 infants in the 5-mg/kg group and 96 in the 20-mg/kg group).
Abbreviation: NCPAP, Nasopharyngeal continuous positive airways pressure.
(Courtesy of Steer P, Flenady V, Shearman A, et al: High dose caffeine citrate for extubation of preterm infants: A randomised controlled trial. *Arch Dis Child Fetal Neonatal Ed* 89:F499-F503, 2004, with permission from the BMJ Publishing Group.)

Conclusion.—Treatment with 20 mg/kg per day of caffeine citrate was effective in reducing the duration of mechanical ventilation and in reducing apnea after extubation in neonates born at fewer than 30 weeks' gestation.

▶ Achieving successful, sustained extubation is one of the highest priorities in clinical care of the very low birth weight infant, yet there are precious few tools to apply to the problem. This study concludes that caffeine citrate may safely be used in doses 4 times higher than typically used. I hope they are right, yet there is reason to hesitate before widespread adoption into clinical practice. The neurologic follow-up data extend only to age 12 months, and there are international, multicenter caffeine trials with long-term outcome measures currently in progress. Caution is indicated at this time.

D. B. DeWitte, MD

Theophylline and Gastric Emptying in Very Low Birthweight Neonates: A Randomised Controlled Trial
Gounaris A, Kokori P, Varchalama L, et al (Regional Gen Hosp of Piraeus, Greece; Charokopion Univ, Athens, Greece)
Arch Dis Child Fetal Neonatal Ed 89:F297-F299, 2004   13–2

Background.—Theophylline treatment causes side effects such as tachycardia, hyperglycaemia, abdominal distension, and vomiting. The latter two are probably the result of delayed gastric evacuation.
Objective.—To study the effect of theophylline on gastric emptying time in preterm infants.

Patients.—The subjects were 18 premature neonates with a mean (SD) birth weight of 1302 (240) g and a mean (SD) gestational age of 28.7 (1.9) weeks.

Main Outcome Measures.—In each case, gastric emptying was measured on two occasions: once when the newborns were being treated with theophylline and once when they were not. Half of the cases were randomised to receive theophylline before the initial measurement. The opposite was applied for the rest. Gastric emptying was assessed ultrasonically by measuring the change in antral cross sectional area (ACSA) at regular intervals over 120 minutes.

Results.—The mean (SD) ACSA half time in the newborns receiving theophylline was 52 (19) minutes compared with 37 (16) minutes in those not receiving theophylline. This difference is significant ($p < 0.05$).

Conclusions.—Treatment with theophylline seems to delay gastric emptying in very low birthweight neonates, and this must be taken into consideration when this drug is used to treat apnoea of prematurity.

▶ Gastric motility and emptying, or lack thereof, is of critical importance in establishing enteral feeding in preterm infants. When you have a toy, the idea is that you play with it. In this case the toy is an US machine to monitor the effects of theophylline on gastric emptying or to study the rates of gastric emptying while on nasal continuous positive airway pressure (CPAP). As would have been anticipated, theophylline delayed gastric emptying. Any experienced neonatal nurse could have informed you of that without resorting to high tech. In the United States theophylline has been replaced essentially by caffeine, but the effects on gastric emptying would be identical. On the other hand most observers would have predicted that nasal CPAP would cause gastric distension and delayed gastric emptying. Gounaris et al[1] found the opposite: gastric emptying was indeed more rapid for the infants on nasal CPAP. This is encouraging for the growing army of proponents for more liberal use of CPAP. For those who like to try erythromycin as a prokinetic agent—it has been done—it is ineffective and potentially harmful. El Hennawy et al,[2] using the same US monitoring technique, reported that erythromycin failed to improve feeding outcome in feeding intolerant preterm infants. Ng et al[3] reported similar results. Treatment with theophylline or caffeine is widespread. The delay in gastric emptying that they produce in very low birth weight neonates must be considered and monitored when these agents are used before extubation or for the treatment of apnea.

A. A. Fanaroff, MD

References

1. Gounaris A, Costalos C, Varchalama L, et al: Gastric emptying in very-low-birthweight infants treated with nasal continuous positive airway pressure. *J Pediatr* 145:508-510, 2004.
2. El Hennawy AA, Sparks JW, Armentrout D, et al: Erythromycin fails to improve feeding outcome in feeding-intolerant preterm infants. *J Pediatr Gastroenterol Nutr* 37:281-286, 2003.

3. Ng SC, Gomez JM, Rajadurai VS, et al: Establishing enteral feeding in preterm infants with feeding intolerance: A randomized controlled study of low-dose erythromycin. *J Pediatr Gastroenterol Nutr* 37:554-558, 2003.

A Multicenter, Randomized, Double-Blind, Placebo-Controlled Trial of the Prokinetic Agent Erythromycin in the Postoperative Recovery of Infants with Gastroschisis

Curry JI, the BAPS Multicentre Research Committee (Great Ormond Street Hosp for Children, London)
J Pediatr Surg 39:565-569, 2004   13–3

Background/Purpose.—The recovery of gut function after repair of gastroschisis is frequently prolonged, and these infants are prone to complications associated with parenteral nutrition. This trial was designed to investigate the effect of the prokinetic agent, erythromycin, on the attainment of full enteral feeding in infants after primary repair of uncomplicated gastroschisis.

Methods.—A multicenter, randomized, double-blind, placebo-controlled trial was used to investigate the effect of enteral erythromycin (3 mg/kg/dose 4 times daily) compared with placebo on the attainment of full enteral feeding tolerance after primary repair of uncomplicated gastroschisis. Eleven neonatal surgical units in the United Kingdom participated in the study. The primary end-point was the time taken to achieve continuous enteral feeding at 150 mL/kg/24 hours sustained for 48 hours.

Results.—Of 70 eligible infants, 62 were recruited and randomly divided. There were 30 patients in group I (placebo) and 32 in group II (erythromycin). The groups were comparable in terms of mean gestational age, mean birth weight, extent of evisceration, and degree of intestinal peel. There was no statistically significant difference between the 2 groups in the time taken to achieve full enteral feeding (27.2 v 28.7 days; $P = .75$). Similarly, no significant differences were found in the incidence of catheter-related sepsis, duration of parenteral nutrition, or time to discharge between the 2 groups.

Conclusions.—Enterally administered erythromycin at a dose of 3 mg/kg 4 times daily conferred no advantage in the time taken to achieve full enteral feeding after primary repair of uncomplicated gastroschisis.

Establishing Enteral Feeding in Preterm Infants With Feeding Intolerance: A Randomized Controlled Study of Low-dose Erythromycin

Ng SC-Y, Gomez JM, Rajadurai VS, et al (Natl Univ Hosp, Singapore; Kandang Kerbau Women's & Children's Hosp; Natl Univ of Singapore)
J Pediatr Gastroenterol Nutr 37:554-558, 2003   13–4

Objective.—A prospective, double-blind, randomized, controlled trial was conducted to evaluate the effect of low-dose erythromycin on the time taken to attain full enteral feedings in preterm infants with very low birth weight and feeding intolerance.

Methods.—Two groups of preterm infants (birth weight $\leq$ 1500 g) with feeding intolerance were randomized to either low-dose erythromycin (5 mg/kg every 8 hours) or 5% dextrose placebo, both of which were discontinued 1 week after full enteral feedings were tolerated. The primary outcome variable was the time taken to attain full enteral feedings of at least 130 mL/kg/d.

Results.—The gestational age at birth was similar in the two groups (erythromycin, 27.1 ± 1.9 weeks; placebo, 27.5 ± 2.9 weeks). The mean birth weight of the erythromycin group was lower (806.3 ± 215.6 g) than the placebo group (981.4 ± 285.4 g; $P = 0.18$), and included more infants who were small for gestational age (4/13 = 31% versus 1/11 = 9%; $P = 0.224$). There was no difference between the two groups with regard to the volume of feedings they were receiving at the time of enrollment. Reduction in symptoms of gastroesophageal reflux was similar in the two groups. 3 of 13 in the erythromycin group and 4 of 11 in the placebo group improved during the study ($P = 0.565$). The mean time to attain full enteral feedings after enrollment was 24.9 + 2.9 days in the erythromycin group and 30.8 ± 4.1 days in the placebo group, a difference that did not reach statistical significance ($P = 0.17$).

Conclusions.—Low-dose erythromycin did not reduce the time taken to attain full enteral feedings in preterm infants with very low birth weight and feeding intolerance. Gastroesophageal reflux decreased as a consequence of maturation of the gastrointestinal tract and not because of erythromycin. These preliminary results justify verification in larger multicenter trials.

▶ The recovery of gut function and duration of hospitalization after repair of gastroschisis is frequently prolonged, and determined by the time it takes to reestablish full enteral nutrition. Erythromycin, a motilin receptor agonist, triggers migrating motor complexes and accelerates gastric emptying in adults with feeding intolerance. Curry et al (Abstract 13–3) therefore speculated that it would shorten the time to full enteral feeds for infants after primary repair of uncomplicated gastroschisis. Alas, in a multicenter trial that included 11 neonatal surgical units and enrolled 62 subjects, erythromycin neither shortened the time to full enteral feeds nor reduced catheter-related sepsis or the duration of parenteral nutrition.

In another small randomized trial Ng et al (Abstract 13–4) accomplished the same negative results. Only 24 preterm infants with feeding intolerance were studied. The mean time to attain full enteral feedings after enrollment was 24.9 ± 2.9 days in the erythromycin group and 30.8 ± 4.1 days in the placebo group, a difference that did not reach statistical significance ($P = .17$). They concluded "These preliminary results justify verification in larger multicenter trials." However, their call may go unheeded after clinicians look at the data generated by El Hennawy et al[1] whose objective was to assess the efficacy of erythromycin in feeding-intolerant infants. They measured gastric emptying, maturation of gastrointestinal motor patterns, and time to achieve full enteral.

Feedings were in a controlled, randomized, double-blinded clinical trial, wherein infants received intragastric erythromycin or placebo for 8 days without crossover. Motor activity was recorded in the antrum and the duodenum during fasting, in response to intragastric erythromycin (1.5 mg/kg) or placebo, and in response to feeding. Gastric emptying at 20 minutes and transit time from duodenum to anus were determined. No differences were found in gastric emptying and the characteristics of antroduodenal motor contractions were similar in the 2 groups, as were transit times from duodenum to anus. Feeding outcomes were comparable in the 2 groups.

Their obvious conclusion, that erythromycin does not improve feeding tolerance in preterm infants with established feeding intolerance because it fails to improve gastrointestinal function in the short or long term, speaks against further trials using this agent. To add fuel to the fire Sorenson et al,[2] on the basis of a population cohort study in Denmark, established that the use of macrolides (including erythromycin) during breast feeding increases the risk of hypertrophic pyloric stenosis 10-fold for girls and 2-fold for boys. Premature infants have enough problems without adding hypertrophic pyloric stenosis to the list. So let's use human milk as the best prokinetic agent for preterm infants.

A. A. Fanaroff, MD

References

1. El Hennawy AA, Sparks JW, Armentrout D, et al: Erythromycin fails to improve feeding outcome in feeding-intolerant preterm infants. *J Pediatr Gastroenterol Nutr* 37:281-286, 2003.
2. Sorensen HT, Skriver MV, Pedersen L, et al: Risk of infantile hypertrophic pyloric stenosis after maternal postnatal use of macrolides. *Scand J Infect Dis* 35:104-106, 2003.

A Randomised Controlled Trial of Morphine Versus Phenobarbitone for Neonatal Abstinence Syndrome

Jackson L, Ting A, Mckay S, et al (Glasgow Royal Infirmary, Scotland)
Arch Dis Child Fetal Neonatal Ed 89:F300-F304, 2004   13–5

Background.—The incidence of neonatal abstinence syndrome (NAS) has increased 10-fold over the last decade in Glasgow. In the Princess Royal Maternity Hospital, it now accounts for 17% of special care baby unit (SCBU) admissions.

Objective.—To compare opiate replacement therapy (morphine sulphate) with the present standard treatment (phenobarbitone) for management of NAS. The primary study end point was duration of pharmaceutical treatment. Secondary end points were the requirement for additional drugs and the requirement for SCBU admission.

Design.—Double blind, randomised controlled clinical trial.

Methods.—Differential diagnoses were excluded, and two consecutive Lipsitz scores > 4 defined NAS requiring treatment. Infants were randomised to receive morphine sulphate or phenobarbitone. Treatments were identical in appearance, odour, and volume. Increments, decrements, and discontinuation of treatments were protocol driven.

Results.—Seventy five infants participated. All mothers received opiate replacement therapy (methadone) during pregnancy and most used other drugs (n = 62, 83%). No significant difference in maternal drug use patterns was observed between treatment groups. Median treatment duration was four days shorter with opiate replacement (8 v 12 days, Mann-Whitney U test, p = 0.02). Phenobarbitone treated infants tended to require second line treatment (47% v 35%, χ^2 test, p = 0.11) and SCBU admission (62% v 30%, χ^2 test, p = 0.04) more often.

Conclusions.—Opiate replacement therapy appears to be superior for management of symptomatic NAS when maternal opiate use is prevalent. The shorter treatment duration and lower requirement for higher intensity nursing may have significant cost implications. Tailoring NAS treatment to local maternal drug use may result in similar benefits.

▶ Although knowledge of abstinence, its treatment, and outcome continues to grow, the neonatal abstinence syndrome (NAS) remains a significant problem. It has become complicated by polydrug use, in addition to exposure to tobacco, alcohol, and psychoactive substances that are frequently prescribed for pregnant women. In the United States from 1996 to 1998, 6.4% of nonpregnant women of childbearing age and 2.8% of pregnant women reported that they used illicit drugs. Of drug users, the relative proportion of women who abstained from illicit drugs after recognition of pregnancy increased from 28% during the first trimester of pregnancy to 93% by the third trimester.[1]

It has never been easy to distinguish an infant with NAS, and with shortened hospital stays the opportunities to do so have been diminished. A high index of suspicion is necessary, together with recognition of specific behaviors that occur in 10% or more of newborns, including excessive sneezing, nasal stuffiness, unsustained suck, tremor, and abnormal nipple latch.[2] Kuschel et al,[3] therefore, assessed the usefulness of cord and serum methadone concentrations at 2 days of age in predicting the severity of NAS in infants whose mothers received methadone during pregnancy. Methadone concentrations taken from cord blood may identify infants at greater risk of neonatal withdrawal and therefore require treatment. All but 1 of the 12 infants who required treatment had undetectable concentrations of methadone in the postnatal sample, whereas the median postnatal methadone concentration in infants who required no treatment was 23 ng/mL (*P* = .002). This is helpful for known abusers, but if the history is negative the staff must observe the babies more carefully.

With regard to therapy for NAS, Jackson et al document that morphine is superior to phenobarbitone. Indeed, the consensus seems to favor opioids and avoidance of diazepam, which is ineffective. Opiate replacement therapy appears to be superior for management of symptomatic NAS when maternal opiate use is prevalent.

A. A. Fanaroff, MD

References

1. Ebrahim SH, Gfroerer J: Pregnancy-related substance use in the United States during 1996-1998. *Obstet Gynecol* 101:374-379, 2003.
2. Elliott MR, Cunliffe P, Demianczuk N, et al: Frequency of newborn behaviours associated with neonatal abstinence syndrome: A hospital-based study. *J Obstet Gynaecol Can* 26:25-34, 2004.
3. Kuschel CA, Austerberry L, Cornwell M, et al: Can methadone concentrations predict the severity of withdrawal in infants at risk of neonatal abstinence syndrome? *Arch Dis Child Fetal Neonatal Ed* 89:F390-F393, 2004.

14 Miscellaneous

Dads as Breastfeeding Advocates: Results From a Randomized Controlled Trial of an Educational Intervention
Wolfberg AJ, Michels KB, Shields W, et al (Brigham and Women's Hosp, Boston; Harvard Med School, Boston; Johns Hopkins Univ, Baltimore; et al)
Am J Obstet Gynecol 191:708-712, 2004   14–1

Objective.—Recognizing that an expectant father may influence a mother's decision to breast- or formula-feed, we tested the effectiveness of a simple, educational intervention that was designed to encourage fathers to advocate for breastfeeding and to assist his partner if she chooses to breastfeed.

Study Design.—We conducted a randomized controlled trial in which expectant fathers (n = 59) were assigned randomly to attend either a 2-hour intervention class on infant care and breastfeeding promotion (intervention) or a class on infant care only (control group). The classes, which were led by a peer-educator, were interactive and informal and utilized different media to create an accessible environment for participants. Couples were recruited during the second trimester from a university obstetrics practice.

Results.—Overall, breastfeeding was initiated by 74% of women whose partners attended the intervention class, as compared with 41% of women whose partners attended the control class (*P* = .02).

Conclusion.—Expectant fathers can be influential advocates for breastfeeding, playing a critical role in encouraging a woman to breastfeed her newborn infant.

▶ The role of husbands in breastfeeding is truly supportive. Wolfberg et al have nicely demonstrated that promoting breast feeding to expectant fathers during antenatal classes had a significant impact on increasing breastfeeding. Indeed, they concluded that the role of the father was critical.

The low prevalence and short duration of breastfeeding in international studies have highlighted the need for more investigations into factors influencing the decision to breastfeed. Furthermore, there has been a call for more baby-friendly hospitals with a goal of a higher incidence and more prolonged breastfeeding. In a study from 13 hospitals in Hong Kong, personal, cultural, social, and environmental factors were identified as common influencing factors in the decision to breastfeed. Mothers' knowledge and attitudes, followed by husbands' support, were identified as important in influencing infant feeding choice.[1] The role of the father has been identified as one of the strongest influences on the initiation and duration of breastfeeding by mothers in the United States.[2] Similarly, in a study of aboriginal women in Perth, breastfeeding at discharge was most positively associated with perceived paternal support of breastfeeding.[3] Hence, prenatal counseling with regard to breastfeeding must include the spouse.

A. A. Fanaroff, MD

References

1. Kong SK, Lee DT: Factors influencing decision to breastfeed. *J Adv Nurs* 46:369-379, 2004.
2. Cohen R, Lange L, Slusser W: A description of a male-focused breastfeeding promotion corporate lactation program. *J Hum Lact* 18:61-65, 2002.
3. Binns C, Gilchrist D, Gracey M, et al: Factors associated with the initiation of breast-feeding by aboriginal mothers in Perth. *Public Health Nutr* 7:857-861, 2004.

Difference in Prevalence of Congenital Cryptorchidism in Infants Between Two Nordic Countries
Boisen KA, Kaleva M, Main KM, et al (Rigshospitalet, Copenhagen; Univ of Turku, Finland)
Lancet 363:1264-1269, 2004   14–2

Background.—Several investigators have shown striking differences in semen quality and testicular cancer rate between Denmark and Finland. Since maldescent of the testis is a shared risk factor for these conditions we undertook a joint prospective study for the prevalence of congenital cryptorchidism.

Methods.—1068 Danish (1997-2001) and 1494 Finnish boys (1997-99) were consecutively recruited prenatally. We also established prevalence data for all newborns at Turku University Central Hospital, Finland (1997-99, n=5798). Testicular position was assessed by a standardized technique. All subtypes of congenital cryptorchidism were included, but retractile testes were considered normal.

Findings.—Prevalence of cryptorchidism at birth was 9.0% (95% CI 7.3-10.8) in Denmark and 2.4% (1.7-3.3) in Finland. At 3 months of age, prevalence rates were 1.9% (1.2-3.0) and 1.0% (0.5-1.7), respectively. Significant geographic differences were still present after adjustment for confounding factors (birthweight, gestational age, being small for gestational age, maternal age, parity, mode of delivery); odds ratio (Denmark vs Finland) was 4.4 (2.9-6.7, $P<0.0001$) at birth and 2.2 (1.0-4.5, $P=0.039$) at three months (Table 4). The rate in Denmark was significantly higher than that reported 40 years ago.

Interpretation.—Our findings of increasing and much higher prevalence of congenital cryptorchidism in Denmark than in Finland contribute evidence to the pattern of high frequency of reproductive problems such as tes-

TABLE 4.—Prevalence and Risk of Cryptorchidism at Expected Date of Delivery in Finnish and Danish Boys, With Respect to Birthweight, Gestational Age, and Weight for Gestational Age

	Number Cryptorchid/ Number Examined		Prevalence		Odds Ratio (95%) Denmark *vs* Finland*
	Denmark	Finland	Denmark	Finland	
BW<2500 g	9/40	5/29	22·5%	17·2%	1·5 (0·4-5·5)†
BW ≥2500 g	85/1006	30/1426	8·4%	2·1%	4·8 (3·0-7·5)†
GA <37 weeks	13/60	4/61	21·7%	6·6%	3·8 (1·1-12·7)‡
GA ≥37 weeks	81/986	31/1394	8·2%	2·2%	4·3 (2·8-6·7)‡
WGA <(−2 SD)	6/39	2/26	15·4%	7·7%	2·2 (0·4-12·5)§
WGA ≥(−2 SD)	88/1007	33/1429	8·7%	2·3%	4·5 (2·9-7·0)§

Note: Birthweight (g), gestational age (days), maternal age (years), and parity were used as continuous variables. Mode of delivery was used as a class variable; being SGA was used dichotomized (SGA/AGA−KGA).

*Finland served as a reference, ie OR=1.00.

†Adjusted for gestational age, being SGA, maternal age, parity, and mode of delivery.

‡Adjusted for birthweight, being SGA, maternal age, parity, and mode of delivery.

§Adjusted for birthweight, gestational age, maternal age, parity, and mode of delivery.

Abbreviations: BW, Birthweight; *GA*, gestational age; *WGA*, weight for gestational age; *SGA*, small for gestational age; *AGA*, average for gestational age; *LGA*, large for gestational age.

(Courtesy of Boisen KA, Kaleva M, Main KM, et al: Difference in Prevalence of Congenital Cryptorchidism in Infants Between Two Nordic Countries. *Lancet* 363:1264-1269, 2004. Reprinted with permission from Elsevier.)

ticular cancer and impaired semen quality in Danish men. Although genetic factors could account for the geographic difference, the increase in reproductive health problems in Denmark is more likely explained by environmental factors, including endocrine disrupters and lifestyle.

▶ These are really striking and somewhat startling findings. Why should the prevalence of cryptorchidism be 4 times greater in Denmark than Finland, when all the potential variables have been taken into consideration? Furthermore, in view of the reportedly high frequency of reproductive problems such as testicular cancer and impaired semen quality in Danish men, the findings are truly ominous. As the authors have attributed these conditions to environmental factors, including endocrine disruptors and lifestyle, there is hope that this could be remedied. Cryptorchidism is the most common genitourinary disorder of childhood, and is usually present at birth in 3% to 5% of term male infants. Note in Boisen's study the incidence in Denmark was 9%. The incidence is higher in preterm and low birth weight infants. In most instances the testes will descend normally in the first months of life. Hack et al[1] has proposed a new classification for undescended testis (UDT), suitable for a clinical setting. UDT is categorized into congenital and acquired forms. Congenital forms include intra-abdominal, intracanalicular, suprascrotal, and ectopic testes, and should be corrected by 1 year of age. Acquired forms can be divided into primary and secondary types.

The 2 most important possible sequelae are infertility (usually with bilateral abdominal testes) and testicular tumor. Diagnostic studies are usually not necessary if the undescended testis is palpable. Laparoscopy has replaced imaging studies for localization of a nonpalpable testis and might also obviate the need for exploration of the groin. Mullerian-inhibiting substance (MIS), also known as anti-Mullerian hormone (AMH), causes Mullerian duct involution during male sexual differentiation and also has a postnatal regulatory role in the gonads. Measurement of serum MIS/AMH helps in the evaluation of children with gonadal disorders. In boys with cryptorchidism (nonpalpable gonads), serum MIS/AMH correlates with testicular tissue. A measurable value is predictive of undescended testes, while an undetectable value is highly suggestive of anorchia.[2]

The recommended age for treatment has progressively decreased. Current practice with a view to maximizing the potential for fertility is to place the testis in the scrotum by 1 year of age. Treatment options include surgical relocation or hormonal therapy. The lower the pretreatment position of the testis, the better the success rate for either method. However, if there is a possibility of a testicular torsion, then a more aggressive approach is recommended. Belman and Rushton[3] reported that the combination of a nonpalpable left testis and an enlarged right testis is highly predictive of perinatal testicular torsion. When both criteria were met, 20 of 22 (91%) consecutive patients had histologic or laparoscopically confirmed perinatal torsion and 1 had only clinical features. This finding supports the concept of scrotal exploration as the initial procedure in the child who has an empty left hemiscrotum and hypertrophied descended right testis. Laparoscopy should be reserved for boys in whom a distinct remnant is not found on scrotal exploration.

A. A. Fanaroff, MD

References

1. Hack WW, Meijer RW, Bos SD, et al: A new clinical classification for undescended testis. *Scand J Urol Nephrol* 37:43-47, 2003.
2. Lee MM, Misra M, Donahoe PK, et al: MIS/AMH in the assessment of cryptorchidism and intersex conditions. *Mol Cell Endocrinol* 211:91-98, 2003.
3. Belman AB, Rushton HG: Is an empty left hemiscrotum and hypertrophied right descended testis predictive of perinatal torsion? *J Urol* 170(Pt 2):1674-1675, 2003.

Voluntary Anonymous Reporting of Medical Errors for Neonatal Intensive Care

Suresh G, for the NICQ2000 and NICQ2002 Investigators of the Vermont Oxford Network (Univ of Vermont, Burlington; et al)

Pediatrics 113:1609-1618, 2004   14–3

Introduction.—Medical errors are responsible for significant morbidity and mortality in patients who are hospitalized. Specialty-based, voluntary reporting of medical errors by health care providers is an important exercise that may improve patient safety. Described is a voluntary, anonymous, Internet-based reporting system for medical errors in neonatal intensive care; its feasibility was evaluated, along with errors that affect high-risk neonates and their families.

TABLE 4.—Factors that Contributed to Events Reported in Phase 2

Factor	No. of Events With Factor Reported	% of All Events ($n = 584$) in Which Factor Was Reported
Practices		
Failure to follow policy or protocol	273	46.8
Communications problem	131	22.4
Error in charting or documentation	78	13.4
Labeling error	56	9.6
Poor teamwork	50	8.6
Calculation error	40	6.9
Error in computer entry	37	6.3
Nursing handoff or shift change	33	5.7
Inadequate protocol	26	4.5
Lack of supervision	19	3.3
Physician handoff or shift change	12	2.1
Wrong protocol used	9	1.5
Inability to contact needed staff	6	1.0
Inadequate security	2	0.3
Human factors		
Inattention	157	26.9
Distraction	69	11.8
Inexperience	59	10.1
Inadequate training	35	6.0
Fatigue	33	5.7
Stress	26	4.5
Confrontational or intimidating behavior	4	0.7
Staffing		
High patient acuity in unit	40	6.9
High census in unit	23	3.9
Low levels of other professional staff	17	2.9
Low nursing staff levels	13	2.2
Consultant or subspecialist unavailable	7	1.2
Low physician staff levels	5	0.9
Low levels of clerical or support staff	2	0.3
Equipment		
Poor equipment design	29	5.0
Equipment failure	20	3.4
Inadequate equipment maintenance	14	2.4
Unfamiliar equipment	11	1.9
Necessary equipment unavailable	6	1.0
Environment		
Lack of space or room	7	1.2
Unfamiliar environment	5	0.9
Noise	1	0.2
Inadequate lighting	1	0.2

(Reproduced by permission of *Pediatrics*, courtesy of Suresh G, for the NICQ2000 and NICQ2002 Investigators of the Vermont Oxford Network: Voluntary anonymous reporting of medical errors for neonatal intensive care. *Pediatrics* 113:1609-1618, 2004.)

Methods.—A total of 739 health professionals from 54 hospitals in the Vermont Oxford Network received access to a secure Internet site for the anonymous reporting of medical errors, near-miss errors, and adverse events. Free-text entry was used during 17 months of phase 1, and a structured form was used during the 10 months of phase 2. The number and types of reported events and factors that contributed to the events were assessed.

Results.—Of 1230 reports submitted, 522 were during phase 1, and 708 were during phase 2. The most common event categories were wrong medi-

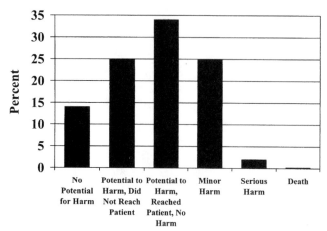

FIGURE 2.—Categories of harm for events reported in phase 2. Outcome of 673 events in which degree of harm was reported. This outcome was not reported in 35 events. Minor harm, which consisted of increased monitoring, treated with intervention, etc, occurred in 167 events (25%). Serious harm, in which there was a threat to life or an impaired outcome, etc, was reported in 13 events (1.9%). Death was reported in 1 event (0.15%). Categories are based on the system used for medication errors by the National Coordinating Council for Medication Error Reporting and Prevention. (Reproduced by permission of *Pediatrics*, courtesy of Suresh G, for the NICQ2000 and NICQ2002 Investigators of the Vermont Oxford Network: Voluntary anonymous reporting of medical errors for neonatal intensive care. *Pediatrics* 113:1609-1618, 2004.)

cation, dose, schedule, or infusion rate (47%) (nutritional agents and blood products were also included in this category); error in administration or method of using a treatment (14%); patient misidentification (11%); other system failure (9%); error or delay in diagnosis (7%); and error in performance of an operation, procedure, or test (4%). The most common contributory factors included failure to follow policy or protocol (47%), inattention (27%), communication problems (22%), error in charting or documentation (13%), distraction (12%), inexperience (10%), labeling error (10%), and poor teamwork (9%) (Table 4). In 24 instances, family members assisted in detection of the medical error, contributed to the cause, or themselves were victims of the errors. In phase 2, 2% of reports noted serious patient harm, and 25% documented minor harm (Fig 2).

Conclusion.—Specialty-based, voluntary, anonymous, Internet-based reporting by health care professionals revealed a wide range of medical errors that occur in neonatal ICUs. This kind of reporting provides an opportunity for multidisciplinary learning. These systems may have the potential to improve patient safety in many different clinical settings.

▶ This article on voluntary anonymous Internet reporting of medical errors in neonatal intensive care is unique in an era in which clinical investigation relies so heavily on rates, confidence intervals, and power estimations. From an analytical perspective, the anonymous and voluntary nature of the system has several disadvantages. For example, it is not possible to calculate error rates or to assess the extent to which the distribution of error types has been distorted by reporting bias. However, from a quality improvement perspective, these disadvantages are greatly overshadowed by the system's ability to character-ize the types of errors encountered in a neonatal ICU setting and the system's ability to provide an approximation of their relative frequency. This information provides an important guide to both individual neonatal ICUs and Quality Collaboratives in setting priorities for assessing and improving the extent to which their existing policies, procedures, and outlooks address the potential for specific types of medical errors. The system also offers a venue for the par-ticipants to share their experience in error prevention and represents an impor-tant quality improvement strategy.

J. B. Gould, MD, MPH

Clinical Outcomes of Near-Term Infants
Wang ML, Dorer DJ, Fleming MP, et al (Harvard Med School, Boston; Massa-chusetts Gen Hosp, Boston; Partners HealthCare, Boston)
Pediatrics 114:372-376, 2004   14–4

Objective.—To test the hypothesis that near-term infants have more med-ical problems after birth than full-term infants and that hospital stays might be prolonged and costs increased.

Methods.—Electronic medical record database sorting was conducted of 7474 neonatal records and subset analyses of near-term (n = 120) and full-

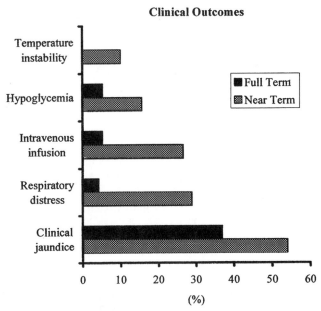

FIGURE 2.—Graph of clinical outcomes in near-term and full-term infants as percentage of patients stud-ied. Near-term newborn data are graphed with *gray bars*, full-term data with *black bars*. (Courtesy of Wang ML, Dorer DJ, Fleming MP, et al: Clinical outcomes of near-term infants. *Pediatrics* 114:372-376, 2004. Re-produced by permission of Pediatrics.)

term (n = 125) neonatal records. Cost information was accessed. Length of hospital stay, Apgar scores, clinical diagnoses (temperature instability, jaundice, hypoglycemia, suspicion of sepsis, apnea and bradycardia, respiratory distress), treatment with an intravenous infusion, delay in discharge to home, and hospital costs were assessed.

Results.—Data from 90 near-term and 95 full-term infants were analyzed. Median length of stay was similar for near-term and full-term infants, but wide variations in hospital stay were documented for near-term infants after both vaginal and cesarean deliveries. Near-term and full-term infants had comparable 1- and 5-minute Apgar scores. Nearly all clinical outcomes analyzed differed significantly between near-term and full-term neonates: temperature instability, hypoglycemia, respiratory distress, and jaundice (Fig 2). Near-term infants were evaluated for possible sepsis more frequently than full-term infants (36.7% vs 12.6%; odds ratio: 3.97) and more often received intravenous infusions. Cost analysis revealed a relative increase in total costs for near-term infants of 2.93 (mean) and 1.39 (median), resulting in a cost difference of 2630 dollars (mean) and 429 dollars (median) per near-term infant.

Conclusions.—Near-term infants had significantly more medical problems and increased hospital costs compared with contemporaneous full-term infants. Near-term infants may represent an unrecognized at-risk neonatal population.

▶ Anyone who is the least bit surprised by Wang et al's report has not been paying attention. Their conclusion that "near-term infants had significantly more medical problems and increased hospital costs compared with contemporaneous full-term infants" merely states the obvious. I found their final sentence, "Near-term infants may represent an unrecognized at-risk neonatal population," distressing because it is high time that health care providers be aware that these near-term infants, masquerading as term infants, are indeed extremely vulnerable. I would almost go so far as to say the near-term infant represents an accident waiting to happen. They are more likely to have thermal instability, feed poorly, and appear to be hypotonic, which prompts a sepsis evaluation and initiation of IV fluids and antibiotic therapy. It goes without saying that they are more likely to develop respiratory distress syndrome on the basis of surfactant deficiency after elective cesarean section. Roth-Kleiner et al,[1] from Switzerland, reported that infants who developed severe respiratory distress syndrome after elective cesarean syndrome without labor were comparable to newborns delivered by cesarean section (after onset of labor or rupture of the membranes) that were 1 week younger. No case of respiratory distress syndrome was found in that population when cesarean section was carried out after 39 completed weeks of gestation.

However, jaundice and the risk of kernicterus chill me most about the near-term infant. Tragically, although as a group they account for less than 10% of all deliveries, they have been responsible for almost 40% of the cases in the kernicterus registry. So be aware: follow the new bilirubin guidelines and ensure that there is close follow-up of all babies, but give special attention to those between 35 and 37 weeks' gestation.[2,3]

A. A. Fanaroff, MD

References

1. Roth-Kleiner M, Wagner BP, Bachmann D, et al: Respiratory distress syndrome in near-term babies after caesarean section. *Swiss Med Wkly* 133:283-288, 2003.
2. American Academy of Pediatrics Subcommittee on Hyperbilirubinemia: Management of hyperbilirubinemia in the newborn infant 35 or more weeks of gestation. *Pediatrics* 114:297-316, 2004.
3. Johnson LH, Bhutani VK, Brown AK: System-based approach to management of neonatal jaundice and prevention of kernicterus. *J Pediatr* 140:396-403, 2002.

Randomized Controlled Trial of Skin-to-skin Contact From Birth Versus Conventional Incubator for Physiological Stabilization in 1200- to 2199- Gram Newborns
Bergman NJ, Linley LL, Fawcus SR (Mowbray Maternity Hosp; Univ of Cape Town, South Africa)
Acta Paediatr 93:779-785, 2004   14–5

Aim.—Conventional care of prematurely born infants involves extended maternal-infant separation and incubator care. Recent research has shown that separation causes adverse effects. Maternal-infant skin-to-skin contact (SSC) provides an alternative habitat to the incubator, with proven benefits for stable prematures; this has not been established for unstable or newborn low-birthweight infants. SSC from birth was therefore compared to incubator care for infants between 1200 and 2199 g at birth.

Methods.—This was a prospective, unblinded, randomized controlled clinical trial; potential subjects were identified before delivery and randomized by computerized minimization technique at 5 min if eligible. Standardized care and observations were maintained for 6 h. Stability was measured in terms of a set of pre-determined physiological parameters, and a composite cardio-respiratory stabilization score (SCRIP).

Results.—34 infants were analysed in comparable groups: 3/18 SSC compared to 12/13 incubator babies exceeded the pre-determined parameters ($p < 0.001$). Stabilization scores were 77.11 for SSC versus 74.23 for incubator (maximum 78), mean difference 2.88 (95% CI: 0.3-5.46, $p = 0.031$). All 18 SSC subjects were stable in the sixth hour, compared to 6/13 incubator infants. Eight out of 13 incubator subjects experienced hypothermia.

Conclusion.—Newborn care provided by skin-to-skin contact on the mother's chest results in better physiological outcomes and stability than the same care provided in closed servo-controlled incubators. The cardio-respiratory instability seen in separated infants in the first 6 h is consistent with mammalian "protest-despair" biology, and with "hyper-arousal and dissociation" response patterns described in human infants: newborns should not be separated from their mothers.

▶ The practice of skin-to-skin care (in which the mother places her diaper-clad infant upright between her breasts in direct skin contact) has gained much notoriety and continues to gain the evidence to support such a practice in both term and preterm infants. Most reports confirm better infant temperature control and neurobehavioral outcomes, greater success with breastfeeding, and positive attachment relationships. Nonetheless, the consensus of 3 reviews[1-3] is that there is much work still needed; the available data are limited because of methodologic quality and variations in the implementation of the intervention as well as outcomes. The reviewers offered advice as to how future trials should be designed. Anderson et al[1] noted that "Early skin-to-skin contact appears to have some clinical benefit especially regarding breastfeeding outcomes and infant crying and has no apparent short- or long-term negative effects. Further investigation is recommended." Ferber and Makhoul,[4] on the basis of a small randomized trial, reported that skin-to-skin contact, which in their study was termed kangaroo care, seems to influence state organization and motor system modulation of the newborn infant shortly after delivery. The kangaroo care infants slept longer, were mostly in a quiet sleep state, exhibited more flexor movements and postures, and showed less extensor movements.[4]

Bergman et al, from Cape Town, concluded on the basis of their unblinded, randomized study that in the first 6 hours after delivery low birth weight infants exposed to skin-to-skin contact on the mother's chest had better physiologic outcomes and stability than infants cared for in a in closed, servo-controlled incubator. They referred to the cardiorespiratory instability seen in infants separated from their mothers by placement in the incubators manifested mammalian "protest despair" biology, with hyperarousal and dissociation response patterns. Their pleas were that newborns should not be separated from their mothers at birth. Bystrova et al[5] reinforced this recommendation when they demonstrated that extended skin-to-skin contact with the mother in the delivery room was superior to swaddling. They concluded that it is the most effective way to maintain the infant's temperature and decrease the "stress of being born." My colleagues Marshall Klaus and John Kennell would utter, "I told you so 30 years ago" or "Amen" to this recommendation.

A. A. Fanaroff, MD

References

1. Anderson GC, Moore E, Hepworth J, et al: Early skin-to-skin contact for mothers and their healthy newborn infants. *Cochrane Database Syst Rev* 2:CD003519, 2003.
2. Carfoot S, Williamson PR, Dickson R: A systematic review of randomised controlled trials evaluating the effect of mother/baby skin-to-skin care on successful breast feeding. *Midwifery* 19:148-155, 2003.
3. Conde-Agudelo A, Diaz-Rossello JL, Belizan JM: Kangaroo mother care to reduce morbidity and mortality in low birthweight infants. *Cochrane Database Syst Rev* 2:CD002771, 2003.

4. Ferber SG, Makhoul IR: The effect of skin-to-skin contact (kangaroo care) shortly after birth on the neurobehavioral responses of the term newborn: A randomized, controlled trial. *Pediatrics* 113:858-865, 2004.
5. Bystrova K, Widstrom AM, Matthiesen AS, et al: Skin-to-skin contact may reduce negative consequences of "the stress of being born": a study on temperature in newborn infants subjected to different ward routines in St. Petersburg. *Acta Paediatr* 92:320-326, 2003.

Proactive Management Promotes Outcome in Extremely Preterm Infants: A Population-Based Comparison of Two Perinatal Management Strategies

Håkansson S, Farooqi A, Holmgren PÅ, et al (Inst of Clinical Science, Umeå, Sweden)

Pediatrics 114:58-64, 2004   14–6

Objective.—There is a need for evidence-based knowledge regarding perinatal management in extreme prematurity. The benefit of a proactive attitude versus a more selective one is controversial. The objective of the present study was to analyze perinatal practices and infant outcome in extreme prematurity in relation to different management policies in the North (proactive) and South of Sweden.

Methods.—A population-based, retrospective, cohort study design was used. Data in the Swedish Medical Birth Register (MBR) from 1985 to 1999 were analyzed according to region of birth and gestational age (22 weeks + 0 days to 27 weeks + 6 days). A total of 3 602 live-born infants were included (North = 1040, South = 2562). Survival was defined as being alive at 1 year. Morbidity in survivors, based on discharge diagnoses of major morbidity during the first year of life, was described by linking the MBR to the Hospital Discharge Register.

Results.—In infants with a gestational age of 22 to 25 weeks, the proactive policy was significantly associated with 1) increased incidence of live births, 2) higher degree of centralized management, 3) higher frequency of caesarean section, 4) fewer infants with low Apgar score (<4) at 1 and 5 minutes, 5) fewer infants dead within 24 hours, and 6) increased number of infants alive at 1 year. There were no indications of increased morbidity in survivors of the proactive management during the first year of life, and the proportion of survivors without denoted morbidity was larger.

Conclusion.—In infants with a gestational age of 22 to 25 weeks, a proactive perinatal strategy increases the number of live births and improves the infant's postnatal condition and survival without evidence of increasing morbidity in survivors up to 1 year of age.

▶ Our approach to the extremely premature infant has evolved in the last 3 to 4 decades from the survival of the fittest to a relatively aggressive, proactive approach. Survival at the limits of viability has improved dramatically over that time, but questions continue about the morbidity and neurodevelopmental outcome of the survivors. The existence of significant differences in the regional strategies for the management of these infants in the north and the south of Sweden allowed these investigators to compare the data in two population-based samples. In the southern region of Sweden, active obstetric intervention for fetal indications was restricted in infants of 25 weeks' gestation or less, and an individualized approach to the resuscitation of these infants was adopted. In the northern region of the country a more aggressive approach was adopted.

The use of a so-called "restrictive attitude" toward obstetric intervention and neonatal resuscitation is, of course, a self-fulfilling prophesy that will inevitability lead to a higher mortality rate in these extremely premature infants. The more proactive and aggressive approach produced a dramatic difference in survival at 22 to 25 weeks of gestation. It is reassuring that this improved survival was not associated with an increase in the proportion of infants with short-term morbidity (chronic lung disease, retinopathy of prematurity, intraventricular hemorrhage), although the absolute number of impaired infants must, inevitably, increase.

M. J. Maisels, MB, BCh

Evaluation of Neonatal Intensive Care for Extremely Low Birth Weight Infants in Victoria Over Two Decades: I. Effectiveness

Doyle LW, for the Victorian Infant Collaborative Study Group (Royal Women's Hosp, Carlton, Victoria, Australia; et al)
Pediatrics 113:505-509, 2004   14–7

Context.—Although individual components of neonatal intensive care have proven efficacy, doubts remain about its overall effectiveness.

Objective.—To determine the changes in effectiveness of neonatal intensive care for extremely low birth weight (ELBW) infants over 2 decades.

Design.—Population-based cohort study of consecutive ELBW infants born during 4 distinct eras: 1979-1980, 1985-1987, 1991-1992, and 1997, all followed to at least 2 years of age.

Setting.—The state of Victoria, Australia.

Patients.—All ELBW live births of birth weight 500 to 999 g in the state in the calendar years indicated (1979-1980 [n = 351]; 1985-1987 [n = 560]; 1991-1992 [n = 429]; 1997 [n = 233]). Survivors were assessed at 2 years of age by pediatricians and psychologists blinded to perinatal details. The follow-up rates were high for each ELBW cohort (1979-1980: 100% [89 of 89]; 1985-1987: 100% [212 of 212]; 1991-1992: 98% [237 of 241]; 1997: 99% [168 of 170]).

Main Outcome Measures.—Survival and quality-adjusted survival rates at 2 years of age.

Results.—The survival rate to 2 years of age improved significantly between successive eras (absolute increase and 95% confidence interval: 1985-1987 vs 1979-1980, 12.5% and 6.3%-18.4%; 1991-1992 vs 1985-1987, 18.3% and 12.1%-24.4%; 1997 vs 1991-1992, 16.8% and 9.2%-23.9%), as did the quality-adjusted survival rate (absolute increase: 1985-1987 vs

■ **Survival**   □ **Quality-adjusted Survival**

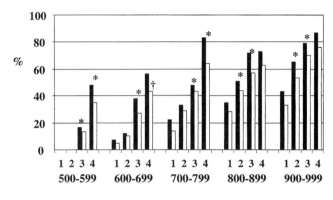

Birthweight sub-group (g)

FIGURE 1.—Survival rates and quality-adjusted survival rates in ELBW survivors in 100-g birth-weight subgroups, contrasted between eras (1979-1980: 1; 1985-1987: 2; 1991-1992: 3; 1997: 4). An asterisk indicates a statistically significant difference in both survival and quality-adjusted survival rates compared with the immediately preceding era within the 100-g birth-weight subgroup. A dagger indicates statistically significant difference in quality-adjusted survival rate compared with the immediately preceding era within the 100-g birth-weight subgroup. (Courtesy of Doyle LW, for the Victorian Infant Collaborative Study Group: Evaluation of neonatal intensive care for extremely low birth weight infants in Victoria over two decades: I. Effectiveness. *Pediatrics* 113:505-509, 2004. Reproduced by permission of *Pediatrics*.)

1979-1980, 12.4%; 1991-1992 vs 1985-1987, 13.8%; 1997 vs 1991-1992, 13.2%) (Fig 1). Overall, the survival rate increased from approximately 1 in 4 (25%) in 1979-1980 to 3 in 4 (73%) in 1997, and the quality-adjusted survival rate also increased threefold, from 19% in 1979-1980 to 59% in 1997. The biggest gains in survival and quality-adjusted survival in the most recent era were in infants in lighter birth-weight subgroups.

Conclusion.—The effectiveness of neonatal intensive care for ELBW infants in Victoria improved progressively from the late 1970s to the late 1990s.

Evaluation of Neonatal Intensive Care for Extremely Low Birth Weight Infants in Victoria Over Two Decades: II. Efficiency
Doyle LW, for the Victorian Infant Collaborative Study Group (Royal Women's Hosp, Carlton, Victoria, Australia; et al)
Pediatrics 113:510-514, 2004   14–8

Context.—Although the increasing effectiveness of neonatal programs for extremely low birth weight (ELBW, birth weight <1000 g) infants has been established from cohort studies, there is a paucity of data on the relationship between the costs and the consequences of neonatal intensive care.

Objective.—To determine the changes in the efficiency of neonatal intensive care for ELBW infants in Victoria, Australia over 2 decades.

Design.—Economic evaluation (cost-effectiveness and cost-utility analyses) in a population-based cohort study of consecutive ELBW infants born during 4 distinct eras (1979-1980, 1985-1987, 1991-1992, and 1997) followed to at least 2 years of age.

Setting.—The state of Victoria.

Patients.—All ELBW live births of birth weight 500 to 999 g in the state in the calendar years indicated (1979-1980: n = 351; 1985-1987: n = 560; 1991-1992: n = 429; 1997: n = 233).

Main Outcome Measures.—Costs were assessed primarily by the consumption of hospital resources. The consequences included survival and quality-adjusted survival rates at 2 years of age.

Results.—The cost-effectiveness ratios (expressed in Australian dollars for 1997) were similar between successive eras at 5270 dollars, 3130 dollars, and 4050 dollars per life-year gained, respectively. The cost-utility ratios were similar between successive eras at 5270 dollars, 3690 dollars, and 5850 dollars per quality-adjusted life-year gained, respectively, and were similar to the cost-effectiveness ratios. The cost-effectiveness and cost-utility ratios were generally higher in lower birth-weight subgroups, but there were consistent gains in efficiency over time in infants of lower birth weight.

Conclusions.—As there have been large increases in effectiveness from the late 1970s to the late 1990s, the efficiency of neonatal intensive care for ELBW infants in Victoria has remained relatively stable.

▶ In the first of these 2 articles (Abstract 14–7), the investigators evaluated the effectiveness of their care of ELBW infants over a 2-decade period. By using a population-based database in a geographically defined region, these authors can tell us whether their program works under "field" conditions. As expected, over 4 eras covering 2 decades, they show significant improvement in overall survival for ELBW infants (500-999 g). Survival increased from approximately 1 in 4 in 1979-1980 to about 3 in 4 by 1997. The quality-adjusted survival rate is calculated by dividing the sum of the utilities by the number of live births. Utilities for survivors are assigned according to the severity of disability: 0.4 for severe, 0.6 for moderate, 0.8 for mild, and 1 for no disability.

Both survival rates and quality-adjusted survival rates increased over the 4 eras. Although the rate of cerebral palsy has remained stable at approximately 10% over the 2 decades, the rate of blindness in survivors fell significantly in this cohort. This is in contrast to the findings from Leicester, UK, where the incidence of severe retinopathy of prematurity appears to have increased (see Abstract 8–21). There were no differences in deafness, developmental delay, or overall neurosensory disability rates in survivors during this study.

Notwithstanding these reassuring data, we now have many more survivors of ELBW with a more or less consistent rate of developmental delay and neurosensory disability. This means that with each successive decade we will have more surviving infants who require more health care, more assistance, and more community resources.

In part 2 of this study (Abstract 14–8), the investigators use a creative and innovative study design to look at the question of whether neonatal intensive care is worth implementing. Because resources are always finite, they ask the important question: how can we show that the money devoted to the cost of neonatal intensive care is being spent wisely? In other words, could this money be better spent in other components of the health care system? The cost represents the consumption of hospital resources and the consequences include survival and quality-adjusted survival rates at age 2 years. Consistent with observations elsewhere, the survival rate for these infants increased by 3-fold from the late 1970s to the late 1990s.

Thus, it is very reassuring to find that the efficiency of neonatal intensive care in this population of infants has not deteriorated but has remained stable. The authors deserve our congratulations for this analysis and they remind us that we must continually re-evaluate the economic consequences and the efficiency of our interventions so that our limited resources can be spent wisely.

M. J. Maisels, MB, BCh

Predictors of Hospital Readmission of Manitoba Newborns Within Six Weeks Postbirth Discharge: A Population-Based Study
Martens PJ, Derksen S, Gupta S (Univ of Manitoba, Winnipeg, Canada)
Pediatrics 114:708-713, 2004   14–9

Background.—Neonatal rehospitalization is associated with significant morbidity and cost burdens. Much of the literature on this issue has focused on associations with early discharge; however, some studies have shown an increased risk with a short length of stay but others have reported no effect. A maternal age of younger than 20 years has also been associated with rehospitalization in normal birth weight infants, as has being a first-time mother. The geographic variation in newborn readmission rates and potential relationships with regional health and socioeconomic status has received less attention, but low income has been identified as a risk factor. The geographic variation in and the proportion and predictors of infant hospital readmission within 6 weeks of postbirth discharge were examined.

Methods.—With the use of hospital discharge data in the Canadian province of Manitoba, a cross-sectional, population-based study was conducted of all infants who were born from 1997 to 2001, linkable to the birth mother, and discharged alive from the hospital. A total of 68,681 infants were included in the study. Logistic regression was used to examine several predictors of readmission, including preterm status, low birth weight, neighborhood income, geographic location, breast-feeding status, length of stay, maternal age, and type of delivery. Ecologic correlations were determined between newborn hospital readmission rates and several factors, including a region's overall health status and a region's socioeconomic risk.

Results.—The proportion of infants readmitted to the hospital at least once a week within 6 weeks of postbirth hospital discharge was 3.95%. The leading cause of readmission was respiratory illness (22.3% of readmissions). The risk of readmission was higher for infants who were born preterm, who were in the 3 lowest income quintiles, who lived in northern or rural southern Manitoba, who were not breast-fed, whose mother was 17 years or younger, whose mother was 18 to 19 years of age, or who were born by cesarean section. Regional readmission rates were correlated with the premature mortality rate.

Conclusions.—Geographic location and income were strongly associated with newborn hospital readmission in this cohort. The modifiable risk factors included increasing breast-feeding rates, decreasing cesarean section rates, and decreasing adolescent pregnancy rates; however, additional study of these risk factors is needed to establish causation.

▶ This Canadian, population-based study of neonatal readmissions in the first 6 weeks demonstrates that nearly a 2-fold difference in readmission rates exists across Manitoba's geographic regions (6.6% in the North vs 3.4% in Winnipeg), despite universal health insurance. Independent risk factors included prematurity, low income, lack of breast-feeding, having a teenage mother, delivery by cesarean, and residing in an impoverished geographic area with a low life expectancy. The study suggests risk reduction as a strategy to decrease readmissions, but, from a broader patient care perspective, it raises the question of what mix of factors, such as infant fragility, quality of perinatal care and discharge planning, quality of postdischarge care, parental practices, and environmental factors, might serve as focal points for intervention. Developing a multidisciplinary readmission review strategy similar to those used for fetal, infant, and maternal mortality may be an efficient approach for identifying specific local factors that result in neonatal readmission.

J. B. Gould, MD, MPH

Factors That Affect Satisfaction With Neonatal-Perinatal Fellowship Training
Pearlman SA, Leef KH, Sciscione AC (Thomas Jefferson Med College, Philadelphia; Christiana Care Health Systems, Newark, Del; Drexel Univ, Philadelphia)
Am J Perinatol 21:371-375, 2004   14–10

This study was designed to assess neonatal fellows' satisfaction with their training and the role of mentorship. A 31-question survey was sent to all second- and third-year fellows in the United States and Canada (n = 304). Responses were received from 201 fellows (66% response rate). Respondents were evenly distributed between second- and third-year fellows. Overall, 75% were satisfied with their training. Eighty percent had a mentor on the neonatal faculty. Only 2.5% believed that they would not fulfill the subboard research requirement, but another 24% were unsure of completion. The presence of a mentor correlated with being prepared for academic practice ($p = 0.013$) and plans to enter academic practice ($p = 0.031$). Correlation between mentorship and completion of the research requirement showed a trend ($p = 0.09$). Twenty-five percent of neonatal fellows are not satisfied with their training and believed that they may not complete their research requirement. Fellows who had a mentor were more prepared for academic practice and were more likely to be satisfied with their fellowship training. Mentorship is important in neonatal training programs.

▶ This report is a sequel to the study by Sciscione in which he demonstrated that a faculty mentor ("a trusted counselor or guide") played a significant role in the training of Maternal Fetal Medicine fellows.[1] In the current study mentorship was the critical factor in the training of neonatal-perinatal fellows. I was surprised to learn that 20% of the fellows did not have an identified mentor. Many would argue, myself included, that mentor-deficient fellowships should not be accredited. Mentors, in addition to serving as counselors and guides, are also role models and friends, and although they are clearly academic family in many instances, they bond like true family. They help mold the character and steer the direction for the fellow. They uplift them when they are down and bring them back to reality when they are overexuberant and getting carried away with their emotions. They become life-long trustees and friends. Choosing the right mentor is a critical decision for the trainee, and there must be a choice for the program to be viable. As Arthur Miller said, "The apple cannot be stuck back on the tree of knowledge; once we begin to see, we are doomed and challenged to see more, not less."

A. A. Fanaroff, MD

Reference

1. Sciscione AC, Colmorgen GH, D'Alton ME: Factors affecting fellowship satisfaction, thesis completion, and career direction among maternal-fetal medicine fellows. *Obstet Gynecol* 91:1023-1026, 1998.

Ultrasound Screening for Developmental Dysplasia of the Hip
Riboni G, Bellini A, Serantoni S, et al (Macedonio Melloni Hosp, Milan, Italy; Local Health Authority, Milan, Italy)
Pediatr Radiol 33:475-481, 2003   14–11

Background.—Clinical examination of newborns has been shown to be inadequate for the early detection of developmental dysplasia of the hip (DDH). It is debatable whether US examination is a valid alternative.

Objective.—To contribute further knowledge to the natural history of DDH; to examine the distribution of hip morphology as classified by Graf according to sex and risk factors in an unselected Italian population; to propose a temporal pattern of US screening of all newborns to detect DDH.

Materials and Methods.—All newborns (n = 8,896) sequentially delivered in the Maternal and Child Health Hospital of Milan underwent US examination in the first week of life and, when findings were within normal limits, in the third month of life. Subjects categorised at birth as Graf type 2a with alpha angle between 50 degrees and 52 degrees, underwent a further US examination at the end of the first month of life. Subjects with ambiguous findings at the 3-month examination were re-examined at the end of the fourth month of life. All infants with abnormal hips abandoned the screening process and underwent treatment.

Results.—Overall, 56 cases of DDH were identified: 34 in the first week of life examination, 10 at 1 month; 10 at 3 months and 2 at 4 months.

Conclusions.—A two-step US screening of newborns is recommended: at the end of the first month and within the fourth month of life.

▶ To reduce the incidence of long-term complications, early diagnosis of DDH is an imperative. But it is generally accepted that clinical examination is inadequate for the early detection of DDH. Riboni et al report the value of sequential US in their quest for early and comprehensive detection of DDH. They detected 56 cases from a population of almost 9000 deliveries and concluded that a 2-step US screening approach was optimal, with the first at the end of the first month and a repeat examination during the fourth month of life. Based on their findings this recommendation is reasonable.

What about other evidence? Puhan et al[1] reviewed all the available observational studies (n = 49) on US screening in unselected newborns. The prevalence of DDH ranged from 0.5% to 30%, largely depending on the various possible definitions of DDH. The encouraging news was that less than 0.1% of patients with DDH were missed by US, regardless of the technique employed. But because of the limitations of the studies, which included incomplete reports, lack of follow-up of newborns with normal findings at the time of screening, lack of controls, and missing clinically meaningful data about outcome, they concluded that the effectiveness of a general US screening cannot be evaluated reliably. "The lack of evidence does not mean that US screening is ineffective, but randomized, controlled trials comparing the effectiveness of different screening regimens are needed."[1] Awareness of risk factors for DDH, which include genetic, developmental, mechanical, and physiologic factors, should trigger careful initial physical examination and US follow-up. Both nonsurgical (Pavlik harness) and surgical options are available for the treatment of DDH and dislocation, but early diagnosis and treatment lead to the best long-term results. Treatments are aimed at concentric reduction and prevention of residual subluxation and dysplasia.

A. A. Fanaroff, MD

Reference

1. Puhan MA, Woolacott N, Kleijnen J, et al: Observational studies on ultrasound screening for developmental dysplasia of the hip in newborns—a systematic review. *Ultraschall Med* 24:377-382, 2003.

Impact of Early Newborn Discharge Legislation and Early Follow-up Visits on Infant Outcomes in a State Medicaid Population

Meara E, Kotagal UR, Atherton HD, et al (Harvard Med School, Boston; Natl Bureau of Economic Research, Cambridge, Mass; Cincinnati Children's Hosp, Ohio; et al)

Pediatrics 113:1619-1627, 2004   14–12

Objective.—Scant information exists on the effects of legislation mandating coverage of minimum postnatal hospital stays on infant health outcomes. There are also gaps in knowledge regarding the effectiveness of early follow-up visits for newborns. The objective of this study was to determine the impact of 1) legislation mandating coverage of minimum postnatal hospital stays and 2) early follow-up visits by the age of 4 days on infant outcomes during the first month of life.

Methods.—A retrospective analysis was conducted of Ohio Medicaid claims data linked with birth certificate data for the period 1991-1998. The impact of the legislation was evaluated using interrupted time-series analysis of health-related utilization. The effects of early follow-up visits for vaginally delivered newborns with short stays were analyzed using the day of the week on which the birth occurred (eg, Monday, Tuesday) as an instrumental variable to account for potential confounding. A total of 155 352 full-term newborns who were born to mothers who receive Medicaid were studied. The main outcomes measured were rehospitalizations, emergency department (ED) visits, and diagnoses of dehydration and infection within 10 and 21 days of birth.

Results.—Few outcomes exhibited significant changes after legislation mandating coverage of minimum postnatal hospital stays. Rates of rehospitalization for jaundice within 10 days of birth fell from 0.78% to 0.47% in the year after legislation was introduced but leveled off after the legislation took effect. Rates of ED visits within 21 days increased from 6.0% to 10.4% during periods of increasing short stay but fell to 8.0% during the year after

TABLE 3.—Impact of Early Follow-up Visit on Adverse Outcomes Within 10 Days of Birth*

	Estimated Effect	95% Confidence Interval	
Any rehospitalization	−6.4%	−12.6%	−0.2%
Rehospitalization for jaundice	−3.5%	−7.9%	1.0%
ED visit	−6.6%	−17.6%	4.3%
Dehydration diagnosis	−0.8%	−3.1%	1.6%
Infection diagnosis	6.1%	−1.1%	13.2%
No. of observations		40 225	

*Estimates based on IVs models using day of week of birth as instrument for early preventive visits (visit within 4 days of birth). Sample restricted to vaginally delivered newborns with short hospital stays. All models control for maternal education, age, marital status, parity, race, number of prenatal care visits, region of birth, and metropolitan area residence.

(Reprinted by permission of *Pediatrics* from Meara E, Kotagal UR, Atherton HD, et al: Impact of early newborn discharge legislation and early follow-up visits on infant outcomes in a state medicaid population. *Pediatrics* 113:1619-1627, 2004.)

introduction of the legislation and leveled off when the legislation took effect. Rates of all-cause rehospitalization, dehydration, and infection diagnoses showed no consistent relationship to Ohio's legislation. Using instrumental variable analysis, newborns who received early follow-up visits were significantly less likely to have rehospitalizations within the first 10 days of life than those who did not (Table 3).

Conclusions.—In this state Medicaid population, legislation mandating coverage of minimum postnatal hospital stays was associated with reductions in the rates of rehospitalization for jaundice and ED visits. For newborns with short stays, early follow-up visits may reduce rehospitalizations in the early postpartum period.

▶ Congress and 43 states passed a law in the late 1990s mandating insurance coverage for a hospital stay of at least 48 hours after a vaginal delivery. This law was well intended but misguided. Of course it is nice to know that insurers must cover a 48-hour stay in the hospital, but if the purpose is to provide appropriate care rather than insurance, then Congress should have required third-party payers to cover the cost of appropriate care for the infant during the first week of life. Whether this care is delivered in the hospital or in the home is probably irrelevant and, of the two, perhaps follow-up care in the home is more important. These authors show that newborns who received early follow-up visits were significantly less likely to be rehospitalized within the first 10 days of life than those who did not, and the effect of early follow-up visits on reducing rehospitalization was significantly larger than simply avoiding early discharges. These results are even more important because they were achieved in a vulnerable population. Both this study and that of Abstract 11–9 provide justification for the current recommendations of the American Academy of Pediatrics regarding the follow-up of newborn infants, particularly those who are discharged before 48 to 72 hours. If safety is our objective, then early follow-up is mandatory.

M. J. Maisels, MB, BCH

The Use of In-line Intravenous Filters in Sick Newborn Infants
van Lingen RA, Baerts W, Marquering ACM, et al (Isala Clinics, Zwolle, The Netherlands)
Acta Paediatr 93:658-662, 2004   14–13

Aim.—This study assesses the improvement in outcome for newborn infants by decreasing major complications associated with intravenous fluid therapy by using an in-line filter, and evaluates the economical impact this might have in relation to daily changing of i.v. lines.

Methods.—In a prospective controlled study, 88 infants were randomly assigned to receive either filtered (except for lipids, blood and blood products) or non-filtered infusions via a central catheter. Main outcome measures such as bacteraemia, phlebitis, extravasation, thrombosis, septicaemia and

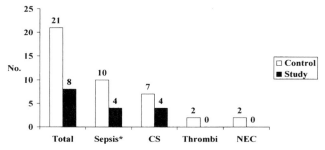

FIGURE 1.—Major complications. CS: clinical sepsis; NEC: necrotizing enterocolitis; *blood-culture positive. (Courtesy of van Lingen RA, Baerts W, Marquering ACM, et al: The use of in-line intravenous filters in sick newborn infants. *Acta Paediatr* 93:658-662, 2004. Published by Taylor & Francis, Ltd. at http://www.tandf.cc.uk/journals/jsp.htm.)

necrosis were all scored. The costs attributable to patients during a standard 8-day stay were also recorded.

Results.—Significant reductions were found in major complications such as thrombi and clinical sepsis (control group (21), filter group (8); $p < 0.05$) (Fig 1). Bacterial cultures of the filters showed a contamination rate on the upstream surface of 15/109 filters (14%). The mean costs of disposables were less in the filter group, showing a reduction from €31.17 to €23.79.

Conclusions.—The use of this in-line filter leads to a significant decrease in major complications and substantial cost savings.

▶ This is a simple and relatively inexpensive intervention that appears to have a very significant benefit for infants in the neonatal ICU. The importance of the reduction in nosocomial infection cannot be over emphasized, particularly in view of the impact of nosocomial infections on cost and length of stay.[1] Because gram-negative bacteria will accumulate on the filter membrane, there is a risk of released endotoxin getting into the baby. Thus, a filtration device used for an extended period must be capable of removing endotoxin.

M. J. Maisels, MB, BCh

Reference

1. Payne NR, Carpenter JH, Badger GJ, et al: Marginal increase in cost and excessive length of stay associated with nosocomial blood stream infections and surviving very low birth weight infants. *Pediatrics* 114:348-355, 2004.

15 Postnatal Growth and Development/ Follow-up

Bias in Reported Neurodevelopmental Outcomes Among Extremely Low
Birth Weight Survivors
Castro L, Yolton K, Haberman B, et al (Univ of Cincinnati, Ohio; Cincinnati Children's Hosp, Ohio; Research Triangle Inst, Research Triangle Park, NC; et al)
Pediatrics 114:404-410, 2004   15-1

Background.—Advances in the care of extremely low birth weight (ELBW) infants have increased the survival rate of this high-risk population. However, long-term follow-up of these infants has been difficult. As many as 10% to 26% of infants are not brought back for follow-up evaluations each year. The inability to evaluate all members of a cohort may result in bias in population-based estimates of long-term outcomes. Many factors are possible causes for this loss of follow-up data. It has been speculated that relatively healthy infants are more likely to participate in longitudinal studies because families with disabled infants may be reluctant to publicly acknowledge the disability. It is also possible that impaired infants are more likely than healthier children to return for follow-up evaluations. Other authors have proposed that lower socioeconomic status or parental education and ethnicity may be important determinants of compliance with follow-up recommendations. Possible biases were investigated in the evaluation of neurodevelopmental and somatic growth in ELBW survivors at 18 to 22 months' postmenstrual age.

Methods.—A retrospective review was conducted of data from a cohort of 1483 ELBW infant survivors (Table 3). Children who were seen for an 18- to 22-month follow-up visit, who visited but were not measured, or who made no visit were compared in terms of 4 outcomes: a score on the Bayley Scales of Infant Development (edition 2) Mental Developmental Index (MDI) of less than 70; a score on the Psychomotor Developmental Index (PDI) of less than 70; the presence or absence of cerebral palsy; and weight less than the 10th percentile for age. Logistic regression models were used to predict the likelihood of these outcomes for children with no follow-up

TABLE 3.—Comparison of Characteristics Among Study Groups

Variable	Compliant (*n* = 1008)	No Visit (*n* = 332)	Visit but Not Measured† (*n* = 143)
Gestational age, wk			
Mean ± 1 SD	26 ± 2	26 ± 2	27 ± 2
Range	19-34	22-34	22-37
Birth weight, g			
Mean ± SD	793 ± 136	797 ± 124	816 ± 122
Range	428-1000	445-1000	483-1000
Mother's age, y			
Mean ± SD	26 ± 7	26 ± 6	26 ± 6
Range	13-45	14-45	16-42
Prenatal care (at least 1 visit; *n* [%])	889 (88%)	284 (86%)	126 (89%)
Mother's marital status (single *n* [%])	581 (60%)	191 (64%)	81 (59%)
Mother's education < high school (*n* [%])	282 (28%)	NA‡	40 (30%)
Annual household income (*n* [%])			
<$20 000	532 (56%)	NA‡	75 (60%)
>$20 000	411 (44%)		51 (40%)
Insurance Medicaid (*n* [%])	639 (64%)	NA‡	83 (61%)
Male gender (*n* [%])	471 (47%)	150 (45%)	69 (48%)
Race (*n* [%])			
Black	516 (51%)	187 (56%)	74 (52%)
White	348 (35%)	100 (30%)	52 (36%)
Hispanic	128 (13%)	38 (12%)	14 (10%)
Other	16 (2%)	7 (2%)	3 (2%)
No. of fetuses >1 (*n* [%])	194 (19%)	44 (13%)§	28 (20%)
Antenatal glucocorticoid use (*n* [%])	379 (38%)	120 (36%)	59 (41%)
Postnatal glucocorticoid use (*n* [%])	445 (44%)	120 (36%)§	67 (47%)
IVH grade 3 or 4 (*n* [%])	224 (22%)	61 (19%)	27 (19%)
SGA (*n* [%])	184 (18%)	56 (17%)	26 (18%)
CLD (*n* [%])	407 (41%)	106 (32%)§	52 (37%)
NEC Bell stage 2 or 3 (*n* [%])	72 (7%)	23 (7%)	10 (7%)

*Children who returned for follow-up and were evaluated for all 4 outcomes (Bayley MDI, Bayley PDI, CP, and weight less than 10th percentile for age).

†Children who returned for follow-up but information is missing for at least 1 of the 4 outcomes. Both MDI and PDI scores are missing for 90 children, PDI scores are missing for 19 more children, and MDI scores are missing for 5 more. CP and/or weight for age are missing for 29 additional children.

‡Information is available only for mothers and children who attended follow-up.

§*P* ≤ .01 between compliant and lost to follow-up groups by Fisher exact test.

Abbreviations: SGA, Small for gestational age; *NA*, not available; *MDI*, Mental Developmental Index; *PDI*, Psychomotor Developmental Index; *CP*, cerebral palsy; *IVH*, intraventricular hemorrhage; *CLD*, chronic lung disease; *NEC*, necrotizing enterocolitis.

(Reproduced by permission of *Pediatrics*, courtesy of Castro L, Yolton K, Haberman B, et al: Bias in reported neurodevelopmental outcomes among extremely low birth weight survivors. *Pediatrics* 114:404-410, 2004.)

evaluations, and predicted probability distributions were compared across the groups.

Results.—Compared with children who were not brought back for follow-up, those children who were compliant with follow-up were more likely to have been 1 of a multiple birth, to have received postnatal glucocorticoids, and to have had chronic lung disease, all of which were factors that were associated with MDI and PDI scores of less than 70 in the compliant group. Chronic lung disease was associated with an increased risk of cerebral palsy. MDI and PDI scores of less than 70 were identified in 37% and 29% of children, respectively, who were identified at follow-up. Prediction models determined that 34% and 26% of infants in the no-visit group would have had scores of less than 70 on the MDI and PDI, respectively. Cerebral

TABLE 4.—Percentage of Children With Each Outcome by Study Group*

	Compliant	No Visit	Visit but Not Measured
MDI <70	37%	34%†	38%
PDI <70	29%	26%	29%
CP	17%	18%‡	15%
Weight <10th percentile	44%	42%	41%

*The observed percentage is reported for the compliant group, whereas the estimated percentage (mean predicted probability) is reported for the other groups.

†$P < .05$ for a comparison between the predicted probability distributions in the lost to follow-up and compliant groups.

‡$P = .05$ for a comparison between the predicted probability distributions in the lost to follow-up and compliant groups.

(Reproduced by permission of *Pediatrics*, courtesy of Castro L, Yolton K, Haberman B, et al: Bias in reported neurodevelopmental outcomes among extremely low birth weight survivors. *Pediatrics* 114:404-410, 2004.)

palsy was identified in 17% of the compliant group and was predicted in 18% of the no-visit group (Table 4). No statistically significant differences were seen in somatic growth among the 3 groups.

Conclusions.—Neurodevelopmental outcomes in ELBW infants who are compliant with follow-up evaluations may have worse scores on the Bayley MDI than do infants with no follow-up visit, which may lead to an overestimation of adverse outcomes in ELBW survivors.

▶ The authors make an important observation that is often assumed to be the case without evidence. The fact that ELBW infant survivors who are compliant with follow-up evaluations may have worse Bayley scores of infant development than do infants with no visits confirms the suspicion and suggests that data resulting from incomplete follow-up care may lead to an overestimation of adverse outcomes in ELBW survivors. Nonetheless, the study points out that the ideal is 100% follow-up. The fact that 100% follow-up most often cannot be achieved leaves open the question of what assumptions can be made about overestimating or underestimating the outcomes for a particular cohort. This is an important matter when trying to understand the resources that might be needed to assist survivors, including those who do not show up at the clinic. Differences in the health care system and in cultures may also contribute to whether those infants not showing up at the clinic are healthy or disabled. In the final analysis, the estimate for outcomes of the no-visit group is dependent on a predictive model. Perhaps it would be better to just approximate the ideal, that is, 100% follow-up.

D. K. Stevenson, MD

Center Differences and Outcomes of Extremely Low Birth Weight Infants

Vohr BR, for the Neonatal Research Network (Women and Infants Hosp, Providence, RI; Natl Inst of Child Health and Human Development, Bethesda, Md; Indiana Univ, Indianapolis; et al)

Pediatrics 113:781-789, 2004   15–2

Background.—Previous multicenter studies of extremely low birth weight infants (ELBW) have shown significant differences in neonatal characteristics and morbidities. Differences in outcomes for ELBW infants (401-1000 g) at 18 to 22 months of age were evaluated by center after adjustment for demographic factors and antenatal interventions. In addition, neonatal interventions associated with any differences in outcomes were identified by center.

Methods.—The outcomes of 2478 liveborn ELBW infants were assessed. All infants were admitted in 1993 and 1994 to the 12 centers that comprise the Neonatal Research Network of the National Institute of Child Health and Human Development. Of these infants, 1483 (60%) survived to 18 to 22 months, and 1151 (78%) had comprehensive evaluations. Logistic regression analyses were conducted to identify center differences and the association of 4 neonatal interventions: active resuscitation, postnatal steroids, ventilator treatment for 27 days or less, and full enteral feedings for 24 days or less. The incidence of adverse outcomes, including cerebral palsy, low Bayley scores, and neurodevelopmental impairment (NDI), were adjusted for demographics and antenatal interventions.

Results.—Bivariate analysis identified significant differences by center for mortality, antenatal and postnatal interventions, social and environmental variables, neonatal morbidities, and neurodevelopmental outcomes for the 12 centers. After adjustment for maternal and infant demographics and antenatal interventions, the percentage of ELBW infants who had died or had NDI at 18 to 22 months ranged from 52% to 85%. Active resuscitation and postnatal steroids were associated with increases in NDI of 11.8% and 19.3%, respectively. In comparison, shorter periods of ventilator support and a shorter time to achieve full enteral feeding were associated with decreases in NDI of 20.7% and 17.3%, respectively.

Conclusions.—Significant and disturbing differences in outcomes for extremely low birth weight infants at 18 to 22 months of age were noted among centers, even after adjustment for demographic and antenatal interventions. Differences among centers in postnatal interventions associated with differences in outcomes can be used to formulate hypotheses for testing ways to improve outcomes in these infants.

▶ This study of risk characteristics, neonatal practices, and neurologic outcomes for infants weighing less than 1000 g at the 12 tertiary care neonatal intensive care centers of the National Institute of Child Health and Human Development network in 1993-1994 demonstrates that heterogeneity is a defining feature of contemporary neonatology. Across these "high profile" neonatal ICUs, vast differences exist in racial composition (percent white, 6%-76%), socioeconomic status (income <$20,000, 33%-80%), prenatal care (81%-97%), antenatal steroid use (16%-61%) and outborn infants (2%-27%). The extent of these differences challenge any attempt to describe the characteristics of a "typical" US level III neonatal ICU. These centers also had marked differences in neurologic outcomes, as would be expected given the wide range in their case mix. However, even after taking differences in demographics, antenatal interventions, and birth weight into account, a 4- to 6-fold difference in the incidence of neurodevelopment problems at 18 to 22 months of age remained. If one considers the risk-adjusted neurodevelopmental outcome to be an indicator of the quality of care, this 4- to 6-fold difference is a very disturbing call to action. But what actions are called for? What are the underpinnings of this quality differential? Although the authors tantalize us with the observation that active resuscitation, postnatal steroid use, duration of ventilator treatment, and time to enteral feedings differ across units and are important predictors of neurologic outcomes, the extent to which the severity of illness (ie, sicker infants are more likely to be resuscitated, to need ventilatory support longer, take longer to reach full enteral feeding) versus differences in practice style (ie, optimizing ventilation, optimizing ELBW nutrition, avoiding postnatal steroids) account for these differences will require further study—study in which clinical trials will play an important role.

J. B. Gould, MD, MPH

Early Physiological Development of Infants With Intrauterine Growth Retardation

Jackson JA, Wailoo MP, Thompson JR, et al (Univ of Leicester, England)
Arch Dis Child Fetal Neonatal Ed 89:F46-F50, 2004   15–3

Background.—Infants who have experienced intrauterine growth retardation (IUGR) have more fatal congenital deformities; thus, they are more likely to die in the neonatal period. As a group, infants with IUGR will have more illnesses in infancy, and more sudden unexplained deaths will occur. Factors associated with IUGR range from poor maternal health and inadequate nutrition to maternal drug use and cigarette smoking; however, the continuing mechanism by which the lasting effects of such an antenatal insult are transmitted into adult life in the infant has not been identified. The patterns of early postnatal physiologic adaptation and maturation in infants with IUGR were assessed by measurement of the changes in sleeping deep body temperature, heart rate, and concentrations of urinary cortisol.

Methods.—The study group was composed of 65 infants with IUGR and 127 control infants matched for sex, social class, and levels of parental smoking.

Results.—Nighttime sleeping deep body temperatures, heart rates, and levels of cortisol excretion declined with age: the infants eventually established an adult-type diurnal rhythm of physiologic functioning. The minimum overnight temperature linearly declined with age, but differences in the intercept and slope were significant between the infants with IUGR and control infants. No such differences were found between the 2 groups in maximum temperature. The infants with IUGR had a mean (SD) age-adjusted minimum overnight heart rate that was 4.2 (1.5) beats/min higher than that of control infants. Overnight cortisol–creatinine ratios declined with age, at a rate of 4.1% per week; however, the ratio for infants with IUGR was, on average, 42% higher than for control infants of the same age. Morning cortisol concentrations did not exhibit a similar pattern.

Conclusions.—Postnatal physiologic adaptation and maturation in infants exposed to IUGR are slower than in normal infants; thus, these infants with IUGR may remain in a physiologically immature state for a longer period. The higher heart rates and greater cortisol excretion in infants with IUGR may be precursors to hypertension and cardiovascular disease in adulthood.

▶ Much emphasis has been placed on the impact of IUGR on the subsequent adult onset of disease. Once an infant with IUGR is born, the metabolic circumstance associated with the impaired growth does not suddenly change; instead, there is a legacy of transitional physiology that distinguishes the infant with IUGR from normally grown infants over the first several postnatal months. The higher minimum heart rates and higher cortisol levels are related to IUGR and remain a telltale sign of a consequential alteration in fetal physiology. However, a behavioral component to this physiology may also exist, with respect to the organization of sleep. This latter phenomenon may be particularly noticeable to caretakers. Thus, it is not only the disposition of fuels and altered growth but also other aspects of physiology that may persist for some time. Whether they predispose to later hypertension, heart disease, and strokes remains an open question.

D. K. Stevenson, MD

Postnatal Growth Retardation: A Universal Problem in Preterm Infants
Cooke RJ, Ainsworth SB, Fenton AC (Univ of Newcastle upon Tyne, England)
Arch Dis Child Fetal Neonatal Ed 89:F428-F430, 2004   15–4

Background.—It has been suggested that postnatal growth retardation (PGR) is inevitable among preterm infants. The postnatal growth of preterm infants discharged from all intensive care and special care baby units in the Northern Region of the United Kingdom was evaluated.

Study Design.—The study group consisted of all preterm infants ($\leq$32 weeks' gestation and $\leq$1500 g) discharged from 4 level III intensive care centers and 10 level I to II special care baby units from January 1998 through December 1999. Those with congenital or chromosomal abnormalities were excluded. Data are continuously and prospectively collected from all of these units. Data included date of birth, birth weight, gestational age, sex, clinical risk index for babies (CRIB), date of hospital discharge, and weight at discharge. Body weight was converted to a z score by using the British

Foundation Growth Standards. To obtain PGR, the z score at birth was subtracted from the z score at discharge.

Findings.—A total of 659 preterm infants were admitted during this 24-month period. There were no differences in birth characteristics, CRIB scores, length of hospital stay, weight gain, weight at discharge, or PGR between infants discharged from level III and level I to II units. There was significant variation in length of hospital stay, weight gain, weight at discharge, and PGR between the level III units. There was even greater variability between the level I to II units.

Conclusions.—These findings support the universal nature of PGR among preterm infants. The lack of variation in outcome between hospitals with different levels of care indicates that the distinction between their patient populations may be more perceived than real. The variation in outcome between hospital units at the same level suggests that nutrient intake and feeding practices vary considerably. The study data suggest that optimal nutritional support for preterm infants has yet to be widely achieved.

▶ Nutritional support in the neonatal ICU (NICU) is a growing concern, with little clinical consensus. It has been clear for sometime that enteral nutrition practice varies widely among NICUs. Concerns about how to minimize the incidence of necrotizing enterocolitis, though certainly understandable, have led to a myriad of different feeding styles, with little "evidence-based medicine" behind them. A "best practice" for enteral nutrition needs to be found and promulgated. Similarly, parenteral nutrition practice is widely varied. Recent data demonstrate that we can advance hyperalimentation safely faster than traditionally has been done. Early addition of amino acids (eg, 2-3 g/kg on day 1) helps eliminate the "protein deficit" seen in small preterm infants. Hopefully, all NICUs will look at these data and be more aggressive with parenteral nutrition. Lastly, feeding practices for our convalescent patients have improved in recent years, but these data again demonstrate further room for improvement. We have focused too much on calories and not enough on the quality of the nutrition. Aberrant growth at this crucial stage of development has the potential for long-term impact on bone density, blood pressure, the metabolic syndrome, etc, and is too important to ignore.

R. S. Cohen, MD

Two-Year Infant Neurodevelopmental Outcome After Single or Multiple Antenatal Courses of Corticosteroids to Prevent Complications of Prematurity
Spinillo A, Viazzo F, Colleoni R, et al (Univ of Pavia, Italy)
Am J Obstet Gynecol 191:217-224, 2004   15–5

Background.—The use of antenatal corticosteroids for the prevention of neonatal complications of prematurity in women at risk of preterm delivery has been supported by many controlled observational studies and meta-analyses. In recent years, it has become common practice for obstetricians to prescribe weekly antenatal steroid courses to women who have not delivered after the first dose. However, some human and animal studies have suggested that repeated antenatal steroid doses could adversely affect the growth and development of the immature brain. The effect of exposure to multiple antenatal steroid courses on short-term neonatal morbidity and 2-year infant neurodevelopmental outcomes was evaluated.

Methods.—This prospective observational study included 201 preterm singleton infants who received 1 or more courses of corticosteroids to prevent complications of prematurity and who were delivered between 24 and 34 weeks' gestation at a single institution. Neurodevelopmental outcomes in these infants were evaluated at 2 years' corrected age. Associations and trends were analyzed with logistic regression analysis and multivariate analyses.

Results.—A total of 138 patients (68.7%) received at least 1 complete course of betamethasone, and 63 patients (31.3%) were treated with dexamethasone. The prevalence of exposure to multiple steroid doses was 26.8% in the betamethasone group and 52.4% in the dexamethasone group (Table 2). The prevalence of infant leukomalacia, including both prolonged echogenicity and cystic leukomalacia, was 25.9% after a complete course of corticosteroids and 40%, 42.3%, and 44.4% after 1, 2, and more than 2 addi-

TABLE 2.—Odds Ratios and 95% Confidence Intervals for Various Neonatal Outcomes in the Groups of Infants Treated Antenatally With Betamethasone or Dexamethasone

	Dexamethasone (n = 63)	Betamethasone (n = 138)	OR (95% CI)*
Neonatal death	4 (6.3%)	7 (5.1%)	2.24 (0.47-10.9)
Respiratory distress syndrome	19 (30.2%)	43 (31.2%)	1.05 (0.51-2.15)
Assisted ventilation	22 (34.9%)	41 (29.7%)	2.06 (0.97-4.37)
Acidosis at birth	19 (30.2%)	22 (15.9%)	2.54 (1.19-5.44)
Acidosis first 24 h	26 (41.3%)	27 (19.6%)	3.73 (1.82-7.67)
Convulsions	2 (3.2%)	2 (1.5%)	2.25 (0.27-19.0)
Sepsis	5 (7.9%)	9 (6.5%)	2.08 (0.65-6.67)
Intraventricular hemorrhage			
No	56 (88.9%)	131 (94.9%)	Referent
Grade I-II	4 (6.3%)	4 (2.9%)	2.13 (0.54-8.4)
Grade III-IV	3 (4.8%)	3 (2.2%)	2.67 (0.46-15.46)
Overall	7 (11.1%)	7 (5.1%)	2.45 (0.77-7.80)
Periventricular leukomalacia			
No	36 (57.1%)	101 (73.2%)	Referent
Prolonged echogenicity	24 (38.1%)	33 (23.9%)	2.53 (1.13-5.65)
Cystic leukomalacia	3 (4.8%)	4 (2.9%)	3.11 (0.57-16.78)
Overall	27 (42.9%)	37 (26.8%)	2.25 (1.07-4.74)
Neurologic outcome			
Normal (n = 134)	39 (69.6%)	95 (81.9%)	Referent
Minor impairment (n = 26)	11 (19.6%)	15 (12.9%)	1.95 (0.73-5.18)
Moderate-severe impairment (n = 12)	6 (10.7%)	6 (5.2%)	2.67 (0.79-9.02)
Overall (n = 38)	17 (30.4%)	21 (18.1%)	2.13 (0.94-4.84)

*As obtained by logistic regression equations containing neonatal outcomes as the dependent variable and gestational age, birth weight ratio (single terms), surfactant use (yes, no), multiple steroid dosages exposure (yes, no), and ritodrine tocolysis (yes, no) as independent variables.

Abbreviation: OR, Odds ratio.

(Reprinted courtesy of the publisher from Spinillo A, Viazzo F, Colleoni R, et al: Two-year infant neurodevelopmental outcome after single or multiple antenatal courses of corticosteroids to prevent complications of prematurity. *Am J Obstet Gynecol* 191:217-224. Copyright 2004 by Elsevier.)

TABLE 4.—Prevalence of Leukomalacia and Overall Neurodevelopmental Abnormalities According to Type of Corticosteroid and Dosage Used

| | Single Dose | | | Multiple Doses | | |
	Dexa (n = 30)	Beta (n = 101)	OR (95% CI)	Dexa (n = 33)	Beta (n = 37)	OR (95% CI)
Leukomalacia						
No	22	75	Referent	14	26	Referent
Yes	8	26	1.05 (0.38-2.87)	19	11	3.21 (1.07-9.77)
	(n = 28)	(n = 81)		(n = 28)	(n = 35)	
Neurodevelopmental abnormalities						
No	23	66	Referent	16	29	Referent
Yes	5	15	0.96 (0.27-3.25)	12	6	3.63 (1.03-13.6)

Abbreviations: Dexa, Dexamethasone; *Beta,* betamethasone; OR, odds ratio.
(Reprinted courtesy of the publisher from Spinillo A, Viazzo F, Colleoni R, et al: Two-year infant neurodevelopmental outcome after single or multiple antenatal courses of corticosteroids to prevent complications of prematurity. *Am J Obstet Gynecol* 191:217-224. Copyright 2004 by Elsevier.)

tional courses, respectively (Table 4). After a complete course and 1, 2, and more than 2 additional courses of steroids, the corresponding prevalences of 2-year infant neurodevelopmental abnormalities were 18%, 21.4%, 29.2%, and 34.8%, respectively. Multivariate analysis of first-grade interactions indicated that the risk of leukomalacia and 2-year infant neurodevelopmental abnormalities associated with exposure to multiple doses was confined to dexamethasone. In comparison with betamethasone exposure, exposure to multiple doses of dexamethasone was associated with an increased risk of leukomalacia and overall 2-year infant neurodevelopmental abnormalities.

Conclusions.—Multiple antenatal courses of dexamethasone, but not betamethasone, were associated with an increased risk of leukomalacia and 2-year infant neurodevelopmental abnormalities.

▶ The Italians have offered their preliminary opinions on the use of 1 or more courses of corticosteroids to prevent complications of prematurity. Weaknesses of the study include its single-institution observational design and limited size, despite the investigators attempts to correct for a variety of confounding factors. Nonetheless, the findings are at least suggestive that multiple courses of steroids do not confer any advantage with respect to avoiding neonatal short- and long-term infant morbidities. However, dexamethasone administration was associated with an increased risk of periventricular leukomalacia and neurodevelopmental abnormalities. The authors speculate, as others have, on the basis of animal data, that perhaps the sulphite ions present in dexamethasone vehicles in combination with peroxynitrite could impair neural cell viability. Other animal studies suggest alternative mechanisms. Nonetheless, the fact that multiple doses of steroids do not confer an advantage and that dexamethasone possibly confers a disadvantage warrants careful consideration of repeatedly administering antenatal corticosteroids to reduce neonatal morbidities. The routine practice of weekly corticosteroid treatment might result in exactly the opposite effect. Perhaps a "rescue" approach for the mother presenting in preterm labor would be the safer alternative, and, if a choice is available, use betamethasone.

D. K. Stevenson, MD

Neurologic and Developmental Disability at Six Years of Age After Extremely Preterm Birth
Marlow N, Wolke D, Bracewell MA, et al (Univ of Nottingham, England; Univ of Bristol, England; Univ of Hertfordshire, Hatfield, England)
N Engl J Med 352:9-19, 2005   15–6

Background.—Birth before 26 weeks of gestation is associated with a high prevalence of neurologic and developmental disabilities in the infant during the first two years of life.

Methods.—We studied at the time of early school age children who had been born at 25 or fewer completed weeks of gestation in the United Kingdom and Ireland in 1995. Each child had been evaluated at 30 months of age.

TABLE 2.—Neurocognitive Function and Degree of Disability at Six Years of Age Among 241 Extremely Preterm Children and 160 Classmates Born at Full Term*

Disability†	Comparison with Standardized Data				Comparison with Classmates			
	Comparison Group		Extremely Preterm Group		Comparison Group		Extremely Preterm Group	
	No.	% (95% CI)	No.	% (95% CI)	No.	% (95% CI)	No.	% (95% CI)
Severe								
Cerebral palsy, nonambulatory	0		15	6 (4-10)	0		15	6 (4-10)
IQ >3 SD below mean								
Range, 39-54	0		27	11 (8-16)	0		50	21 (16-26)
Profound sensorineural hearing loss	0		7	3 (1-6)	0		7	3 (1-6)
Blind	0		6	2 (1-5)	0		6	2 (1-5)
Any severe disability	0		32	13 (9-18)	0		53	22 (17-28)
Moderate								
Abnormal neurologic findings with functional loss but ambulatory	0		17	7 (4-11)	0		17	7 (4-11)
IQ >2 to 3 SD below mean								
Range, 55-69	0		23	10 (6-14)	0		48	20 (15-26)
Sensorineural hearing loss corrected with hearing aids	1	1 (0-3)	7	3 (1-6)	2	1 (0-4)	7	3 (1-6)
Impaired vision but ability to see	0		11	5 (2-8)	1	1 (0-3)	11	5 (2-8)
Any moderate disability	1	1 (0-3)	27	11 (8-16)	2	1 (0-4)	57	24 (18-30)
Mild								
Neurologic signs, minimal functional impairment	0		26	11 (7-15)	0		26	11 (7-15)
IQ >1 to 2 SD below mean								
Range, 70-84	3	2 (0-5)	61	25 (20-31)	23	14 (9-21)	75	31 (25-37)
Mild hearing impairment	2	1 (0-4)	10	4 (2-7)	2	1 (0-4)	10	4 (2-7)
Squint or refractive error	7	4 (2-8)	69	29 (23-35)	7	4 (2-8)	69	29 (23-35)
Any mild disability	9	6 (3-10)	71	29 (24-36)	28	18 (12-24)	83	34 (29-41)
No disability	150	94 (89-97)	111	46 (40-53)	120	75 (68-81)	48	20 (15-25)

*IQ scores for extremely preterm infants were classified with the use of the original test standardization norms or results obtained for classmates. IQ scores are presented as ranges of the overall cognitive scores in each category; for standardization norms, these are scores with a standardization mean (±SD) of 100±15, and for classmates a standardization mean of 106±12. Among extremely preterm children, 50 had scores more than 2 SD below the mean as compared with the standardized data and 98 had scores more than 2 SD below the mean as compared with classmates.

†A severe disability was defined as one that was likely to make the child highly dependent on caregivers; a moderate disability as one that would probably allow a reasonable degree of independence to be reached; and a mild disability as the presence of neurologic signs with minimal functional consequences or with other impairments, such as squint or refractive error.

(Courtesy of Marlow N, Wolke D, Bracewell MA, et al: Neurologic and developmental disability at six years of age after extremely preterm birth. N Engl J Med 352:9-19, 2005. Copyright Massachusetts Medical Society; all rights reserved.)

TABLE 3.—Severity and Type of Disability at Six Years of Age Among Extremely Preterm Children, According to Gestational Age at Birth and Sex*

Domain	Boys (N = 7)	≤23 Wk Girls (N = 17)	All (N = 24)	Boys (N = 37)	24 Wk Girls (N = 36)	All (N = 73)	Boys (N = 78)	25 Wk Girls (N = 66)	All (N = 144)	Total (N = 241)
					Number of Children (Percent)					
Overall cognition										
No disability (score, >94)	0	6 (35)	6 (25)	4 (11)	11 (31)	15 (21)	20 (26)	27 (41)	47 (33)	68 (28)
Mild disability (score, 82-94)	1 (14)	3 (18)	4 (17)	13 (35)	12 (33)	25 (34)	24 (31)	22 (33)	46 (32)	75 (31)
Moderate disability (score, 70-81)	3 (43)	5 (29)	8 (33)	6 (16)	7 (19)	13 (18)	16 (21)	11 (17)	27 (19)	48 (20)
Severe disability (score, ≤69)	3 (43)	3 (18)	6 (25)	14 (38)	6 (17)	20 (27)	18 (23)	6 (9)	24 (17)	50 (21)
Neuromotor										
No disability	5 (71)	13 (76)	18 (75)	21 (57)	30 (83)	51 (70)	58 (74)	56 (85)	114 (79)	183 (76)
Abnormal signs, minimal functinal loss	2 (29)	2 (12)	2 (8)	4 (11)	4 (11)	8 (11)	11 (14)	5 (8)	16 (11)	26 (11)
Cerebral palsy with disability, ambulatory	0	1 (6)	3 (12)	6 (16)	0	6 (8)	5 (6)	3 (5)	8 (6)	17 (7)
Cerebral palsy, nonambulatory	0	1 (6)	1 (4)	6 (16)	2 (6)	8 (11)	4 (5)	2 (3)	6 (4)	15 (6)
Hearing										
No diability	6 (86)	15 (88)	21 (88)	32 (86)	30 (83)	62 (85)	73 (94)	61 (92)	134 (93)	217 (90)
Mild hearing loss	1 (14)	1 (6)	2 (8)	3 (8)	2 (6)	5 (7)	2 (3)	1 (2)	3 (2)	10 (4)
Use of hearing aid, but hears	0	0	0	0	2 (6)	2 (3)	2 (3)	3 (5)	5 (3)	7 (3)
Profound hearing loss	0	1 (6)	1 (4)	2 (5)	2 (6)	4 (5)	1 (1)	1 (2)	2 (1)	7 (3)
Vision										
No disability	5 (71)	6 (35)	11 (46)	20 (54)	20 (56)	40 (55)	53 (68)	51 (77)	104 (72)	155 (64)
Squint or refractive error	2 (29)	7 (41)	9 (38)	11 (30)	14 (39)	25 (34)	21 (27)	14 (21)	35 (24)	69 (29)
Visually impaired, not blind	0	2 (12)	2 (8)	4 (11)	1 (3)	5 (7)	3 (4)	1 (2)	4 (3)	11 (5)
Severe blindness	0	2 (12)	2 (8)	2 (5)	1 (3)	3 (4)	1 (1)	0	1 (1)	6 (2)
Overall disability										
None	0	3 (18)	3 (12)	2 (5)	8 (22)	10 (14)	16 (21)	19 (29)	35 (24)	48 (20)
Mild	1 (14)	5 (29)	6 (25)	11 (30)	15 (42)	26 (36)	24 (31)	27 (41)	51 (35)	83 (34)
Moderate	3 (43)	6 (35)	9 (38)	9 (24)	7 (19)	16 (22)	19 (24)	13 (20)	32 (22)	57 (24)
Severe	3 (43)	3 (18)	6 (25)	15 (41)	6 (17)	21 (29)	19 (24)	7 (11)	26 (18)	53 (22)

*Cognitive impairment was defined with the use of contemporary classmates as a reference group.
(Courtesy of Marlow N, Wolke D, Bracewell MA, et al: Neurologic and developmental disability at six years of age after extremely preterm birth. *N Engl J Med* 352:9-19, 2005. Copyright Massachusetts Medical Society, all rights reserved.)

The children underwent standardized cognitive and neurologic assessments at six years of age. Disability was defined as severe (indicating dependence on caregivers), moderate, or mild according to predetermined criteria.

Results.—Of 308 surviving children, 241 (78 percent) were assessed at a median age of six years and four months; 160 classmates delivered at full term served as a comparison group. Although the use of test reference norms showed that cognitive impairment (defined as results more than 2 SD below the mean) was present in 21 percent of the children born extremely preterm (as compared with 1 percent in the standardized data), this value rose to 41 percent when the results were compared with those for their classmates (Table 2). The rates of severe, moderate, and mild disability were 22 percent, 24 percent, and 34 percent, respectively; disabling cerebral palsy was present in 30 children (12 percent) (Table 3). Among children with severe disability at 30 months of age, 86 percent still had moderate-to-severe disability at 6 years of age. In contrast, other disabilities at the age of 30 months were poorly predictive of developmental problems at 6 years of age.

Conclusions.—Among extremely preterm children, cognitive and neurologic impairment is common at school age. A comparison with their classroom peers indicates a level of impairment that is greater than is recognized with the use of standardized norms.

▶ This is one of the first reports on the outcomes of extremely immature and low birth weight infants born in the 1990s. It serves as a model for perinatal outcome studies since it consists of a geographically based population (the United Kingdom), is gestational age specific, the children were followed to 30 months of corrected age rather than just into the second year, disability was functionally described, results were compared with the normal population, and there was a good follow-up rate.

The authors realistically described how less than 26 weeks' gestation children born in the mid-1990s functioned at school age and what can be expected as they proceed through schooling and adolescence.

However, now 10 years later, one wonders whether these results are applicable to current survivors since survival has doubled in the mid-2000s. At least 20% to 30% of 23-week, 50% of 24-week, and 80% of 25-week gestation infants currently survive. The authors do not examine the predictors of their outcomes; however, during the 1990s many infants received postnatal steroid therapy to prevent or treat chronic lung disease. This had a deleterious effect on development. Since this treatment is now used less often, one hopes that the current rates of neurodevelopmental impairment will be less than those described by Marlow et al.

M. Hack, MD

Cognitive Outcomes of Preschool Children With Prenatal Cocaine Exposure

Singer LT, Minnes S, Short E, et al (Case Western Reserve Univ, Cleveland, Ohio; Cleveland State Univ, Ohio; Ohio State Univ, Columbus)
JAMA 291:2448-2456, 2004   15–7

Background.—Only a few prospective studies have assessed the long-term cognitive effects of prenatal cocaine exposure, and their results were inconsistent. The effects of prenatal cocaine exposure and the quality of the caregiving environment on 4-year cognitive outcomes were assessed.

Methods.—Four hundred fifteen infants identified from a high-risk population screened for drug use were enrolled in the longitudinal, masked comparison cohort study. Screening included clinical interview, urine testing, and meconium testing. At 4 years of age, 190 cocaine-exposed and 186 unexposed children were available for follow-up (93% of survivors in the original sample). Assessment included the Wechsler Preschool and Primary Scales of Intelligence–Revised.

Findings.—After adjustment for covariates, prenatal cocaine exposure was unassociated with lower full-scale IQ scores, summary verbal scores, or performance IQ scores at 4 years of age. However, prenatal cocaine exposure correlated with small but significant deficits on several subscales, including visual-spatial skills, general knowledge, and arithmetic skills. In addition, prenatal cocaine exposure correlated with a lower likelihood of achievement of an IQ score above normative means. The strongest independent predictor of outcomes was the quality of the caregiving environment.

Cocaine-exposed children in nonrelative foster or adoptive care lived in homes with more stimulating environments and had caregivers with better vocabulary scores. Children in such environments achieved full-scale and performance IQ scores comparable to those of unexposed children in biological maternal or relative care. Also, children in such environments had higher scores than did cocaine-exposed children in biological maternal or relative care.

Conclusion.—Prenatal exposure to cocaine does not appear to be associated with lower full-scale, verbal, or performance IQ scores at 4 years of age. However, it apparently is associated with an increased risk for specific cognitive impairments and a lower likelihood of an IQ above the normative mean. Cocaine-exposed children in better home environments had IQ scores comparable to those of the unexposed control group in this study.

▶ While there were a number of significant limitations in this study, which the authors point out, it remains a very important and well-designed prospective analysis of the impact of prenatal cocaine exposure on the developing child. The 2 most important conclusions were (1) prenatal cocaine exposure increases the risk for specific cognitive impairments and (2) the environment in which the child grows up can have significant positive moderating effects on the child and dramatically decrease the risk for cognitive impairment.

This study confirms what we have known for a long time: Developmental-behavioral outcomes are multifactorial, and the environment can have a re-demptive effect if the biological risk factors are not overwhelming. It also re-minds us that we should turn our attention to strengths and redemptive factors when considering intervention strategies for high-risk infants and children. The presence of risk factors does not warrant pessimism. Children have amazing resilience in a nurturing environment.

E. F. Krug III, MDiv, MD

The Relationship Between Birth Weight and Childhood Asthma: A Population-Based Cohort Study
Sin DD, Spier S, Svenson LW, et al (Univ of Alberta, Edmonton, Canada; Univ of Calgary, Alberta, Canada; Alberta Health and Wellness, Edmonton, Canada)
Arch Pediatr Adolesc Med 158:60-64, 2004   15–8

Background.—The prevalence and severity of childhood asthma are growing, especially among children 5 years of age or younger. At the same time that the asthma hospitalization rate in these young children has in-creased, a substantial increase in birth weight among neonates born in the Western world has occurred. Whether low or high birth weight changes the risk for childhood asthma beyond the effect of prematurity, whether a rela-tionship exists between birth weight and childhood asthma, and whether age, sex, race, income status, and similar factors also influence the develop-ment of childhood asthma were determined in a large population-based co-hort study.

Methods.—A relationship was sought between the occurrence of high birth weight and the risk of emergency visits for asthma during childhood. Neonates were all born at term (at or beyond 37 weeks' gestation) and were placed into categories of low (<2.5 kg), normal (2.5-4.5 kg), or high (>4.5 kg) birth weight. Evaluation was carried out prospectively for 10 years.

Results.—The 83,595 term neonates were followed up for 10 years. Their mean birth weight was 3.44 kg. Just under half of the neonates (48.8%) were girls, 4.8% were aboriginal, and 14.6% were born into a low-income family. At least 1 emergency visit for asthma was made by 6.5% of the children; the total number of emergency visits was 15,634. High birth weights were more likely to be found among aboriginal children than among nonaboriginal children. Children who had high birth weights also had a higher risk of emer-gency visits for asthma within the first 10 years of life than did children with normal birth weights. After adjustment was made for gestational age, sex, maternal age, aboriginal status, and low-income status, high birth weight children showed a statistically significant association with an increased risk of needing emergency department care for asthma during childhood when compared with normal birth weight children. Children with the highest birth weight had the greatest risk, and an additional 10% increase in risk was seen for every 0.10-kg increase in birth weight above 4.5 kg. No signifi-cant relationship was found between low birth weight and the risk of emergency visits for asthma during childhood. Other factors accompanying high birth weight and related to a higher risk for emergency visits for asthma during childhood were male sex, aboriginal race, and low-income family.

Conclusions.—High birth weight had a significant relationship to the development of asthma during childhood that was sufficiently severe to require an emergency department visit. Low birth weight carried no similar risk. An increased risk was also noted for male, aboriginal, and low-income children with high birth weights compared with children with normal or low birth weights.

▶ This is a population-based cohort study on all neonates born at term (≥37 weeks) between April 1, 1985 and March 31, 1988 in Alberta, Canada (N = 83,595). This is a fascinating article that has a statistical basis for concluding that neonates with a high birth weight (≥4.5 kg), followed for more than 10 years, had a significantly increased risk of emergency visits for asthma during childhood compared with neonates of normal birth weight (relative risk [RR], 1.16; 95% CI, 1.04-1.29). This relationship was linear with each increment of 0.10 kg in birth weight. Other significant factors were male sex (RR, 1.26; 95% CI, 1.22-1.30), aboriginal status (RR, 1.20; 95% CI 1.11-1.29), and low-income status (RR, 1.11; 95% CI, 1.06-1.16). In their discussion, the authors compare these data to literature for and against this hypothesis and point out that their data focus on term infants and does not mix data with preterm infants. The biological mechanism of this association is unclear, but the authors offer evidence that large neonates are more likely to be obese adolescents. Furthermore, adiposity has a negative effect on lung functioning, and a proinflammatory state related to obesity may also be a contributory factor. Read the article to get all these details. In summary, evidence is accumulating for long-term outcomes associated with birth weight and, perhaps, associated with the pregnancy (my editorial). Although this article did not find an association between asthma and low birth weight, it is becoming more evident that being too large or too small may have life-long implications.

R. L. Ariagno, MD

Prematurity and Reduced Body Fatness at 8-12 y of Age
Fewtrell MS, Lucas A, Cole TJ, et al (Inst of Child Health, London)
Am J Clin Nutr 80:436-440, 2004   15–9

Background.—Body composition is an important influence on morbidity and mortality in adult life, and evidence is increasing that body composition might be programmed by early growth and nutrition. Breast-feeding, delayed introduction of solid foods, and lower protein intake at age 10 months are associated with reduced fatness in adulthood. Several studies have shown that growth and body composition in preterm infants in the neonatal period are influenced by their diet, and preterm children are known to be shorter and lighter than children born at term throughout childhood and adolescence. However, it is unclear whether the size difference is associated

TABLE 1.—Anthropometric and Body-Composition Data
According to Cohort[1]

	Preterm ($n = 497$)	Term ($n = 95$)
Age (y)	$11.2 \pm 0.89^{2,3}$	10.6 ± 0.86
Boys [% (n)]	51 ± 256	55 ± 52
Attained puberty[4] [% (n)]	30 ± 151	23 ± 22
Weight (kg)	35.4 ± 8.5^5	37.6 ± 8.9
Height (cm)	141.6 ± 9.0	142.9 ± 7.7
BMI (kg/m²)	17.5 ± 2.8^5	18.2 ± 3.0
Waist circumference (cm)	60.8 ± 7.2^6	62.3 ± 7.6
Skinfold thickness (mm)		
Biceps	7.2 ± 3.3^5	7.9 ± 3.7
Triceps	11.6 ± 4.2^3	13.8 ± 5.0
Subscapular	8.4 ± 4.2	9.3 ± 5.7
Suprailiac	10.5 ± 6.4^5	12.5 ± 8.2
MUAC (cm)	21.5 ± 2.7^6	22.1 ± 2.9
TUA (cm²)	37.5 ± 10.1	39.4 ± 10.8
AFA (cm²)	12.9 ± 6.3^3	15.7 ± 7.9
AMA (cm²)	252.5 ± 56.6	249.8 ± 49.5
Slaughter equations		
Percentage fat (%)	18.4 ± 5.9^3	20.5 ± 7.0
Fat mass (kg)	6.84 ± 3.70^7	8.20 ± 4.68
Fat-free mass (kg)	28.6 ± 5.5	29.4 ± 5.0
FMI (kg/m²)	3.34 ± 1.62^7	3.93 ± 2.01
FFMI (kg/m²)	14.1 ± 1.5	14.3 ± 1.3
Deurenberg equations		
Percentage fat (%)	18.8 ± 5.2^7	20.5 ± 5.8
Fat mass (kg)	6.88 ± 3.36^8	8.09 ± 4.07
Fat-free mass (kg)	28.3 ± 5.5^9	29.5 ± 5.3
FMI (kg/m²)	3.38 ± 1.46^8	3.89 ± 1.74
FFMI (kg/m²)	14.1 ± 1.5	14.3 ± 1.5
DXA[10]		
Percentage fat (%)	20.1 ± 8.3^7	23.3 ± 8.3
Fat mass (kg)	7.14 ± 4.32^3	9.31 ± 5.23
Fat-free mass (kg)[11]	26.4 ± 4.9^3	28.4 ± 5.0
BMC (g)	1061 ± 245^3	1162 ± 254
FMI (kg/m²)	3.59 ± 1.99^3	4.47 ± 2.30
FFMI (kg/m²)	13.5 ± 1.4^5	13.8 ± 1.3

[1]*BMI*, Body mass index; *MUAC*, midupper arm circumference; *TUA*, total midupper arm area; *AFA*, arm fat area; *AMA*, arm muscle area; *FMI*, fat mass index; *FFMI*, fat-free mass index; *DXA*, dual-energy x-ray absorptiometry; *BMC*, bone mineral content.
[2]$\bar{x} \pm$ SD (all such values).
[3,5,7,8]Significantly different from term: [3]$P \leq .001$, [5]$P < .05$, [7]$P < .005$, [8]$P < .01$.
[4]Tanner stage ≥ 2.
[6,9]Nearly significantly different from term: [6]$P = .06$, [9]$P = .05$.
[10]$n = 200$ in the preterm cohort and 95 in the term cohort.
[11]Including BMC.
(Courtesy of Fewtrell MS, Lucas A, Cole TJ, et al: Prematurity and reduced body fatness at 8-12 y of age. Copyright *Am J Clin Nutr* 80:436-440, 2004. American Society for Clinical Nutrition.)

with altered body composition. Whether fat mass (FM) and fat-free mass (FFM) are proportionately lower in children born preterm than in children born at term was determined.

Methods.—A total of 497 children born preterm and 95 term children were studied at age 8 to 12 years of age. Body composition was determined with the use of skinfold thickness measurements and, in 200 preterm and 95 term children, dual-energy x-ray absorptiometry. FM and FFM were normalized for height to give the fat mass index (FMI) and the fat-free mass index (FFMI), respectively.

Results.—The preterm children were significantly lighter than those born at term and had lower FM and FFM. However, the FMI was significantly lower in preterm children, whereas the FFMI was not. The FMI was also significantly lower in boys than in girls and in children with higher activity levels (Table 1). Additional data obtained in the preterm group showed no association between birth weight, gestational age, or neonatal diet and later FMI or FFMI.

Conclusions.—The smaller size of preterm children compared with term children at birth is associated with a lower FM but not a lower FFM when data were normalized for height. This could result in a reduction in the risk of obesity and related diseases in adulthood.

▶ Most of the time, we are concerned about how infant growth and nutrition might adversely affect long-term adult health. The authors have previously reported smaller body size at 8 to 12 years of age for children born preterm compared with children born at term, but this article suggests that preterm infants may be predisposed to a lower FMI, which might possibly have a beneficial impact on the adult circumstance because of a reduced risk of obesity and related diseases during adult life. However, no such direct advantage is demonstrated, and further investigation is required to establish such a relationship. The lack of effect of gestational size or age at birth on either the FMI or the FFMI remains mysterious, but the later leanness of prematurely born people may reflect a more global consequence of the disruption of the critical period for fat deposition during the last trimester by preterm birth. The impact of such a disruption on leptin receptors in the hypothalamus and the sensitivity to leptin later in life are also topics for further inquiry. Nonetheless, on the surface, it looks like being born preterm may predispose to being a less fat adult, although these individuals will also probably be smaller.

D. K. Stevenson, MD

Behavioral Outcomes and Evidence of Psychopathology Among Very Low Birth Weight Infants at Age 20 Years
Hack M, Youngstrom EA, Cartar L, et al (Case Western Reserve Univ, Cleveland, Ohio; Kent State Univ, Ohio)
Pediatrics 114:932-940, 2004   15–10

Introduction.—Little information is available concerning the mental health of very-low birth weight (VLBW; <1500 g) infants in young adulthood. Sex-specific behavior outcomes were investigated, together with evidence of psychopathologic behavior in VLBW young adults.

Methods.—The study included 241 survivors of VLBW (1180 g; mean gestational age at birth, 29.7 weeks; male, 116; females, 125) who were compared with 233 control subjects (males, 108; females, 124) from the same population with normal birth weights (NBW). Young adult behavior was evaluated at 20 years of age using the Achenbach Young Adult Self-Report and the Young Adult Behavior Checklist for Parents. Sex-specific outcomes were adjusted for socioeconomic status.

Results.—The VLBW males reported significantly fewer delinquent behaviors, compared with those of NBW control subjects. No differences were observed on the Internalizing, Externalizing, or Total Problem Behavior scales. Parents of VLBW males reported significantly more thought problems for male children than did parents of control subjects. The VLBW females reported significantly more withdrawn behaviors and fewer delinquent behaviors, compared to the control group. The rates of VLBW females on internalizing behaviors (including anxious/depressed and withdrawn behaviors) above the borderline clinical cutoff were 30%, compared to 16% for the NBW females (odds ratio [OR]: 2.2; 95% confidence interval [CI], 1.2-4.1). Parents of VLBW females reported significantly higher scores for their child on the anxious/depressed, withdrawn, and attention problem subscales, compared with those reported by control parents. The ORs for parent-reported rates above the borderline-clinical cutoff among females for the anxious/depressed subscale was 4.4 (95% CI, 1.4-13.5); for thought problems, it was 3.7 (95% CI, 1.2-11.6); and for attention problems, it was 2.4 (95% CI, 1.0-5.5). No difference was noted in the young adult self-report of attention-deficit/hyperactivity disorder (ADHD). Parents of VLBW males reported higher mean scores on the attention subtype of ADHD, yet did not indicate higher rates of ADHD.

Conclusion.—The increase in psychopathologic behavior among VLBW survivors in young adulthood indicates a need for anticipatory guidance and early intervention that may help prevent or ameliorate potential psychopathology.

▶ Hack et al have provided important information about the incidence of psychopathologic behavior among VLBW survivors in young adulthood. Comparing a cohort of survivors among VLBW infants born between 1977 and 1979 to a sociodemographically similar control group (NBW) they found less risk-taking among VLBW subjects and possibly higher levels of behavioral inhibition with anxious-inattentive behavior in males and anxious-depressed mood in females. The hyperactivity manifest at 8 years of age in the VLBW cohort did not meet clinical criteria for ADHD (based on questionnaire data from subjects and their mothers) at 20 years of age. The apparent increased incidence of thought problems in these subjects is, I suspect, secondary to anxiety, rather than a prepsychotic state, but this requires further research. Of particular importance is the fact that early intervention with cognitive-behavioral therapy may reduce the morbidity associated with the problem behaviors identified and warrants mental health surveillance for VLBW infants as they reach adulthood.

E. F. Krug III, MDiv, MD

Cerebral Palsy and Intrauterine Growth in Single Births: European Collaborative Study

Jarvis S, for the Surveillance of Cerebral Palsy in Europe (SCPE) collaboration of European Cerebral Palsy Registers (Univ of Newcastle, England; et al)
Lancet 362:1106-1111, 2003   15–11

Background.—Cerebral palsy seems to be more common in term babies whose birthweight is low for their gestational age at delivery, but past analyses have been hampered by small datasets and Z-score calculation methods.

Methods.—We compared data from ten European registers for 4503 singleton children with cerebral palsy born between 1976 and 1990 with the number of births in each study population. Weight and gestation of these children were compared with reference standards for the normal spread of gestation and weight-for-gestational age at birth.

Findings.—Babies of 32-42 weeks' gestation with a birthweight for gestational age below the 10th percentile (using fetal growth standards) were 4-6 times more likely to have cerebral palsy than were children in a reference band between the 25th and 75th percentiles. In children with a weight above the 97th percentile, the increased risk was smaller (from 1.6 to 3.1), but still significant. Those with a birthweight about 1 SD above average always had the lowest risk of cerebral palsy. A similar pattern was seen in those with unilateral or bilateral spasticity, as in those with a dyskinetic or ataxic disability. In babies of less than 32 weeks' gestation, the relation between weight and risk was less clear.

Interpretation.—The risk of cerebral palsy, like the risk of perinatal death, is lowest in babies who are of above average weight-for-gestation at birth, but risk rises when weight is well above normal as well as when it is well below normal. Whether deviant growth is the cause or a consequence of the disability remains to be determined.

▶ This is an impressive collaboration among 10 European registers that yields a cohort of 4503 singleton births with cerebral palsy (CP). CP refers to a group of disorders that involve disordered movement, posture, or both, as well as motor dysfunction. It is a permanent condition that can change but is not progressive. There can be no criticism about the sample size. However, there are a limited number of questions that can be posed to a registry database. The analyses prove beyond a shadow of doubt that term infants with a birth weight below the tenth percentile are 4 to 6 times more likely to have CP. At the other end of the spectrum the macrosomic infants (more than 97th percentile) are also at greater risk for CP. The risk of CP was lowest in children whose birth weights were approximately 1 standard deviation above average. Almost like Goldilocks and the 3 bears with the porridge, too big is not good, too little is worse, and above the norm (but within 1 standard deviation) is just right. The million-dollar question is what comes first? Poor growth leading to CP, or is it an in utero brain insult that triggers the aberrant growth? We can but speculate as we bear in mind that there are many causes of CP. Nelson's[1] comments in her editorial last year are an apt summary of the current status with regard to

CP: "The known causes of cerebral palsy account for only a minority of the total cases. Even for most of those cases, however, evidence of the preventability of the disorder is lacking." She concludes "Can we now prevent cerebral palsy? Apart from our ability to avoid exposure to a few associated risk factors in a small minority of cases, there is little evidence at present that we can."

A. A. Fanaroff, MD

Reference

1. Nelson KB: Can we prevent cerebral palsy? *N Engl J Med* 349:1765, 2003.

Behavioral and Emotional Adjustment of Teenagers in Mainstream School Who Were Born Before 29 Weeks' Gestation
Gardner F, for the ELGA (Extremely Low Gestational Age) Steering Group (Univ of Oxford, England; et al)
Pediatrics 114:676-682, 2004   15-12

Background.—Very preterm infants are known to be at increased risk for physical, sensory, and learning disabilities, but less is known about these children in their teen years. Children aged 16 years, in mainstream school, who were born at extremely low gestational age (ELGA, before 29 weeks of gestation) were evaluated for behavioral and emotional problems and positive adjustment from the perspective of parents, teachers, and teenagers.

Study Design.—The study group consisted of 179 adolescents aged 16 years who were born ELGA. A control child of the same gender and similar birth date was selected by each school. Goodman's Strengths and Difficulties Questionnaire was completed by the teenagers, their parents, and their teachers.

Findings.—Of the 179 teenagers from the ELGA cohort, 82% were in mainstream high schools. Parents were more likely to rate these teens as having problems with hyperactivity, peer relationships, and emotions than control peers (Table 3). Teachers' ratings were similar to parents' ratings. Those from the ELGA cohort did not rate themselves as having more hyperactivity and relationship problems than their peers. They did report more emotional problems, but less delinquency, alcohol, cannabis, and other drug use than control peers.

Conclusions.—ELGA children who were in mainstream schools had higher levels of parent- and teacher-reported emotional, attentional, and peer problems at 16 years of age than peers born at term. However, they did not show signs of delinquency, conduct disorders, or drug abuse.

▶ Slowly, investigators are turning their attention to the long-term consequences of "successful" newborn intensive care for the most immature preterm infants, in the case of this report, those before 29 weeks of gestational age. The good news is that a majority of these infants who are in mainstream school are functioning well and do not show major emotional or behav-

TABLE 3.—Behavioral and Emotional Problems of ELGA and Control Teenagers, Reported by Parents, Teachers, and Teenagers

Teenagers in Abnormal Range*	ELGA Group	Control Group	Difference in % Between Groups (95% CI)	P Value for Differences
Parent report	N = 145	N = 100		
Hyperactivity	12 (8)	1 (1)	7 (2 to 12)	.017
Conduct problems	15 (10)	5 (5)	5 (−1 to 12)	.16
Emotional problems	26 (18)	7 (7)	11 (3 to 19)	.014
Peer problems	27 (19)	5 (5)	14 (6 to 21)	.002
Teacher report	N = 120	N = 92		
Hyperactivity	14 (12)	3 (3)	8 (2 to 15)	.039
Conduct problems	7 (6)	8 (9)	−3 (−10 to 4)	.43
Emotional problems	12 (10)	1 (1)	9 (3 to 15)	.008
Peer problems	18 (15)	1 (1)	14 (7 to 21)	.0004
Teenager report	N = 147	N = 108		
Hyperactivity	11 (8)	4 (4)	4 (−2 to 10)	.28
Conduct problems	10 (7)	7 (6)	0 (−6 to 7)	1.00
Emotional problems	11 (8)	2 (2)	6 (1 to 11)	.047
Peer problems	3 (2)	1 (1)	1 (−2 to 4)	.64
Teenager report, other feelings and behaviors†	N = 147	N = 108		
Uses alcohol	45 (31)	62 (57)	−27 (−39 to −14)	<.0001
Ever used cannabis	12 (8)	26 (24)	−16 (−25 to −7)	.0007
Ever used other drugs	2 (1)	8 (7)	−6 (−11 to −1)	.021
Depression score, mean (SD)	3.8 (5.0)	3.9 (4.4)	−0.1 (−1.3 to 1.1)	.86
Delinquency score, mean (SD)	3.5 (3.0)	4.4 (2.9)	−0.9 (−1.6 to −0.1)	.023
Parent report of impact of problems	N = 41‡	N = 16		
Mean (SD)	5.4 (3.3)	3.9 (1.9)	1.6 (0.2 to 3.0)	.029
Teacher report of impact of problems	N = 52	N = 19		
Mean (SD)	3.8 (2.1)	2.9 (2.0)	0.9 (−0.2 to 2.0)	.12

Values are n (%) of teenagers unless stated otherwise.
* Based on Strengths and Difficulties Questionnaire (Goodman). Two ELGA teenagers did not respond.
† For sources, see "Methods." Higher scores mean more problems. Missing responses: alcohol: 1 ELGA; depression: 4 ELGA, 1 control; delinquency: 5 ELGA, 1 control.
‡ For impact rating, N based only on those showing problems.
Abbreviations: ELGA, Extremely low gestational age; CI, confidence interval.
(Courtesy of Gardner F, for the ELGA [Extremely Low Gestational Age] Steering Group: Behavioral and emotional adjustment of teenagers in mainstream school who were born before 29 weeks' gestation. *Pediatrics* 114:676-682, 2004. Reproduced by permission of *Pediatrics*.)

ioral adjustment problems. Nonetheless, the data clearly can be interpreted to show that extremely preterm birth is associated with an increased propensity for higher levels of parent- and teacher-reported emotional, attentional, and peer problems compared with mainstream classmates. One of the most important things to remember is that whatever behaviors are observed in a person is a reflection of a brain that may, in fact, be functioning differently. As we learn more about the development of the brains of extremely premature infants and how they grow subsequently after preterm birth and function later in life, perhaps there can be a better understanding about the biology and physiology underlying what is now only observed "from the outside." If the differences in brain anatomy and function can be identified at an early enough point in the developmental history after birth, then perhaps interventions would be undertaken that can alter long-term behavior and diminish further persistent conduct problems. Neuroscience needs to explore further the relationships between the anatomy, biology, and physiology of the recovering premature infant brain, as well as later behavioral and emotional dispositions. Such information could have an impact on how we understand our children in general, as well as how we interpret the application of the laws of our society to their behaviors.

D. K. Stevenson, MD

Long-term Outcome Following Extracorporeal Membrane Oxygenation for Congenital Diaphragmatic Hernia: The UK Experience
David PJ, Firmin RK, Manktelow B, et al (Glenfield Hosp, England; Univ of Leicester, England; Great Ormond Street Hosp for Children, London)
J Pediatr 144:309-315, 2004   15–13

Objective.—We evaluated the long-term outcome of neonates receiving extracorporeal membrane oxygenation (ECMO) for congenital diaphragmatic hernia (CDH).

Study design.—A retrospective review of all 73 neonates with CDH supported with ECMO in the United Kingdom between 1991 and 2000, with follow-up to January 2003. Information was from hospital charts and from communication with family doctors and pediatricians. Median follow-up period for survivors was 67 months.

Results.—46 infants (63%) were weaned from ECMO, 42 (58%) survived to hospital discharge, and 27 (37%) survived to age 1 year or more. A higher birth weight, higher 5-minute Apgar score, and postnatal diagnosis were "pre-ECMO" predictors of long-term survival. Comorbidity was common in long-term survivors: 13 (48%) had respiratory symptoms, 16 (59%) had gastrointestinal problems, and 6 (19%) had severe neurodevelopmental problems. Only 7 children were free of significant neurodevelopmental deficit and required no further medical or surgical intervention.

Conclusion.—Using the current referral criteria, ECMO can be used to support the sickest neonates with CDH. However, there is significant mortality in the first year of life, and long-term physical and neurodevelopmental morbidity remains in the majority of survivors.

▶ This article offers very little in the way of encouraging news. In a retrospective analysis of all neonatal CDH cases treated with either ECMO in the United Kingdom over 9 years, only 37% of the initial 73 infants survived beyond 1 year, and only 10% were free of any physical problems. The same predictors associated with favorable outcome in earlier publications hold up in this series as well; namely, higher birth weight, a higher 5-minute Apgar score, and postnatal diagnosis. Pulmonary, gastrointestinal (GI), and neurodevelopmental problems were noted in the majority of survivors.

ECMO remains a marker for disease severity in CDH. In the United States, less than 50% of CDH cases require ECMO support, but the mortality in this special cohort exceeds 40%.[1]

What can be done to improve outcome in this condition? In a prospective, randomized trial fetal surgery neither improved survival nor decreased morbidity among survivors, although 90-day survival exceeded 70% in both arms of the study.[2]

Surfactant treatment and inhaled nitric oxide also failed to improve outcome despite early testimonials of efficacy.[3,4] There is some good news on the North American front, however. Permissive hypercapnea has shown promise in the acute management of CDH. In the United States studies when this ventilatory strategy has been used, survival to discharge exceeded 80% in infants with isolated diaphragmatic hernia.[5,6]

Paradoxically, improved survival may translate into increased morbidity as borderline cases survive. We have seen this parallel in extremely low birth weight premature infants as their survival improved. The CDH survivors face a daunting list of serious sequelae, including chronic lung disease, residual pulmonary hypertension, gastroesophageal reflux, oral feeding aversion, poor weight gain, hernia recurrence, hearing loss, and neurodevelopmental delay, not to mention late scoliosis.[7]

This is scary stuff! Still the outcome of most CDH infants who make it through the first 2 years is surprisingly good, our pediatric surgical colleagues tell us. What we need is more data on school-age outcome of CDH survivors emerging from the gentle ventilation era.

Stay tuned—hopefully for better news!

A. A. Fanaroff, MD

References

1. ELSO Registry.
2. Harrison MR, Keller RL, Hawgood SB, et al: A randomized trial of fetal endoscopic tracheal occlusion for severe fetal congenital diaphragmatic hernia. *N Engl J Med* 349:1916-1924, 2003.
3. Van Meurs KP, the Congenital Diaphragmatic Hernia Study Group: Is surfactant therapy beneficial in the management of the term newborn with CDH. *J Pediatr* 145:312-316, 2004.
4. Finer N for the Neonatal Inhaled Nitric Oxide Study Group (NINOS): Inhaled nitric oxide and hyperoxic respiratory failure in infants with CDH. *Pediatrics* 99:838, 1997.

5. Boloker J, Batewan D, Wung J-T, et al: Congenital diaphragmatic hernia in 120 infants treated consecutively with permissive hypercapnea/spontaneous respirations/elective repair. *J Pediatr Surg* 37:357, 2002.
6. Kays DW, Langham MR Jr, Ledbetter DJ, et al: Detrimental effects of standard medical therapy in CDH. *Ann Surg* 230:340, 1999.
7. Bohn D: Congenital diaphragmatic hernia [clinical commentary]. *Am J Respir Crit Care Med* 166:911-915, 2004.

16 Ethics

Neonatal Research: The Parental Perspective
Stenson BJ, Becher J-C, McIntosh N (Royal Infirmary, Edinburgh, Scotland)
Arch Dis Child Fetal Neonatal Ed 89:F321-F324, 2004   16–1

Background.—Written parental consent is generally required before any child is enrolled in a clinical trial. This policy may safeguard the child's interests, but it is associated with numerous difficulties. Concerns have been expressed regarding the additional stress that neonatal clinical trials place on the parents and the parents' ability to process information and make informed decisions under these conditions. Alternatives to the consent process have been proposed, but these alternatives may be unacceptable to parents whose consent would otherwise be sought. There are few data on the experiences of parents who have been approached for consent. The recollections of parents who consented to enrollment of their infants in research studies were investigated, and their opinions were determined regarding the need for informed consent.

Methods.—The study was conducted among the parents of 199 infants enrolled in a randomized controlled trial of pulmonary function testing conducted in Edinburgh, Scotland, from August 1991 to June 1993. A questionnaire was mailed to the parents 18 months after the trial's end. Parents who did not respond to the initial questionnaire were sent a second questionnaire and a letter.

Results.—The response rate was 64%. Some of the parents (12%) did not recall being asked to consent to their babies' participation in the pulmonary function testing study, and another 6% of parents were unsure as to whether they had been asked for such consent. Most of the respondents (79%) were happy, 13% were neutral, and 8% were unhappy with their decision to give consent. None of the parents believed that they had experienced heavy pressure to agree to enroll their babies in the trial. Enrollment of their children in the trial caused 24% of respondents to feel more anxious and 20% to feel less anxious about their babies; 56% indicated they felt neutral. Most of the respondents (83%) would be unhappy to forgo the consent process passed by the institutional ethics committee for trials.

Conclusions.—A significant proportion of parents who give written consent for enrollment of their infants in a trial in the early neonatal period do not later recall having done so. Parents who have had experience with neonatal research would disapprove of their babies' enrollment in a study without their consent.

▶ Investigators should realize, similar to what has been observed by those interacting with mothers during labor, that parents who give written consent for a trial in the early neonatal period may not remember having done so. Fortunately, most parents are satisfied with their experience of neonatal research, but they would also be generally unhappy to have their babies included in a study that had ethics committee approval but that did not require parental permission. Taken altogether, and with the understanding that informed consent is never obtained in its fullest sense, an effort to continually communicate with parents about their infants' participation in a study for which the parents have given consent will contribute to the increased participation of parents and their infants in the important effort of randomized controlled trials involving newborns.

D. K. Stevenson, MD

Factors That Influence Parents' Assessments of the Risks and Benefits of Research Involving Their Children
Tait AR, Voepel-Lewis T, Malviya S (Univ of Michigan, Ann Arbor)
Pediatrics 113:727-732, 2004   16–2

Objective.—The ability to assess accurately the risks and benefits of a study are important to ensure that the subject can make an informed decision regarding his or her own or his or her surrogate's participation. This study was designed to examine factors that influence parents' assessments of the risks and benefits of anesthesia and surgery research involving their children.

Methods.—The study population consisted of parents of 505 children who had been approached to participate in 1 of several ongoing clinical studies. Regardless of their decision to allow or decline their child's participation in a study, parents completed a questionnaire that elicited information regarding their perceptions of the risks and benefits of the study and factors that had influenced their decision.

Results.—Factors that influenced positive risk/benefit assessments by the parents included use of a placebo, the designated risk category of the study, the clarity of information given, the parents' perceptions of the amount of time provided to make a decision, and the amount of privacy afforded them in making a decision. Furthermore, positive risk/benefit assessments were associated with low decisional uncertainty and greater trust in the medical system.

Conclusions.—Identification of factors that influence parents' perceptions of the risks and benefits of a research study is important as a means to optimize the manner in which consent information is disclosed and to ensure that parents and subjects can assess accurately the relative importance of the risks and benefits.

▶ Examination of a research study's risks and benefits is very important for clinicians and researchers, but perception of these risks and benefits has also been found to be an important determinant of parents' decisions to allow their child to participate.[1] Despite the importance of determining these risks and benefits, previous studies have shown that these are often poorly understood. Thus, identification of the factors that influence positive risk/benefit assessments by parents, even relatively simple ones such as the amount of time they were given to make their decision regarding research participation, are very important and should lead to more truly informed consent.

A. Moore, MB, MD, FRCPC, MHSc

Reference

1. Tait AR, Voepel-Lewis T, Robinson A, et al: Priorities for disclosure of the elements of informed consent for research: A comparison between parents and investigators. *Paediatr Anaesth* 12:232-236, 2001.

Neonatal Research and the Validity of Informed Consent Obtained in the Perinatal Period
Ballard HO, Shook LA, Desai NS, et al (Univ of Kentucky; Univ of Arkansas, Little Rock)
J Perinatol 24:409-415, 2004   16–3

Background.—Consent for participation in clinical research is considered valid if it is informed, understood, and voluntary. In the case of minors, parents give permission for their child to participate in research studies after being presented with all information needed to make an informed decision. Although informed consent is a vital component of clinical research, there is little information evaluating its validity in neonatal intensive-care populations. The objective of this project was to determine the validity of informed consent obtained from parents of infants enrolled in the multicenter randomized research study, neurologic outcomes and pre-emptive analgesia in the neonate (NEOPAIN).

Design/Methods.—Parents of infants who survived to discharge and had signed consent for their newborn to participate in the NEOPAIN study at the University of Kentucky were asked 20 open-ended questions to determine their level of understanding about the NEOPAIN study. The NEOPAIN consent form, which had been approved by the University of Kentucky Medical Institutional Review Board (IRB), was used to formulate these questions. Questions addressed the timing of consent, parental understanding of the purpose, benefits, and risks of the study, the voluntary nature of the project, and their willingness to enroll in future studies if the opportunity presented. Answers were scored on a Likert scale, with 1 for no understanding and 5 for complete understanding.

Results.—Five of 64 parents (7.8%) had no recollection of the NEOPAIN study or of signing consent. Of those who remembered the study, only 67.8% understood the purpose of the study, with a higher proportion of the mothers than fathers knowing the purpose of the study (73.3% vs 57.1%), ($p = 0.029$). Of those who understood the purpose of the study 95% were able to verbalize the benefits, but only 5% understood any potential risks. No parents reported feeling pressured or coerced to sign consent for the project and all parents reported they would enroll their child in additional studies if asked.

Conclusions.—Valid consent in the antenatal/perinatal population is difficult, if not impossible, to obtain. To maximize validity of consent in the antenatal/perinatal population every effort should be made to include mothers in the consent process. Additional attention during the consent process should be given to possible risks of the study.

▶ Neonatologists are probably sobered, but not too surprised, at the findings in this study. We all recognize that the neonatal ICU stay is extremely stressful for parents and that much given information cannot be recalled. Among the parents interviewed, 7.8% could not remember that they had granted permission, including signing a consent form, for their infant to take part in a study. Of those who did remember, only 68% could describe its purpose. More worrying, only 5% of the parents could recollect any risks associated with the study, and the final conclusion is that only 3% of parents had given truly valid consent. One wonders again if parents can ever give fully informed consent during this vulnerable time, or if the whole process is just an "elaborate ritual".[1] Previous research has also shown poor validity of consent obtained from adult populations consenting for themselves to take part in clinical research.[2]

In the original NEOPAIN study, there was a well-organized educational program for those obtaining consent, and a number of checks and balances were in place within the neonatal unit. So if anything, these findings are optimistic. No one is suggesting abandoning the consent process for difficult situations, such as the perinatal population; however, some findings of this study, such as being more careful to point out study risks and including mothers in the consent process, may help researchers obtain more valid informed consent.

A. Moore, MB, MD, FRCPC, MHSc

References

1. Mason S: Obtaining informed consent for neonatal randomized controlled trials: An "elaborate ritual"? *Arch Dis Child Fetal Neonatal Ed* 76:F143-F145, 1997.
2. Lantos J: Informed consent. The whole truth for patients? *Cancer* 72 (suppl 9):2811-2815, 1993.

Delivery Room Decision-making at the Threshold of Viability
Peerzada JM, Richardson DK, Burns JP (Harvard Med School, Boston; Beth Israel Deaconess Hosp, Boston; NIH, Bethesda, Md)
J Pediatr 145:492-498, 2004   16–4

Introduction.—The decision to provide or withhold delivery-room resuscitation for extremely preterm infants is associated with complex ethical

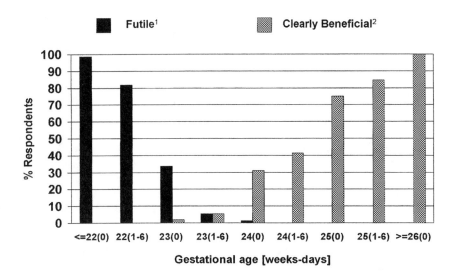

1Futile: "Treatment that will not significantly extend life or postpone death."

2Clearly Beneficial: "A situation where the potential medical benefits of treatment clearly outweigh the risks."

FIGURE 1.—The percentage of neonatologists who considered treatment clearly beneficial or futile at each gestational age. (Reprinted by permission of the publisher from Peerzada JM, Richardson DK, Burns JP: Delivery room decision-making at the threshold of viability. *J Pediatr* 145:492-498. Copyright 2004 by Elsevier.)

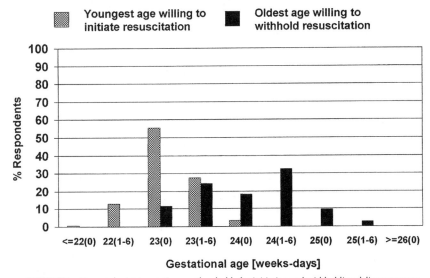

FIGURE 2.—Neonatologists' gestation age thresholds for initiating and withholding delivery room resuscitation at parental request. (Reprinted by permission of the publisher from Peerzada JM, Richardson DK, Burns JP: Delivery room decision-making at the threshold of viability. *J Pediatr* 145:492-498. Copyright 2004 by Elsevier.)

TABLE 3.—Percentage of Respondents Who Rated Each Factor "Very Important" in Decision Making When the Benefit of Treatment is Uncertain

Factor	N	%
		(Total = 149)
Condition of the infant at delivery	100	68
Likelihood of death	93	63
Potential long-term suffering of the infant	87	58
Likelihood of mental retardation (IQ <70)	64	43
Likelihood of severe cerebral palsy (unable to walk)	56	38
Potential burden on parents of caring for infant	57	38
Federal or state child protection regulations	7	5

(Reprinted by permission of the publisher from Peerzada JM, Richardson DK, Burns JP: Delivery room decision-making at the threshold of viability. *J Pediatr* 145:492-498. Copyright 2004 by Elsevier.)

considerations. The attitudes of neonatologists toward parental wishes in delivery-room resuscitation decisions at the threshold of viability were analyzed in a cross-sectional survey that tsed the conceptual framework provided by the President's Commission 2 decades ago.

Methods.—Between May and September 2002, an anonymous self-administered survey was sent to all 175 practicing level II/III neonatologists in 6 New England states. The survey began with the caveats that (1) gestational age was accurate; (2) the infant's weight was appropriate for gestational age; and (3) no severe congenital anomalies were present. A scenario was presented which demonstrated the impending delivery of a preterm infant in whom the benefit of treatment was uncertain. Respondents were queried regarding the resuscitation decisions they would make when (1) parents asked resuscitation be withheld; (2) parents asked that everything possible be done; and (3) parents were unsure of their wishes. They were then asked to rate the following 7 factors in delivery room resuscitation decisions when treatment was of uncertain benefit: (1) condition of the infant at delivery; (2) likelihood of death; (3) potential long-term suffering; (4) likelihood of mental retardation; (5) likelihood of severe cerebral palsy; (6) potential burden on parents; and (7) federal or state child protection regulations.

Results.—Of 175 neonatologists, 149 (85%) responded. At 24 1/7-6/7 weeks' gestation, 41% of respondents considered treatment clearly beneficial; at 25 1/7-6/7 weeks' gestation, 84% regarded treatment as clearly beneficial (Fig 1). When respondents considered treatment clearly beneficial, 91% indicated they would resuscitate in the delivery room despite parental requests to withhold. At or below 23 0/7 weeks' gestation, 93% of respondents considered treatment futile (Fig 2) (Table 3). Thirty-three percent indicated they would provide what they considered futile treatment at parental request. When respondents considered treatment to be of uncertain benefit, all indicated they would resuscitate upon parental request; 98% indicated they would resuscitate when parents were unsure, and 76% indicated they would follow parental requests to withhold.

Conclusion.—Most neonatologists indicated attitudes toward parental wishes concerning treatment for their extremely preterm infants in accordance with a decision-making framework for critically ill children released by a President's Commission more than 20 years ago. Thus, most respondents indicated they would provide treatment they considered clearly beneficial, withhold treatment they considered futile, and defer to parental wishes for either initiation or withholding of resuscitation when the benefit of treatment is uncertain.

▶ Peerzada et al provide a very useful report of neonatologists' attitudes toward parental wishes regarding delivery-room resuscitation of their newborns at the threshold of viability. Using the framework of the 1983 President's Commission for the study of Ethical Problems in Medicine, the authors determined the thresholds for "Clearly Beneficial" and "Futile" treatment and the response of neonatologists to parental wishes in each category. Physicians, as a general rule, have a clear notion of what "futility" is when they see it, although the term is often problematic for parents. Of the 149 neonatologists who responded to this study, 93% felt treatment under 23 0/7 weeks gestation was futile. Eighty-four percent felt that treatment at 25 1/7-6/7 weeks' gestation was clearly beneficial, rising to 100% at 26 0/7 weeks. A majority of respondents would provide treatment they considered clearly beneficial, withhold treatment considered futile, and defer to parents for initiation or withholding resuscitation when the benefit of treatment was uncertain, consistent with the recommendations of the President's Commission. Ninety percent considered treatment benefit uncertain at 23 1/7 -6/7 weeks' gestation and more than 50% felt that way for 24 1/7-6/7 weeks' gestation. Only 13% of respondents were willing to resuscitate below 23 weeks' gestation. Of particular note was the fact that 90% considered the condition of the infant at the time of delivery "important" or "very important" in the decision making. This is very revealing in light of the Miller case in which the Supreme Court of Texas affirmed the validity of assessing an infant's condition at delivery rather than making an irrevocable predelivery decision. This remains controversial, since some ethicists affirm the parents' right to make a decision about resuscitation before delivery when the incidence of morbidity and mortality is high. If parents wish not to provide treatment for their infant under 23 weeks gestation, they would, it appears, have no argument with any neonatologist, at least none in this study. For 23 weeks' gestation infants who are responsive to initial stabilization, the correct course of action is problematic. Respect for parental autonomy would dictate allowing the parents to make the choice about providing treatment, given the high incidence of mortality and morbidity at that gestation period, but it is unlikely, in light of Miller, that any neonatologist would lose a case if sued for resuscitating a responsive neonate.

Can one fault the professionalism of a neonatologist who tries to resuscitate a neonate whom he feels can be helped to live? What if gestational age is less than certain? On which side should one err? This is an area of competing ethical claims, and involvement of parents in the decision to treat when the benefit of treatment is unclear is essential.

Neonatologists should share with parents statistics about survival rates and later disability for survivors. Neonatologists are encouraged to give parents the opportunity to consent to treatment while explaining that an infant may make its own claim upon the neonatologist at delivery. To resuscitate an unresponsive or weakly responsive neonate of 23- or perhaps even 24-weeks' gestation may not be appropriate ethically if the parents feel the burdens of treatment outweigh the potential benefits.

E. F. Krug III, MDiv, MD

▶ We are seeing a more aggressive management approach being applied to smaller and smaller babies.[1,2] Lucey[3] has termed this "therapy creep"— with >4000 infants between 401 and 500 grams with mean gestational age of 23.3 ± 2.1 weeks entered into the Vermont Oxford Data Base between 1996 and 2003. Because of the tremendous difficulty and hesitancy to define lower limits of viability, it is no wonder that neonatologists like to see what fellow practitioners would do in similar circumstances. So another comprehensive survey, with 85% response rate, this time of 149 level II/III neonatologists in six New England states, seeking responses to all the difficult questions: the gestational age thresholds for initiating and withholding treatment, responses to parental requests at different gestational ages, and the factors neonatologists see as most important in decision making when benefit is uncertain. There does seem to be some consensus at or below 230/7 wks (93% of respondents considered treatment futile) and from 25 weeks (few would agree with parental requests not to resuscitate). However, it is clearly in the 23 plus 1 to 24 plus 6 days gestation period that there is not consensus, with variable numbers of respondents considering treatment to be of uncertain benefit and willing or not willing to accept parental requests not to resuscitate within this age range. The authors' conclusion is that in the absence of broad consensus neonatologists should make the reasoning behind their approach explicit, as this has a major impact upon the way they present information and discuss options. One cannot argue with the plea for transparency in a shared decision making process.

With regard to what to do in the 23 weeks plus gestational age group, it is well worth reading both George Annas and Paris et al's commentaries on the ruling of the Texas Supreme Court in the case of Sidney Miller (23.1 weeks' gestation), where there was a clear parental request not to attempt treatment.[4,5] The Court created a very narrow ruling limited to physician discretion at the moments immediately after birth. Paris et al state that this "emergent circumstance" standard "does not mandate the resuscitation of all newborns showing signs of life. It merely permits providing life sustaining treatment over parental refusal when the physician judges the infant to be potentially viable." They go on to caution that "the danger is that authorization for unconsented to touching formulated in this tort litigation might be transformed into standard practice. Trying to resuscitate all potential salvageable newborns indifferent to the known data on mortality and morbidity would be poor medicine. It would also be tragic for infants, parents and society alike."[5] Annas, too, found some implications of the Court ruling troubling, and cautions that "the neonatologist who always resuscitates newborns, no matter how premature or how unlikely their survival is without disabilities is not exercising any medical judgment or making a 'split-second' decision."

What are the underlying reasons for this downward gestational age trend: a lack of consensus amongst neonatologists, a lack of legal clarity or professional guidelines, the availability of the technology and the pursuit of "progress," reluctance to make quality of life decisions regarding how much morbidity is "too much," the method of non-directive information-giving by physicians, the demands of parents, or some other factor[s]? Surveys do give us an idea of what neonatologists would do in certain circumstances, but in so doing raise the issue of what the underlying reasons are behind the divergence of opinions expressed.

J. Hellmann, MBBCh, FCP(SA), FRCPC

References

1. Lucey JF, Rowan CA, Shiono P, et al: Fetal infants: The fate of 4172 infants with birth weights of 401 to 500 grams—the Vermont Oxford Network experience (1996-2000). *Pediatrics* 113:1559-1566, 2004.
2. Hintz SR, Poole WK, Wright LL, et al: Changes in mortality and morbidities among infants born at less than 25 weeks during the post surfactant era. *Arch Dis Child Fetal Neonatal Ed* 90:F128-F133, 2005.
3. Lucey JF: Fetal infants: Thoughts about what to do. *Pediatrics* 113:1819, 2004.
4. Annas G: Extremely preterm birth and parental authority to refuse treatment-the case of Sidney Miller. *N Engl J Med* 351: 2118-2123, 2004.
5. Paris JJ, Schreiber MD, Reardon F: (Commentary) The "emergent circumstances exception to the need for consent: The Texas Supreme Court ruling in Miller v. HCA. *J Perinatol* 24:337-342, 2004.

End-of-Life After Birth: Death and Dying in a Neonatal Intensive Care Unit
Singh J, Lantos J, Meadow W (Univ of Chicago; MacLean Ctr for Clinical Med Ethics, Chicago)
Pediatrics 114:1620-1626, 2004
16–5

Objective.—In canonical modern bioethics, withholding and withdrawing medical interventions for dying patients are considered morally equivalent. However, electing not to administer cardiopulmonary resuscitation (CPR) struck us as easily distinguishable from withdrawing mechanical ventilation. Moreover, withdrawing mechanical ventilation from a moribund infant "feels" different from withdrawing mechanical ventilation from a hemodynamically stable child with a severe neurologic insult. Most previous descriptions of withdrawing and withholding intervention in the neonatal intensive care unit (NICU) have blurred many of these distinctions. We hypothesized that clarifying them would more accurately portray the process of end-of-life decision-making in the NICU.

Methods.—We reviewed the charts of all newborn infants who had birth weight >400 g and died in our hospital in 1988, 1993, and 1998 and extracted potential ethical issues (resuscitation, withdrawal, withholding, CPR, do-not-resuscitate orders, neurologic prognosis, ethics consult) surrounding each infant's death.

Results.—Using traditional definitions, roughly half of all deaths in our NICU in 1993 and 1998 were associated with "withholding or withdrawing." In addition, by 1998, >40% of our NICU deaths could be labeled "active withdrawal," reflecting the extubation of infants regardless of their physiologic instability. This practice is growing over time. However, 2 important conclusions arise from our more richly elaborated descriptions of death in the NICU. First, when CPR was withheld, it most commonly occurred in the context of moribund infants who were already receiving ventilation and dopamine. Physiologically stable infants who were removed from mechanical ventilation for quality-of-life reasons accounted for only 3% of NICU deaths in 1988, 16% of NICU deaths in 1993, and 13% of NICU deaths in 1998. Moreover, virtually none of these active withdrawals took place in premature infants. Second, by 1998 infants, who died without CPR almost always had mechanical ventilation withdrawn. Finally, the median and average day of death for 100 nonsurvivors who received full intervention did not differ significantly from the 78 nonsurvivors for whom intervention was withheld.

Conclusions.—In our unit, a greater and greater percentage of doomed infants die without ever receiving chest compressions or epinephrine boluses. Rather, we have adopted a nuanced approach to withdrawing/withholding NICU intervention, providing what we hope is a humane approach to end-of-life decisions for doomed NICU infants. We suggest that ethical descriptions that reflect these nuances, distinguishing between withholding and withdrawing interventions from physiologically moribund infants or physiologically stable infants with morbid neurologic prognoses, provide a more accurate reflection of the circumstances of dying in the NICU.

▶ One of the most objective measures used to assess the outcome of NICU care is the neonatal mortality rate, allowing benchmarking and comparisons to be made between hospitals, regions, and even countries. We therefore require accuracy and agreed-upon terminology for reporting how these deaths and related decisions occur. This frank review of 1 unit's practice in end-of-life (EOL) decisions provides detailed and textured insight into their changing practice, particularly in the management of dying extremely low birth weight infants. It also raises the need for agreed-upon methods of categorization of NICU deaths so that differences in philosophy and practice can be determined and underlying reasons explored. There is a need for agreement in defining terms, for example, withdrawal of life-sustaining medical treatment: is this "terminal" or "active"/elective withdrawal? Can the reasons for withdrawal be categorized in a standardized manner, such as "death inevitable in short term, death likely in longer term, or survival possible but with poor predicted quality of life"? Similarly, how are decisions to withdraw/withhold life-sustaining medical treatment implemented, and what components of treatment are involved?

Classification of deaths and EOL decisions in the NICU is clearly a highly complex, nuanced issue and very dependent on individual characteristics of baby, physician, parents, unit, and country. Gathering of these types of data in a systematic way will facilitate meaningful benchmarking and allow internationally valid comparisons. Of related interest, see the proposed classification of EOL decisions by the Belgian and Dutch group.[1]

A. A. Fanaroff, MD

Reference

1. Provoost V, Deliens L, Cools F, et al: A classification of end-of-life decisions in neonates and infants. *Acta Paediatrica* 93:301-305, 2004.

Decision Making and Modes of Death in a Tertiary Neonatal Unit
Roy R, Aladangady N, Costeloe K, et al (Homerton Univ, London; Royal London Hosp)
Arch Dis Child Fetal Neonatal Ed 89:F527-F530, 2004   16–6

Aims.—To study the frequency and reason for withdrawal/withholding of life sustaining treatment (LST) and do not resuscitate (DNR) orders in infants who died in a tertiary neonatal unit.

Methods.—Infants who died at Homerton University Hospital between January 1998 and September 2001 were studied by retrospective analysis of patient records.

Results.—The case notes of 71 (84%) of 85 infants who died were studied. Mode of death was withdrawal of LST in 28 (40%), DNR in 11 (15%), withholding of LST in two (3%), and natural in 30 (42%) infants. Withdrawal of LST was discussed with the parents of 39 seriously ill infants; 28 (72%) parents agreed (Table 2). There was no difference in birth weight and gestational age of babies whose parents agreed or refused withdrawal of LST. White and Afro-Caribbean parents and those from the Indian subcontinent (20 of 23) were more likely to agree to withdrawal of LST than Black African or Jewish (eight of 16, p = 0.015) parents (Table 3). The median age at withdrawal of LST was 4 days (range 1-57). The median duration between discussion and the parents agreeing to withdrawal of LST was 165 minutes (range 30-2160), and median duration between withdrawal of LST

TABLE 2.—Withdrawal of Life Sustaining Treatment

Category	Accepted (n = 28)	Refused (n = 11)	*P* Value
Gestational age (weeks)	24 (22-40)	24 (23-40)	0.57
Birth weight (g)	645 (445-2336)	680 (460-3225)	0.70
Age at death (days)	4 (1-57)	7 (2-134)	0.26
Male/female	17/11	7/4	0.58*
Duration of discussion (min)†	165 (30-2160)	Not applicable	—
Time to death (min)‡	22 (5-210)	Not applicable	—

Values are median (range). p Values were obtained using Student's *t* test except where indicated.
*Fischer's exact test.
†Duration between discussion and parent agreeing to withdrawal.
‡Duration between withdrawal of care and death.
(Courtesy of Roy R, Aladangady N, Costeloe K, et al: Decision making and modes of death in a tertiary neonatal unit. *Arch Dis Child Fetal Neonatal Ed* 89:F527-F530, 2004, with permission from the BMJ Publishing Group.)

TABLE 3.—Ethnicity and Parents Agreeing to or Refusing
Withdrawal of Life Sustaining Treatment (n = 39)

Ethnicity	Agreed (n = 28)	Refused (n = 11)
White	13 (87)	2 (13)
Black African	7 (54)	6 (46)
Afro-Caribbean	4 (80)	1 (20)
Jewish	1	2
Indian subcontinent	3	0

Values in parentheses are percentages.
(Courtesy of Roy R, Aladangady N, Costeloe K, et al: Decision making and modes
of death in a tertiary neonatal unit. *Arch Dis Child Fetal Neonatal Ed* 89:F527-F530,
2004, with permission from the BMJ Publishing Group.)

and death was 22 minutes (range 5-210). The most common reason for withdrawal of LST was complications of extreme prematurity (68%) (Fig 1).

Conclusion.—The most common mode of death was withdrawal of LST, and the most common reason was complications of extreme prematurity (Table 1). The ethnic and cultural background of the parents influenced agreement to withdrawal of LST.

▶ An informal survey of units throughout Western Europe and the United States would likely find results that are very similar to those reported from this London Hospital and they are, indeed, quite similar to those recently published from the University of Chicago.[1] Many units have developed criteria for when they will or will not resuscitate a newborn, and most would agree that infants

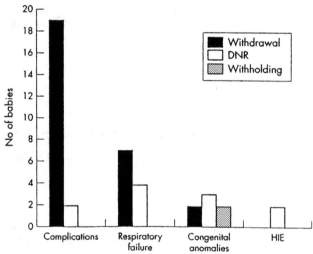

FIGURE 1.—Diagnosis in 41 babies who died after withdrawal or withholding of life sustaining treatment or do not resuscitate (DNR) orders. HIE, Hypoxic ischaemic encephalopathy; complications, complications of extreme prematurity. (Courtesy of Roy R, Aladangady N, Costeloe K, et al: Decision making and modes of death in a tertiary neonatal unit. *Arch Dis Child Fetal Neonatal Ed* 89:F527-F530, 2004, with permission from the BMJ Publishing Group.)

TABLE 1.—Mode of Death in 71 Newborn Babies

Mode of Death	Number of Infants
Withdrawal of LST	28 (40)
DNR orders	11 (15)
Withholding LST	2 (3)
Natural	30 (42)

Values in parentheses are percentages.
LST, Life sustaining treatment; DNR, do not resuscitate.
(Courtesy of Roy R, Aladangady N, Costeloe K, et al: Decision making and modes of death in a tertiary neonatal unit. *Arch Dis Child Fetal Neonatal Ed* 89:F527-F530, 2004, with permission from the BMJ Publishing Group.)

who are delivered at 22 weeks of gestation or earlier will not be resuscitated. Some will extend this to 23 weeks, but most neonatal ICUs in the United States adopt the principle of resuscitating first and asking questions later for infants of 24 weeks and older. In addition, we recognize the potential for an error in the assessment of gestation or birth weight that might lead to a change in plan in the delivery room. Whatever decisions are made in the delivery room, we reassure parents that if the outlook is futile or the chances of reasonably intact survival are very low, then they will be offered the option of withdrawing support.

These data show that, today, the leading cause of death in a tertiary neonatal ICU is withdrawal of life support (including DNR orders or withholding of support). These categories accounted for 58% of the deaths in this study. In only 42% of infants was death "natural." Although the samples are small, they also identify some ethnic differences in parental attitudes to this question. Most families with whom this was discussed agreed to the withdrawal, although some did not.

M. J. Maisels, MB, BCh

Reference

1. Singh J, Lantos J, Meadow W: End-of-life after birth: Death and dying in a neonatal intensive care unit. *Pediatrics* 114:1620-1626, 2004.

How Do Institutional Review Boards Apply the Federal Risk and Benefit Standards for Pediatric Research?

Shah S, Whittle A, Wilfond B, et al (NIH, Bethesda, Md; Emmes Corp, Bethesda, Md)
JAMA 291:476-482, 2004   16–7

Context.—Federal regulations allow children in the United States to be enrolled in clinical research only when the institutional review board (IRB) determines that the risks are minimal or a minor increase over minimal, or that the research offers a prospect of direct benefit. Despite this reliance on IRBs, no data exist on how IRBs apply the risk and benefit categories for pediatric research.

Objective.—To determine how IRB chairpersons apply the federal risk and benefit categories for pediatric research.

Design, Setting, and Participants.—Telephone survey, conducted between May and August 2002 of 188 randomly selected chairpersons of IRBs in the United States. The survey consisted of 21 questions to assess the application of federal risk standards to research procedures, whether certain interventions offer a prospect of direct benefit to participating children, and the extent to which IRBs use the federal definition of minimal risk when categorizing the risks of research procedures in children.

Main Outcome Measures.—Responses regarding categorization of the risk level and direct benefits of pediatric research procedures.

Results.—A single blood draw was the only procedure categorized as minimal risk by a majority (152 or 81%) of the 188 respondents. An electromyogram was categorized as minimal or a minor increase over minimal risk by 100 (53%) and as more than a minor increase over minimal risk by 77 (41%). Allergy skin testing was categorized as minimal risk by 43 IRB chairpersons (23%), a minor increase over minimal risk by 81 (43%), and more than a minor increase over minimal risk by 51 (27%). Regarding benefits, 113 chairpersons (60%) considered added psychological counseling to be a direct benefit, while participant payment was considered a direct benefit by 10% (n = 19).

Conclusions.—Application of the federal risk and benefit categories for pediatric research by IRB chairpersons is variable and sometimes contradicted by the available data on risks and the regulations themselves. To protect children from excessive risks while allowing appropriate research, IRB chairpersons need guidance on applying the federal risk and benefit categories and also need data on the risks children face in daily life and during routine physical or psychological tests.

▶ Neonatologists understand very well the benefits clinical research has made to our patient population. It is very important to protect children from excessive risks, while on the other hand allowing important research to be conducted. In the United States, research on children is only allowed when it "offers a prospect" of direct benefit to the child or infant, or the IRB determines that the risks are "minimal" or a "minor increase over minimal."[1] The federal regulations define minimal risks as the risks ordinarily encountered in daily life. However, researchers and IRB members alike grapple frequently with the concept of minimal risk. For example, is sedating an infant for an MRI greater than minimal risk? In contrast, for research with competent adults, researchers can explain the study clearly and get truly informed consent, even for higher risk projects such as the Navy or Air Force need to conduct. Minimal risk means different things to different people, so it is no surprise that when the authors surveyed IRB Chairs, they found application of the federal risk and benefit categories to be highly variable and sometimes contradictory. Thus, further debate and federal guidance on applying these regulations, rather than having to rely on individual IRB decisions, would be very helpful for those who conduct and review pediatric research.

A. Moore MB, MD, FRCPC, MHSc

Reference

1. Department of Health and Human Services. 45 CFR 46.404-406. Revised June 18, 1991.

Autonomy Gone Awry: A Cross-Cultural Study of Parents' Experiences in Neonatal Intensive Care Units
Orfali K, Gordon EJ (Univ of Chicago; Loyola Univ of Chicago, Maywood, Ill)
Theor Med Bioeth 25:329-365, 2004   16–8

This paper examines parents' experiences of medical decision-making and coping with having a critically ill baby in the Neonatal Intensive Care Unit (NICU) from a cross-cultural perspective (France vs U.S.A.). Though parents' experiences in the NICU were very similar despite cultural and institutional differences, each system addresses their needs in a different way. Interviews with parents show that French parents expressed overall higher satisfaction with the care of their babies and were better able to cope with the loss of their child than American parents. Central to the French parents' perception of autonomy and their sense of satisfaction were the strong doctor-patient relationship, the emphasis on medical certainty in prognosis versus uncertainty in the American context, and the "sentimental work" provided by the team. The American setting, characterized by respect for parental autonomy, did not necessarily translate into full parental involvement in decision-making, and it limited the rapport between doctors and parents to the extent of parental isolation. This empirical comparative approach fosters a much-needed critique of philosophical principles by underscoring, from the parents' perspective, the lack of "emotional work" involved in the practice of autonomy in the American unit compared to the paternalistic European context. Beyond theoretical and ethical arguments, we must reconsider the practice of autonomy in particularly stressful situations by providing more specific means to cope, translating the impersonal language of "rights" and decision-making into trusting, caring relationships, and sharing the responsibility for making tragic choices.

▶ Although one might be less inclined toward ethnographic studies (somewhat difficult to define, but a qualitative research methodology that focuses on the cultural aspects of social phenomena), we cannot deny the powerful observations made by researchers who conducted interviews with 60 clinicians and 75 mothers and who extracted data from more than 85 cases over an 18-month observation period in each of 3 units—2 in France and 1 in the United States. The depth of exploration of mothers' lived experiences warrants our attention. The essential question the study raises is does a system that emphasizes parents' autonomy enable them to cope better with the neonatal ICU experience, and decision making in particular, as some studies and the bioethical theoretical literature strongly suggest? Although one might quibble with the use of the term "parental autonomy," rather than "authority" in the context of parents making decisions for their infants and not themselves, it does focus our attention on the dominant principle of autonomy and its enactment (or not) in practice.

The authors state that it is misleading to bluntly define the 2 models as totally paternalistic or as completely respectful of parental autonomy; however, there are clear differences in approach in the units to warrant comparison, despite very similar technology, equipment, and patient populations. In spite of the obvious societal differences and methods of health care delivery, the similarity of the parental narratives are striking, such that the authors' view that it is possible to talk of a common "neonatal ICU experience" in diverse countries is compelling.

The prevailing view in the French units was that the doctors essentially determined the best interests of the infant, that parents want the same "good" for their baby, that parental consent is therefore implicit, and that parents should not be allowed to decide themselves because of the burden of guilt. In the second French unit there were some differences in the degree of parental participation, but parental opposition would still rarely be taken into account. The U.S. unit was seen as an autonomy-based model in which informed consent was explicit and where physicians offered information and choices that parents would or would not choose to consent to (although there were restrictions on parents' requests for withholding treatment). The striking finding was that in the French units, despite parents' exclusion or very limited role in decision making, they were more satisfied than mothers in the U.S. unit. The key features were the strong doctor-parent relationship, the continuity of care, the presentation of information with little ambiguity, the demonstration of emotional empathy by the physicians, and the belief instilled in mothers that whatever was best for their baby was being done. The contrast in the U.S. unit was that mothers perceived much information was provided, but medical uncertainty was emphasized, there was little emotional support to deal with the information, there was a lack of continuity and inconsistency in communication, and strong relationships with the physicians were not developed. The study showed that the French mothers coped better with the loss of their infants; guilt was almost never mentioned in the 2 French units.

How much of these differences are caused by the different health care systems and differences in regard and trust in physicians in those countries? Or is this really a test of the parental autonomy model of decision making? The larger societal context obviously plays some role, but many of the differences appear to be related to the nature of the practice within each unit, and is, I believe, a valid comparison of the different philosophies regarding parental roles. In a way it does test a model in which physicians provide information and empower parents to exercise their autonomy, but with less emphasis on relationship building and "emotional work" between doctors and parents.

Do these findings mean the autonomy model is insufficiently responsive to the needs of mothers of critically ill babies in neonatal ICUs, wherever they are? The findings would suggest this to be the case, and that decision making may have become too principle driven. Perhaps replacing paternalism and trust with informed consent may not always be the right model; somewhere along the line the "sentimental/emotional" work needs to be done, relationships between parents and physicians need to be developed, and organizational systems of frequent staff changes need to be examined The authors make a good point that "empiric data such as this needs to inform ethical theory" in decision making in the neonatal ICU.

J. Hellmann, MBBCh, FCP(SA), FRCPC

Subject Index

A

Adrenocorticotropic hormone (ACTH)
  circulating concentrations in normal
    newborns vs. those with sepsis and
    respiratory distress, 252
Amniotic fluid
  preterm meconium staining, associated
    findings and risk of adverse
    outcome, 53
  preterm premature rupture of
    membranes and inflammation of,
    24
Asthma
  childhood, birth weight and, 305
Auditory brainstem maturation
  long chain polyunsaturated fatty acid
    supplementation and, 184
Autism spectrum
  terminal 22q deletion syndrome as
    cause of speech and language
    disability, 48
Autoimmune disorders, maternal
  heart block in children and, 91

B

Bacterial vaginosis
  interaction with genetic susceptibility in
    risk of preterm birth, 26
Bartter's syndrome
  with sensorineural deafness and salt
    wasting, chloride channel defects
    and, 185
Behavioral outcomes
  and psychopathology of very low birth
    weight survivors at age 20, 308
  of very low birth weight survivors at
    age 16 in mainstream schools, 311
Betamethasone
  antenatal in preterm infants, 2-year
    neurodevelopmental outcome, 297
Birth asphyxia
  (see also Encephalopathy, neonatal)
  multiorgan dysfunction and, 155
  neuroimaging of cerebellar injury, 154
  neuropathologic and clinical features
    with and without prelabor damage,
    139
  prognostic significance of
    amplitude-integrated EEG, 156
Birth weight
  cerebral palsy risk and, 310
  childhood asthma and, 305

Blood pressure
  newborn, maternal age and other
    predictors of, 97
Blood transfusion
  functional capillary density in skin of
    anemic preterm infants after, 229
Bowel perforation
  in very low birth weight infants,
    surgical approach and outcomes,
    226
Brain function and structure
  brain volumes in adult survivors of very
    low birth weight, 170
  early experience and, 142
  iodothyronine levels and fetal brain
    development, 245
  MRI and T2 relaxometry of cerebral
    white matter and hippocampus in
    children born preterm, 163
  sex differences in brain volumes of
    8-year-olds born preterm, 168
Brain injury
  birth asphyxia and, 139
  frequency, natural history, and obstetric
    factors of subdural hematomas in
    term neonates, 148
  perinatal in term infants, comparison
    with site of lesion and time from
    birth on diffusion-weighted MRI,
    164
  risk factors for neonatal cerebral white
    matter injury, 152
  swaddling vs. massage in management
    of excessive crying with, 191
Breast feeding
  (see also Human milk)
  factors influencing initiation among
    urban women, 214
  fathers as advocates for, 269
  in preterm infants
    effects of bottles, cups, and dummies,
    210
    effects of prenatal consultation with a
    neonatologist, 213
Bronchopulmonary dysplasia
  increased lung water and tissue damage
    in, 124
  physiologic definition and impact on
    rates, 121
  plasma 8-isoprostane levels in, 125

C

Caffeine citrate
  high-dose, for extubation of preterm
    infants, 261

Author Index

A

Abernethy LJ, 163
Adams EW, 124
Adams KM, 41
Adcock K, 73
Ahmed K, 217
Ahola T, 125
Ainsworth SB, 296
Akiyama T, 191
Aladangady N, 327
Allen A, 194
Allen U, 135
Allsop J, 164
Als H, 142
Ambalavanan N, 205
Amory JH, 41
Anand KJS, 197
Andersen AN, 29
Annibale DJ, 118
Anwar M, 217
Arisawa K, 191
Arnold JH, 162
Aster RH, 230
Atherton HD, 287
Austin MT, 133
Aynsley-Green A, 246
Azimi PH, 81
Aziz D, 50

B

Badger GJ, 87
Baerts W, 288
Bahado-Singh RO, 3
Baldwin DN, 108
Ballantyne M, 199
Ballard HO, 319
Bar J, 32
Barkovich AJ, 158
Barnett A, 159
Battin MR, 102
Bauer K, 189
Beauchamp GK, 171
Becher JC, 139
Becher J-C, 317
Bell JE, 139
Bellini A, 285
Ben-Haroush A, 32
Bergman KA, 156
Bergman NJ, 277
Beyene J, 155
Binquet C, 177
Bissonette EA, 93
Björkqvist M, 80
Bo S, 250

Bodin L, 80
Bohnhorst B, 94
Boisen KA, 270
Bokiniec R, 219
Bouwmeester NJ, 200
Bracewell MA, 300
Brankston GN, 20
Bruner JP, 14
Burns JP, 320

C

Carpenter JH, 87
Cartar L, 308
Cartwright DW, 100
Cassidy L, 131
Cassidy SB, 48
Castro L, 291
Cha DH, 43
Chen C-Y, 239
Chen H-L, 239
Chen S-C, 3
Cheng AM, 257
Cheng C-C, 3
Christ F, 229
Christensen K, 47
Cimiotti J, 68
Clark R, 37
Clark RE, 237
Clegg SK, 53
Clericuzio C, 48
Coats DK, 174
Cohen B, 68
Cohen MS, 6
Cole TJ, 306
Coleman MM, 233
Colleoni R, 297
Collin MF, 58
Collins CT, 210
Combs CA, 37
Cook JV, 12
Cooke RJ, 296
Cooper ME, 45
Costeloe K, 327
Cotter AM, 19
Counsell S, 164
Counsell SJ, 124
Cox S, 194
Crowther CA, 210
Curry JI, 264
Curtis BR, 230

D

David PJ, 313
Davoren A, 230

Dehaene-Lambertz G, 146
Demissie K, 38
Derksen S, 283
Desai NS, 319
de Silva A, 76
de Vries LS, 166
Dezerega V, 8
Dhamrait S, 72
Diondo DJ, 255
Dionne K, 199
Dördelmann M, 94
Dorer DJ, 275
Downe L, 116
Doyle LW, 280, 281
Drewett RF, 219
Duffy FH, 142
Dyke M, 115

E

Edwards L, 134
Edwards MS, 78
Edwards WH, 83
Ehrenberg HM, 58
Elkousy M, 26
Engle WD, 77
Erdem G, 234
Eriksson M, 190
Ewald U, 55, 56, 57

F

Farooqi A, 55, 56, 57, 279
Fawcus SR, 277
Fearon P, 170
Fellman V, 125, 179
Fenton AC, 296
Ferber SG, 196
Feurer ID, 133
Fewtrell MS, 306
Finer N, 63
Finer NN, 64
Finkelstein M, 233
Finnström O, 190
Firmin RK, 313
Fitz CR, 10
Fleming MP, 275
Flenady V, 261
Flidel-Rimon O, 213, 223
Flom L, 10
Fonfé GJ, 53
Foulder-Hughes L, 163
Fouron J-C, 1
Franck LS, 194
Frangou S, 170

347

The year's best literature in one convenient volume!

YES! Please start my subscription to the *Year Book(s)* checked below with the current volume according to the terms described below.* I understand that I will have 30 days to examine each annual edition.

Please Print:

Name _____

Address _____

City _____ State _____ ZIP _____

Method of Payment

❑ Check (payable to **Elsevier**; add the applicable sales tax for your area)

❑ VISA   ❑ MasterCard   ❑ AmEx   ❑ Bill me

Card number _____ Exp. date _____

Signature _____

❑ **Year Book of Allergy, Asthma and Clinical Immunology (YALI)**
$110.00 (Avail. November)

❑ **Year Book of Anesthesiology and Pain Management (YANE)**
$115.00 (Avail. August)

❑ **Year Book of Cardiology® (YCAR)**
$115.00 (Avail. August)

❑ **Year Book of Critical Care Medicine® (YCCM)**
$110.00 (Avail. June)

❑ **Year Book of Dentistry® (YDEN)**
$105.00 (Avail. August)

❑ **Year Book of Dermatology and Dermatologic Surgery™ (YDER)**
$115.00 (Avail. October)

❑ **Year Book of Diagnostic Radiology® (YRAD)**
$115.00 (Avail. November)

❑ **Year Book of Emergency Medicine® (YEMD)**
$115.00 (Avail. May)

❑ **Year Book of Endocrinology® (YEND)**
$115.00 (Avail. July)

❑ **Year Book of Family Practice™ (YFAM)**
$99.00 (Avail. June)

❑ **Year Book of Gastroenterology™ (YGAS)**
$110.00 (Avail. December)

❑ **Year Book of Hand Surgery® (YHND)**
$115.00 (Avail. April)

❑ **Year Book of Medicine® (YMED)**
$110.00 (Avail. July)

❑ **Year Book of Neonatal and Perinatal Medicine® (YNPM)**
$115.00 (Avail. September)

❑ **Year Book of Neurology and Neurosurgery® (YNEU)**
$110.00 (Avail. January)

❑ **Year Book of Nuclear Medicine® (YNUM)**
$110.00 (Avail. June)

❑ **Year Book of Obstetrics, Gynecology, and Women's Health® (YOBG)**
$115.00 (Avail. February)

❑ **Year Book of Oncology® (YONC)**
$115.00 (Avail. November)

❑ **Year Book of Ophthalmology® (YOPH)**
$115.00 (Avail. September)

❑ **Year Book of Orthopedics® (YORT)**
$120.00 (Avail. October)

❑ **Year Book of Otolaryngology—Head and Neck Surgery® (YOTO)**
$105.00 (Avail. July)

❑ **Year Book of Pathology and Laboratory Medicine® (YPAT)**
$115.00 (Avail. March)

❑ **Year Book of Pediatrics® (YPED)**
$105.00 (Avail. January)

❑ **Year Book of Plastic and Aesthetic Surgery® (YPRS)**
$115.00 (Avail. March)

❑ **Year Book of Psychiatry and Applied Mental Health® (YPSY)**
$105.00 (Avail. March)

❑ **Year Book of Pulmonary Disease® (YPDI)**
$110.00 (Avail. April)

❑ **Year Book of Rheumatology, Arthritis, and Musculoskeletal Disease™ (YRHE)**
$115.00 (Avail. January)

❑ **Year Book of Sports Medicine® (YSPM)**
$110.00 (Avail. December)

❑ **Year Book of Surgery® (YSUR)**
$110.00 (Avail. September)

❑ **Year Book of Urology® (YURO)**
$115.00 (Avail. November)

❑ **Year Book of Vascular Surgery® (YVAS)**
$115.00 (Avail. April)

© **Elsevier 2005** *Offer valid in U.S. only. Prices subject to change without notice.*   MO 8025 DA 3744

Order your Year Book today! Simply complete and detach this card and drop it in the mail to receive the latest information in your field.

Your Year Book service guarantee:

When you subscribe to a **Year Book**, you will receive notice of future annual volumes about two months before publication. To receive the new edition, do nothing—we'll send you the new volume as soon as it is available. (Applicable sales tax is added to each shipment.) If you want to discontinue, the advance notice allows you time to notify us of your decision. If you are not completely satisfied, you have 30 days to return any **Year Book**.

VISIT OUR HOME PAGE!
www.us.elsevierhealth.com/periodicals

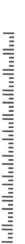

ELSEVIER
MOSBY